# Consciousness

How it is that anything so remarkable as a state of consciousness comes about as a result of irritating nervous tissue, is just as unaccountable as the appearance of Djin when Aladdin rubbed his lamp.

Thomas Huxley, 1886

# Consciousness:

## creeping up on the hard problem

**Professor Jeffrey Gray**

Department of Psychology
Institute of Psychiatry
Denmark Hill
London

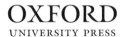

OXFORD
UNIVERSITY PRESS

# OXFORD

UNIVERSITY PRESS

Great Clarendon Street, Oxford OX2 6DP

Oxford University Press is a department of the University of Oxford.
It furthers the University's objective of excellence in research, scholarship,
and education by publishing worldwide in

Oxford  New York

Auckland  Cape Town  Dar es Salaam  Hong Kong  Karachi
Kuala Lumpur  Madrid  Melbourne  Mexico City  Nairobi
New Delhi  Shanghai  Taipei  Toronto

With offices in

Argentina  Austria  Brazil  Chile  Czech Republic  France  Greece
Guatemala  Hungary  Italy  Japan  South Korea  Poland  Portugal
Singapore  Switzerland  Thailand  Turkey  Ukraine  Vietnam

Published in the United States
by Oxford University Press Inc., New York

First published 2004
Reprinted 2005

A catalogue record for this title is available from the British Library

ISBN 0 19 852090 5 (Hbk)

10 9 8 7 6 5 4 3 2

Typeset by EXPO Holdings, Malaysia
Printed in Great Britain
on acid-free paper by
Biddles Ltd., King's Lynn, Norfolk

# Preface

Consciousness has become a very fashionable topic. It wasn't always so. A paper I wrote in 1971 about what is now called the 'Hard Problem' (David Chalmers' catchy phrase, gratefully borrowed for the title of this book) received a grand total of two reprint requests. Indeed, at that time, with behaviourism still dominant in psychology and positivism in philosophy, the topic of consciousness was virtually taboo. My 1971 paper questioned the then popular view ('mind-brain identity theory') that states of consciousness could simply be identified with brain states, so bringing to a peaceful close problems that had bothered philosophers ever since they had begun putting their concerns onto papyri. To me, alas, this solution was simply a philosophical cop-out from what, in the long run, was bound to become the scientific version of the Hard Problem: how do states of consciousness fit into neuroscience (since they seem to be created by the brain) and into psychology (since they seem to be related to behaviour)?

The long run may now be over. The problem of consciousness has entered science with a bang, celebrated in a spate of recent books by eminent authors (not to mention new scientific associations, new journals and hundreds upon hundreds of articles). Yet much of this revived interest is based upon premises that grapple with the fundamental issues—the Hard Problem—no better now than did mind-brain identity theory in the '70s. Today's dominant view is functionalism: the doctrine that states of consciousness can be identified with sets of functional (input-output) relationships that hold between a behaving organism and the environment in which it behaves. Like mind-brain identity theory, functionalism promises a swift end to philosophical debate, since all we now need do is describe input-output functions (difficult, to be sure, but nonetheless part of the 'Easy Problem' of normal science). Alas, this doctrine too is a cop-out: it 'solves' the problem of consciousness by eliminating it.

Nonetheless, there have been real advances. It is now widely accepted that the problem of consciousness indeed falls properly within the remit of natural science. And accumulating data, in both psychology and neuroscience, are beginning to provide strong empirical constraints upon the form any future theory of consciousness must take. So heady, indeed, is current enthusiasm for empirical 'consciousness studies' that we are in danger of overlooking the deep conceptual issues uncovered by generations of philosophers. This book, in contrast, supposes that these issues need to be squarely faced in any serious attempt to fit consciousness into the framework of natural science.

I am not so deluded as to suppose that I have a solution to the Hard Problem. But solutions first require a clear understanding of the questions, and this in turn requires a thorough clearing out of wrong or empty answers that lull theorist and experimentalist alike into a false sense of security. This book aims to contribute to the work of ground-clearing. In so doing, it comes up with conclusions that many readers will find surprising. They surprised me.

In writing this book I had the inestimable advantage of a year (2001–2) spent as a Fellow in the tranquil beauty of the Center for Advanced Study in the Behavioral Sciences, Stanford University. I cannot sing too warmly the praises of the Center, its staff, the class of 2002, or the deer and jack-rabbits who closely observed my writing efforts. It was a marvellous year. I hope this book goes some way to evening the score.

From my time at the Center, among so many excited and exciting discussions, I single out those with Patrick Goebel, John Bargh, Alan Baddeley, Per Aage Brandt, Deborah Gordon and Lynn Gale. I benefited also from detailed replies to importunate questions and from comments on drafts of parts (or even all) of the book, unstintingly given by Susan Hurley, Stuart Hameroff, Max Velmans, Dominic ffytche, Galen Strawson, Guy Claxton, Derek Bolton, Philip Corr, Steve Lehar, Stevan Harnad, John Mollon, Tom Troscianko and Rupert de Borchgrave. Key points in my thinking turn upon data garnered in demanding experiments by colleagues at the Institute of Psychiatry (David Parslow, Sue Chopping, Michael Brammer, Steve Williams, Lloyd Gregory, Mary Phillips, Maike Heining and Catherine Herba) and elsewhere (Julia Nunn, Goldsmith's College; Simon Baron-Cohen, Cambridge; Andy Young, York; Leanne Williams, Sydney). Carol Steen allowed her beautiful painting, *Runs Off in Front, Gold*, based upon one of her synaesthetic experiences, to serve as the cover of the book; and Peter Cresswell provided the stunning image reproduced here as Figure 2.3. I had excellent secretarial help from Deanna Knickerbocker at the Center and Gail Millard at the Institute of Psychiatry. My especial thanks to all these friends and colleagues.

The longest running and most demanding discussions of all are those I have with my wife and fiercest critic, Venus. They have lasted through four children and three grandchildren. I still haven't convinced her. But I can at least dedicate this book to her and to the family with which she has massively rewarded me. They keep me (I think) sane.

Jeffrey Gray
Emeritus Professor Psychology
Institute of Psychiatry, King's College London

# Contents

# Colour Plates

**Plate 2.1** The regions of increased cerebral blood flow in the human brain when subjects view (a) a multi-coloured Mondrian (see Plate 7.2) display and (b) a pattern of moving squares. Highest increases are shown in white, red and yellow. The regions of high cerebral blood flow are indicated in horizontal slices throughout the cerebral cortex. Note the difference in location between the area activated by the colour stimulus (human V4) and the one activated by the motion stimulus (human V5). Note that area V1 and the adjoining area V2 were active with both stimuli, suggesting that both colour and motion signals reach V1 and are distributed from it to the specialized visual areas V4 and V5. From Zeki (1993).

**Plate 4.1** The location of visual areas in the human cortex (cf. Plate 2.1). From Zeki (1999).

**Plate 6.1** (a) Grating patterns of orthogonal orientation that are usually employed in the study of binocular rivalry. Varying the strength of the patterns (e.g. as shown here, their degree of contrast) changes the predominance of each stimulus. Strong stimuli remain suppressed for shorter periods. (b) Rivalling complex patterns. The strength of such stimuli can be manipulated, as shown, by the degree of blurring. (c) 'Caneja' patterns, used to demonstrate that rivalry does not occur just between the two eyes or the two hemispheres but at a higher level of perceptual integration. When these patterns are presented dichoptically, rivalry occurs between percepts of concentric circles or lines (horizontal in the top display, radial in the bottom). (d) Exclusive dominance of a pattern during rivalry depends on both the size and spatial frequency of the stimulus. Stimuli of low spatial frequency (*left*) that are much larger than patterns of higher spatial frequency (*right*) can still yield frequent phases of exclusive dominance. (e) Distribution of alternation phases for human and monkey subjects. (f, g) Both humans and monkeys (see Plate 6.2) show the same predominance-strength functions for two different stimulus types. From Logothetis, Single units and conscious vision. *Philosophical Transactions of the Royal Society B*, 353, 1801–18 (1998).

**Plate 6.2** (a) Non-rivalry; (b) rivalry. The monkeys were taught to pull and hold the left lever whenever a sunburst-like pattern ('left object') was displayed, and to pull and hole the right lever upon presentation of other figures ('right objects'). In addition, they were trained not to respond on presentation of a physical blend of different stimuli ('mixed objects'). During the behavioural task, individual observation periods consisted of random transitions between presentations of left, right and mixed objects. A juice reward was delivered only after the successful completion of an entire observation period. During rivalry periods, the monkeys indicated alternating perception of the left and right objects (see Plate 6.1e–g). From Logothetis, Single units and conscious vision. *Philosophical Transactions of the Royal Society B*, 353, 1801–18 (1998).

**Plate 7.1** (b) The sensitivities of the long-wave (L), middle-wave (M) and short-wave (S) photopigments found in the retinae of humans and of Old World primates. (a) The sensitivities of the pigments thought to have been present in ancestral mammals. From Mollon (1999).

**Plate 7.2** A 'Mondrian' design. *Right*: If the polygon marked by a white circle is viewed in isolation through a small aperture, with the rest of the design obscured, it is seen as white or grey. *Left*: Viewed with the rest of the design visible, the polygon is seen as green. From Zeki (1993).

**Plate 7.3** The two subsystems of primate colour vision. A schematic of the photoreceptor matrix shows the S, M and L cones (see Plate 7.1) in blue, green and orange, respectively. The phylogenetically ancient subsystem (*left*) draws opposed inputs from the S cones, on the one hand, and from the L and M cones on the other. Its signals are carried by the small bistratified ganglion cells and the koniocellular laminae of the lateral geniculate nucleus (LGN). The recent subsystem (*right*) compares the signals of the L and M cones. Its signals are thought to be carried by midget ganglion cells and the parvocellular layers of the LGN. From Regan *et al.*, Fruits, foliage and the evolution of primate colour vision. *Philosophical Transactions of the Royal Society B*, 356, 229–83 (2001).

**Plate 7.4** (a) Fruits of *Manilkara bidentata* (Sapotaceae) photographed in the forest canopy at Les Nouragues. The species *Alouatta seniculus*, *Ateles paniscus* and *Cebus apella* all eat these fruits. (b) Typical stimulus array from a laboratory visual search task: the task might be to press one button if the orange circle is present, and a different button if the orange circle is absent. The chromaticity of the orange target circle is the same as the chromaticity of a fruit in (a), and the chromaticity of the distractors were drawn from the chromaticities of leaves in (a). The same photograph as it would appear (c) to a protanope (a colour-blind individual who lacks the L or red photopigment) and (d) a deuteranope (who lacks the M or green photopigment), illustrating the importance of trichromatic colour vision for locating the fruit. From Regan *et al.*, Fruits, foliage and the evolution of primate colour vision. *Philosophical Transactions of the Royal Society B*, 356, 229–83 (2001).

**Plate 10.1** The displays used by Ramachandran and Hubbard (2001) to demonstrate visual 'pop-out' in coloured grapheme synaesthetes. (a) When presented with a matrix of 5s in which a triangle composed of 2s is embedded, control subjects find it difficult to discern the triangle. (b) However, coloured grapheme synaesthetes who see, for example, the 5s in green and the 2s in red detect the embedded triangle much more rapidly.

**Plate 10.2** (a) Activation maps of coloured-hearing synaesthetes and controls in response to heard words, combined with the results of a colour activation mapping study (Howard *et al.*, 1998). The data shown are 5.5-mm axial slices, between Talairach z planes –13 and +8 mm, for synaesthetes (*upper row*) and controls (*lower row*). Yellow: heard words *minus* tones. Blue: coloured Mondrian (see Plate 7.2) patterns *minus* monochrome Mondrians. Red: cluster common to both heard words and coloured Mondrians. The coordinates of this cluster correspond very closely with those reported by Hadjikhani *et al.* (1998) for V8, the colour selective region of the visual system. The right side of the image corresponds to the left hemisphere of the brain. STG: superior temporal gyrus. IFG: inferior frontal gyrus. (b) Orthogonal views of the site of overlap (red cluster in A) between activation in coloured hearing synaesthetes by heard words, and in non-synaesthetes by coloured Mondrian patterns. Left to right: coronal, sagittal and axial planes. From Nunn *et al.* (2000).

**Plate 12.1** A hierarchy of visual areas in the macaque, based on laminar patterns of interconnections. From Van Essen *et al.* (1992).

**Plate 13.1** An illusion of motion. *Enigma*, by Isia Levant. Palais de la Découverte, Paris. From Zeki (1999).

**Plate 16.1** Microtubule structure shown at left: a hollow tube of 25 nm diameter, consisting of 13 columns of tubulin dimers arranged in a skewed hexagonal lattice. Each tubulin molecule can switch between two (or more) conformations (top right: blue, red), coupled to London forces in a hydrophobic pocket. Each tubulin can also exist in quantum superposition of both conformational states (bottom right: gray). According to the Orch OR model, dipole interactions among tubulin states in the microtubule lattice process information classically and by quantum computation. From Woolf and Hameroff (2001).

**Plate 16.2** Linking isolated microtubule quantum computation to neural membrane mechanisms. From Woolf and Hameroff (2001).

**Plate 17.1** The image from the retina is projected into the perceptual sphere from the centre outward in the direction of gaze, as an inverse analogue of the cone of light that enters the eye in the external world, taking into account eye, head, and body orientation in order to update the appropriate portion of perceptual space. From Lehar (in press).

# CHAPTER 1

# Stances towards the problem of consciousness

We are about to embark on an exploration of the 'Hard Problem of consciousness': how, scientifically and philosophically, should one situate conscious experience in relation to behaviour and the brain?[1] This first chapter might be expected, therefore, to start with a definition of 'consciousness'. But useful definitions come along *after* problems are solved, not before. How might one usefully have defined 'electricity', when all one knew about it was that flashes of bright light tend to appear in the sky just after loud rumbling noises during rain? Scientifically speaking, that is about where we are in our understanding of consciousness. So I shall offer you no definitions. Instead, I shall just point to the phenomena in question—to the lightning—and say: *this* is what we are talking about.

Fortunately, everyone knows these phenomena, from their own experience. For that, precisely, is what they are: our experience—*all* of it.

Imagine yourself waking from sleep. The first things you experience might be some rather vague sensations—a feeling of warmth or cold, some tension in your arms or relaxation in the legs, maybe some words in your own voice and in your own head ('I wonder what time it is?'), a metallic taste in your mouth. You open your eyes: you see the room around you, the light coming in through the window, hear someone talking in the next room. All of this is in stark contrast with the period just before, when you were asleep experiencing nothing (or at least nothing that you can now recall), a period that may have lasted just a few minutes or many hours. You get up: there is a whole, solid, three-dimensional world around you, which you can see, touch, hear, smell, feel, taste, navigate in. *All* of these phenomena make up your conscious experience: from the most vague sensation that only you are aware of (that initial feeling of relaxation in the legs), to the entire solid world that you share with others. For, just like those inner sensations, that world out there is constructed by our brains and exists within our consciousness. In a very real sense, the world as we consciously experience it is not out there at all: it is *inside* each and every one of us. This statement may strike many of you as distinctly odd. But I hope to convince you that it is accurate.

---

[1] If you wish to see in advance where this exploration will take us, you may prefer to read Chapter 20 first.

Not giving definitions is not the same as not making distinctions. We have just met one that will be important as the argument of this book unfolds: the distinction between conscious experiences of which only you are aware (feelings inside your body, thoughts in your head, remembered images and so on), and experiences which construct the perceived external world—the very same external world (or, at any rate, almost so) that other people too construct. It is on the latter kind of experiences that shared language and communication rest (the ability to pick out for commentary, say, 'the red book on the shelf above the mantelpiece'). I shall call these two different forms of consciousness—experiences of which only you are aware versus those that make up the external world—its 'private' and 'public' spaces, respectively.

A second distinction, one that will also be of great importance, is that between consciousness of inner bodily experiences and consciousness of the external world. This is not the same as the private/public space distinction, though the two distinctions overlap. For there are private space experiences that do not depend upon the inner bodily senses (words in your head, images of remembered scenes and so on), as well as experiences that do (feeling warm, hungry, sick or sexy). Nor do the *inner* bodily senses include all conscious experience of the body. When you see your arm move or inspect your face in the mirror you experience your body from the outside, just as others experience it (though, of course, from a different perspective). Perception of your body by this route, therefore, forms part of the experience of the external world.

To describe this second distinction in the most obvious way, as one between consciousness of the inner body and consciousness of the external world, risks confusion, because of the multiple ambiguities that surround the concept of the external world. A different term is therefore needed. Consciousness of the external world typically involves a much greater degree of cognitive processing than does inner body consciousness, a matter to which we devote attention later in the book. I shall therefore distinguish between, on the one hand, 'cognitive consciousness' (of the external world in either the public or private spaces) and 'inner bodily consciousness' (located exclusively in private space).

These distinctions, which will gradually be refined throughout the book, are summarised in Fig. 1.1.

We must also distinguish between the *contents* of consciousness and *states* of consciousness[2]. So far, I have concentrated on the former (what one is conscious *of*): aspects of the external world, images or memories of that world, bodily feelings and so on. 'States of consciousness', in contrast, refer chiefly to the continuum ranging from waking to sleeping. At first sight, study of the differences between these states and the brain mechanisms that produce them offers a royal road to

---

[2] Confusingly, philosophers sometimes make this distinction by referring to 'states of consciousness' (my 'contents') as opposed to 'states of the creature that is conscious' (my 'states').

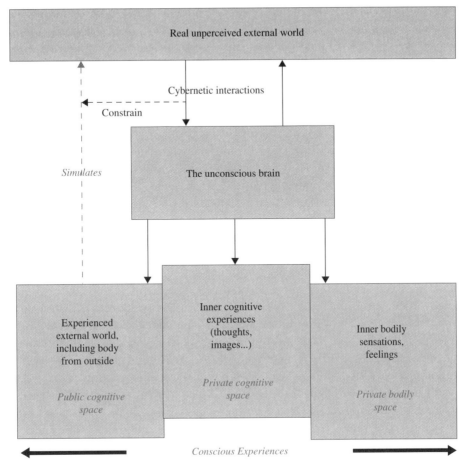

**Fig. 1.1** The different spaces of conscious experience. It will take the entire book for the full exposition of the concepts illustrated by this figure. In brief, however, the brain interacts unconsciously, continuously and cybernetically with the real, unperceived, external world. Constrained by these interactions, the brain at the same time constructs a consciously perceived simulation of the world, experienced as though it were the real thing. The constructed world of consciousness can usefully be divided into three 'spaces': the 'public cognitive space', containing the experienced external world in all its visible and tangible glory, including the body as perceived from the outside; the 'private cognitive space', containing inner cognitive experiences, such as thoughts, memories and images; and the 'private bodily space', containing inner bodily sensations and feelings.

insight into the neurobiology of consciousness. But, seductive as this prospect is, it is a mirage, for two main reasons. First, the differences between waking and sleeping involve far more than just the difference between having and not having conscious experiences. For the range of the brain's *unconscious* capacities is vastly extended in waking compared to sleep. And disentangling what the brain achieves consciously from what it can do unconsciously presents, as we shall see, formidable problems. Second, sleep cannot be taken as a state devoid of consciousness for, as we all know, it is regularly punctuated by those extraordinarily rich conscious experiences known as dreams. So, not anticipating much light from that direction, I shall have relatively little to say in this book about states of consciousness.

A final distinction that sometimes pops up to cause trouble is between consciousness in general and consciousness of the self in particular. Now, the Hard Problem of consciousness concerns how and why one is conscious of anything at all—it does not become either more or less tractable when one considers conscious experience of the self. For the most part, therefore, we can ignore this distinction (but see Chapters 17 and 18, which deal specifically with consciousness of the self).

These, then, are the 'conscious experiences' that this book is about; and 'consciousness' refers to the (unknown) process by which they come about. Conscious experiences constitute the most important aspect of our lives. Without them, existence would be, literally, meaningless. Conscious experiences appear to stand in a very intimate relationship to our behaviour. We think (that is, hear words in our head spoken in our own voice) 'I'm thirsty', pour a glass of water, and enjoy the slaking of our thirst. The conscious experiences and the actions in this chain of events are, it seems, indissolubly linked. Conscious experiences also stand in an intimate relationship to the brain. If you suffer damage to one specific region of your brain, you will lose for ever the ability to see colours: your visible world will be reduced entirely to shades of black, grey and white. Suffer damage to another region, and you will lose the ability to smell. Let a brain surgeon electrically stimulate a third, and you will experience vivid memories—there is virtually no limit to possible examples.

Science has made enormous progress in understanding behaviour, the brain and how the brain controls behaviour. Given the close relationships that brain and behaviour jointly have to conscious experience, surely we have made equally good progress in understanding consciousness? Some scientists and philosophers indeed think so, but others are more sceptical. Which camp you belong to depends upon the view you take of the so-called 'Hard Problem' of consciousness (this useful term is due to David Chalmers).

Broadly speaking, there are four different points of view ('stances') that one can adopt towards the problem of consciousness.

The first ('naïve') stance is taken by all of us before we have thought much about consciousness. This stance takes conscious experience for granted: as the firm ground from which to approach all other problems. Consciousness itself is not seen as posing a problem at all. This stance is not merely naïve. Within philosophy it was, famously and influentially, set forth in great detail and sophistication by René Descartes. And even those who believe that consciousness poses a very deep problem nonetheless go about their everyday business holding firmly onto this first stance. Indeed, if they didn't, they would find great difficulty in going about their daily business at all.

The second ('normal science') stance is taken by a large number of scientists and philosophers, some of whom have thought about consciousness very little, others a great deal. They agree with the naïve stance that consciousness does not pose any particularly hard problem. But that is not because they see consciousness as the grounds for all other beliefs, as did Descartes. On the contrary, it is the sciences—neuroscience, cognitive science, computational science and so on—that they see as primary. Consciousness is then something that will easily be explained (one day) within the conceptual framework that these sciences are busy creating. To be sure, they concede, there is much detail that still needs filling in. We need to know more about how the brain works, about the computations carried out in the brain, about how the brain controls behavioural interactions with the environment, and so on. And, no doubt, filling this detail in will be experimentally and theoretically difficult. But these difficulties—so the 'normal science' stance holds—are of perfectly ordinary kinds that science is used to handling. There is no special 'hard problem' beyond this.

The third ('new theory') stance accepts the importance of these normal-science problems. Solution of these problems will undoubtedly give us valuable new understanding of the workings of brain and behaviour, within the existing scientific framework. But this stance supposes that there is, in addition, a theoretical *Hard Problem* that also needs to be solved, one whose solution is likely to take us beyond the bounds of current scientific orthodoxy. To put this Hard Problem into a preliminary nut-shell: it arises because nothing in our current theoretical models of brain and behaviour accounts for the existence of conscious experience, still less for its detailed properties. Or, to put the other side of what is essentially the same coin: despite the fact that everyone knows it as an empirical fact (in each of our personal lives), conscious experience has no scientifically understood links with the concepts of neuroscience or behavioural science. And, without such links, consciousness lacks any comprehensible causal powers that would enable it to interact with the physical world. To fill this gaping hole, this stance holds, a new scientific theory is needed.

There are one or two candidates around for such a new theory, as we shall see later in the book, though none that yet show much promise. However, it is very early days to give up trying to create a theory. It is after all only in the last few decades that even the dimensions of the Hard Problem have begun to come clear. So we are perhaps in a situation like the one that confronted physics in the late nineteenth century. It was known that there were problems that the existing physics could not solve. Most scientists supposed that solutions would emerge from additional data, plus some tinkering with then standard theory. Eventually, however, it turned out that these problems found a solution only in the radically new theories of relativity and quantum mechanics. Before these theories were constructed, it would have been impossible to imagine what they would be like, still less the kind of data (for example, wave/particles being in more than one place at a time) by which they would be supported. The 'new theory' stance similarly supposes that our current theories about brain and behaviour are in critical respects incomplete or inaccurate (because they cannot account for conscious experience), but that it is impossible to imagine what form the necessary new theory will take (because this has not yet been constructed).

The fourth ('non-scientific') stance agrees with the new-theory stance that there is a Hard Problem, but rejects the likelihood that this will find a solution within science. The non-scientific stance comes in two versions. The first version is philosophical. It accepts that there is an apparently Hard Problem, but attributes it entirely to sloppy thinking. What looks like a Hard Problem will cease to be one when we have understood the errors in our ways of speaking about the issues involved. If this route were successful, we would rejoin the normal science stance: once our heads have been straightened out, science could again just get on with the job of filling in the details of empirical knowledge. The second version holds that the Hard Problem is real (not just due to bad language habits), but not a scientific one at all; and it finds comfort in this conclusion for a variety of spiritual beliefs, both traditional and exotic. Dan Dennett has coined the useful phrase 'New Mysterians' for those who take this stance. Less usefully, the same term is often used to pour scorn on proponents of the third, new-theory, stance. This scorn is misguided. There is nothing 'mysterian' about recognising an unsolved problem, while not foreclosing on the possibility of solving it. To be a true mysterian, you need to rejoice (and many do) in the lack of solution.

This book takes a version of the third, new theory, stance: there *is* a Hard Problem, it is a problem for science not philosophy, and it will almost certainly require a radically new theory for its solution. We don't yet know what form that solution will take, but there is absolutely no reason to think that it is beyond the powers of scientific enquiry to discover it.

# CHAPTER 2

# The illusory narrative of consciousness

The first difficulty in discussing consciousness is to convince people that there is a real problem at all. There are two lines of enquiry that I shall pursue in the attempt to persuade you of this. The first, in this chapter, turns more upon observation; the second, in the next, more upon theory.

The authority that our conscious experiences hold over us is immense. We doubt anything rather than the evidence of our senses. Yet this trust is profoundly misplaced, as has been demonstrated in countless experiments. So be prepared to discover that much of your conscious life is illusory. But cling, nonetheless, to that fundamental rock upon which Descartes built his great conceptual edifice (no matter how unsatisfactory it turned out to be in other respects): whatever else may be an illusion, the fact that you have a conscious life cannot be. For it is *in* consciousness that illusions are created: no consciousness, no possibility of illusion.

Conscious experience has a strong narrative structure. The key figure in the narrative is an actor (yourself) who is in continuous interaction with a world outside. The story line of the narrative generally takes this archetypal form: *I perceived* (consciously saw, heard, tasted, etc.) *this* out *there*, and so *I* then *did* (consciously formed the intention to do, and then did) *that*. Sometimes, things indeed follow, more or less, the lines of this narrative; but most often they do not, they just seem to do so.

Here are some major faults with the archetypal story line.

## 2.1 Consciousness comes too late

First, most behaviour takes place too quickly for it to depend upon conscious perception. This takes time. Estimates of just how much time vary somewhat, depending upon particular experimental designs, but a common estimate is that it takes about 250 millseconds (a full quarter of a second) after an event has impinged upon one of the sense organs before you become consciously aware of it.

Now, apply that length of time to any fast-moving activity, grand-slam tennis, for example. The speed of the ball after a serve is so great, and the distance over which it has to travel so short, that the player who receives the serve must strike it back *before* he has had time consciously to see the ball leave the server's racket. Conscious awareness comes too late to affect his stroke. The same applies to the perception by the receiver of his own return stroke. Consciously, he neither sees nor feels his arm move before the stroke is completed. Now, of course, the *brain* receives information about the visual trajectory of the serve before the return stroke is made; and also information, both visual and proprioceptive (the feel of the arm moving), while it is being made. Without that information, the return stroke could not be accomplished. But the brain's use of this information to compute and perform the return stroke is performed *unconsciously*, that is, without the accom- paniment of conscious awareness. Some (but by no means all) of this information becomes available to consciousness after the event. When it does so, it retains (usually) the same, veridical temporal structure as the events to which it relates: so one has the conscious perception of the ball leaving the server's racket and then the conscious perception of making the return stroke. Where the illusion lies is in the appearance that it was your *conscious* seeing of the ball that made it possible for you *consciously* to strike it.

In case you doubt this (as well you may!), here is a more detailed analysis, from John McCrone's book *Going Inside* (pp. 145–6).

> Facing a fast serve, players have barely 400 milliseconds in which to see whether the ball is headed for their forehand or backhand, and then to make any late adjustments for unexpected skids or jumps of the ball off the court surface. Given that simply turning the shoulders and lifting the racket back occupies a third of a second, and that it takes about half a second to reach wide for a ball... even if awareness were actually instant, it still would not be fast enough to get a player across the court in time.

The only way in which the player can return such a fast serve at all—*consciously or unconsciously*—is by anticipating the ball's trajectory well before it actually occurs. And, sure enough, skilled players do just this. In experiments in which they were shown film clips of a person serving, professional tennis players 'were able to guess the direction of a serve with fair accuracy if the film was halted forty milliseconds *before the ball was struck'*. Similar experiments have shown that skilled cricket players step forward in anticipation of a short-pitched delivery some 100 milli- seconds before the bowler releases the ball. You might think that this observation saves the role of consciousness. But it doesn't:

> None of the top players could explain what they were actually looking at to get their clues. When questioned, they said that they did not feel they were watching anything in particular. Indeed, most said they had not even been aware they were making guesses ahead of time. They believed they had simply been concentrating hard and making sure they watched the ball right on to their bat or racket, so were conscious of the shots pretty much as they happened (*loc. cit.*).

So anticipating the ball's trajectory is achieved *unconsciously*. This is a theme I shall develop more fully later in the book (Chapters 7 and 8).

You may also think that this is an exceptional case that occurs only under the extreme conditions of modern high-speed athletics. But it is in no way exceptional. In 1991 Max Velmans reviewed a large experimental literature from which he concluded that all of the following processes are capable of being, and normally are, completed unconsciously before we have any conscious awareness of what is being carried out: analysis of sensory input; analysis of emotional content of input; phonological and semantic analysis of heard speech; semantic and phonological preparation of one's own spoken words and sentences; learning; the formation of memories; choice and preparation of voluntary acts; planning and execution of movements. That is a formidable list (specific examples are presented throughout the book). The degree to which one is unconscious of what is going on varies somewhat from case to case. Generally, however, one is aware, after the process is completed, only of the perceived result of the process, not of how it was carried out: the meaningful words spoken by others or by ourselves, the form of the move-ment after we have made it, and so on. To take a striking example, one that brings us back to the earth of simpler functions, consider pain: accidentally touch a heated hotplate on the stove and you will withdraw your hand long before you feel the pain.

The survival of our ancestors, human and pre-human, depended upon the ability to out-run, out-fight and out-smart a range of big, fast-moving predators. Today, a tenth of a second makes the difference between being the winner or loser of a hundred-metre sprint. In the past, that same tenth of a second often made the difference between coming home to dinner or being the lion's dinner. Waiting around for a quarter of a second to become consciously aware of the lion would not have been a good idea. That one does become consciously aware of fast-moving lions and tennis balls is undeniable; but that conscious awareness should guide immediate behavioural reactions to them is—on the experimental evidence—impossible.

## 2.2   The world is inside the head

The second major fault with the archetypal story line is the assumption that there exists a world *out there* to which our senses give us more or less direct, conscious access. Not so: our brains *construct* the world, and it exists *inside* them (see Fig. 1.1).

I make this counter-intuitive claim as forcefully as I can, precisely because it is so counter-intuitive that I need fully to capture your attention. (It is made even more forcefully by Steve Lehar; see his illustration of the idea, reproduced here as Plate 17.1.) However, I should at once qualify the claim, lest you abandon reading a book apparently written by a madman. I do not mean that there is no real exter-nal world out there at all: there is one, and it is not located inside the skull. But our knowledge of the real external world is indirect only; and, despite all appear-ances to the contrary, the consciously perceived world is *not* that real world.

Rather, as I shall justify throughout the book, it is a simulation of the real world—one so effective that we take it to be the real world. And that simulation is made by, and exists within, the brain.

Our mental life is so dominated by vision that it is tempting to centre the argument around a case like seeing the cat on the mat. Am I seriously proposing that the (perceived) cat and the mat are in the viewer's head? Well, yes, I am proposing that; but I would rather start with a different, non-visual example.

You are in a concert hall. Someone opens up some pages on the music stand, strikes successive keys on a piano, and you hear a Beethoven sonata: *where is the sonata?* Physically, what is happening is that the keys cause the piano strings to vibrate; this causes vibrations in the air, and these strike your ear-drums, where they are translated into electrical pulses travelling along nerve cells into your brain. Do you directly perceive a piece of music that is *out there* in the vibrations in the piano strings or those in the air? Vibrations are not music. If the Beethoven sonata was played on a gramophone and no-one was there to listen, there would be no music—just vibrations in the air. Music is what you experience in your head, when it is constructed by the brain (in response to the pattern of nerve impulses reaching the brain from the ears). But that's not the only place where the music is located. All the other concert-goers are also experiencing the Beethoven sonata, and in a sufficiently similar manner that, afterwards, you can all have a lively discussion of the merits of the pianist's performance. So their brains construct music much as yours does. Then there is the pianist himself, who perhaps imagines the phrases he plays just before playing them. Indeed, if Beethoven himself were playing one of his late sonatas, this is the only way he could have experienced the music, as he was by then stone deaf. For him, vibrations in the air didn't count at all. And how did he communicate that sonata to us, the concert-goers of today? Not by producing vibrations in the air, but by writing squiggles on paper, forming the instructions for future pianists to strike the keys. Those squiggles provide the *potentiality* for a sonata realisable by any pianist with the skill to strike the keys aright, or anyone sufficiently good at sight reading to recreate in musical imagination what the stone-deaf Beethoven created in his. Vibrations in the air, whether made by a pianist, a CD player, a radio or an audio-tape, similarly provide only the potentiality for the rest of us to experience the sonata. But, in each case, the experience is constructed—on the basis of, and constrained by, what the real external world affords—by the brains inside our heads. And only when the experience is constructed does consciousness—and with it the Hard Problem—enter the story. (This example, by the way, does not turn on the fact that music is a sophisticated cultural artefact; exactly the same points can be made about a clap of thunder.)

This analysis raises the question: if the music isn't out there in the world, but constructed by each and every listener's brain, then what guarantees that each of us experiences the same music? To which a first answer is: there is no guarantee.

Indeed, it is a commonplace that experience of 'the same' piece of music differs greatly between individuals.

But, when we come to the solid world of objects, this answer won't do. It is equally commonplace that, by and large, we do not have radically different experiences of brick walls or motor-cars. And, even in the case of music, if we stick to the group of people who enjoy Beethoven piano sonatas, it is unlikely that they do not have rather similar experiences when they listen to the same performance of the same piece. If each of these experiences is separately constructed by a separate brain, where does the similarity come from? If one *directly* perceived[1] an outside world that is independently there in just the way we perceive it, then the similarity would lie in the properties of that which is perceived. Clearly, this remains to some extent the case even on the 'constructivist' view of perception that I am advancing here. If the aerial vibrations initiating the train of events from ear to brain that eventuate in the experience of a Beethoven piano sonata are changed, then we experience something different. But a further account is needed of why the constructions that different brains put upon the same aerial vibrations end up (roughly) the same. To this question the answer must be: because our brains are all built in roughly the same way, with similar tendencies to construct similar experiences given similar inputs from the world outside.

Let's pass on from the example of music to the sense of vision. It is this sense, above all, that gives the impression that we directly perceive a world outside ourselves. Even if I convince you that the brain constructs musical experiences, you may well remain resistant to the generalisation of such notions from these will o' the wisps to the tangible world of solid objects located in three-dimensional space. The weakest point in this resistance, and where I shall begin my attack, is the experience of colour. This appears to be as much an integral part of the objects around you as their shape, three-dimensional extension or solidity. But it is beyond dispute that colour is not directly determined by the physical properties of these objects. To be sure, the experience of colour normally depends upon physical stimuli emanating from objects: to be precise, upon the mixture of wavelengths of light they reflect onto the retina. But this dependence is very indirect.

The wavelength of light changes smoothly and continuously from long to short (going from the infrared to the ultraviolet part of the spectrum). There are no sudden jumps in wavelength corresponding to the transitions that people see between the different colours—from red to orange, green to blue, and so on. These transitions are the result of the ways in which separate pigments in different cells

---

[1] I use 'direct perception' in the philosophical sense (also termed 'direct realism'), to mean unmediated perception of the external world just as it really is, not (as is common in psychology and neuroscience) to refer to J. J. Gibson's theory that all the information we need to see distance, depth and optic flow are available in the pattern of retinal sensory input, and that you do not need additional representations of these attributes in higher brain centres.

of the retina respond to light falling upon them, followed by an intricate web of further transformations as the resulting electrical signals are sent deeper and deeper into the brain. Usually, there are three such 'photopigments', with closely similar properties in all human beings—so most people respond to differently coloured materials in much the same way. However, some individuals have pigments with slightly different properties; and some lack one or even two pigments entirely. Individuals like these experience colours in radically different ways from the norm—giving rise to the well-known phenomena of colour blindness. So, the colours one sees are clearly *not* inherent in the objects whose surfaces one sees as coloured: they are made by the brain.

The brain does not even need visual stimuli impinging upon the retina in order to construct colours. There are many everyday examples of this, such as dreaming in colour with the eyes closed. A more dramatic example, now well-documented experimentally, lies in a group of individuals (nearly always women) known as 'coloured hearing synaesthetes'. These individuals report that, upon hearing or seeing specific words, they experience specific colours, always the same for a given individual but differing widely between them. I shall spend some time on this phenomenon, as it will later be important for a general argument about the way in which conscious experiences are linked to behavioural functions (see Chapter 10).

We have used a method (functional magnetic resonance imaging) to visualise the activity of the brain in a group of such synaesthetes when they were listening to words. The words activated just and only that part of the visual system (known as 'V4') which is activated in normal individuals by the sight of coloured patterns, as distinct from the same patterns presented in black and white (see Plate 2.1). Now, if V4 is damaged, say in a car accident, there is a complete loss of all sense of colour: the unfortunate individual henceforth experiences the world only in varying shades of grey. So activity in V4 is both necessary (brain damage case) and sufficient (coloured hearing synaesthesia) for the experience of colour. It is here, not on the surface of objects, that colour is constructed. Just as the world lacks all music if there is no-one (having an appropriately built brain) to listen to it, so it lacks all colour if there is no-one (having an appropriately built brain) to see it.

By now you may be worried that, like Bishop Berkeley, I shall shortly make the real world out there vanish entirely. But that is not my objective. Of course, as I have already accepted, there is a real world out there. But it is not the world as we perceive it. It is a world best described, to an astonishingly high degree of accuracy and predictability, by the science of physics. Our perceptions of that world need to be good enough to guide us through it, that is, to ensure Darwinian survival of the perceiving creatures and hence the survival of those very mechanisms of perception. But percepts do not need to be better than this. The ability to discriminate between wavelengths of light in the jumpy fashion that colours superimpose upon the underlying continuous variable of wavelength of light has evidently been conducive to our survival. But it hasn't been useful to the survival of all species, not even all mammalian species, most of which lack trichromatic colour vision. The evolution of colour vision took place in monkeys, presumably because it helped them pick out fruit, often coloured red or orange, amid the green foliage of the bushes where it hung (see Section 7.4 for a more detailed discussion). No doubt for this same reason, colours of these kinds are generally found to be pleasing; for evolution, as well as giving us the power to locate those things which are good for our survival, has conferred upon us the capacity to delight in them and the desire to approach, taste and ingest them.

Let me summarise this part of the argument (Fig. 1.1 may help). There are two worlds: the world as described by physics, and the world we consciously perceive. There is a chair as it is described in physics, in all its atomic and quantum mechanical glory; and there is the chair that I can see, smell, touch and so on. The chair that I sit in is an amalgam of the two. I could not sit in it unless it had physical properties enabling it to bear my weight; but the perception I have of it as a chair is a construct of my brain. The perceived chair may under some conditions play little if any role in my interactions with the chair of physics. So, if it is a familiar chair in familiar surroundings, I may sit down in it with little if any guidance from conscious perception. But under other conditions—if, say, I am admiring a Chippendale—the consciously perceived chair plays a much more important role.

Fortunately, the correspondence between the perceived chair and the chair of physics is close enough for my behaviour in relation to the chair to be usually pretty successful. For that, we have evolution to thank. Brains have evolved so as to perform the computations needed for a good fit (good enough, that is, to aid survival) between perception, behaviour and the world of physics. It is also evolution we have to thank for the fit between your perception and mine. The same constraints upon survival in the environments in which human beings evolved have acted via the same pool of genes to create brains which, in their essentials, do the same things in the same way. So we all see (roughly) the same chair and hear (roughly) the same sonata.

I can, of course, also *imagine* a chair as well as see or sit in it. The imagined chair is different from both the chair I sit in and the chair of physics. The imagined chair, too, is part of my conscious experience, but no more so than the chair I see in my drawing room. The problem of consciousness is far more extensive than just those portions of our experience that are private to our imaginations.

For these arguments to hold, I must convince you that other properties of the entities that populate the perceived world, besides their colour, are similarly 'all in the mind'. (Or, which comes to the same thing, 'all in the brain', 'mind' being simply—or not so simply—the brain in action.) To do this we must overcome the brain's own powerful efforts to convince us of just the opposite: that all these properties are *out there*. For 'projection' of conscious experience into a three-dimensional outside world is precisely what consciousness does best, even perhaps part of what it is *for*.

Take again the example of music. Music has no externally definable location in space. Even if one adopts a determinedly externalist approach to perception, the aerial vibrations that are the physical trigger to the experience of music are located in the ear-drums. But that is not where you hear the trumpet in the concert hall: you hear it as being located where the trumpeter is. If the trumpet sounds come from the loud-speakers in your living room, you hear them as coming from a trumpeter whose position in the room varies depending on the relative loudness at each speaker. Only under the special conditions of hearing the trumpet through ear-phones (and not always then), do you hear the trumpet sounds as being produced—where they have in fact been produced all along—in the space between your ears. These special conditions eliminate the information in the pattern of sound waves at the ear-drums that the brain normally uses to construct a three-dimensional acoustic space and to insert into it a trumpet. The predictable relations that hold in the world of physics (given the acoustics of the concert hall) between sound waves leaving the trumpet and those arriving at your ear permit the brain to use that information to make a pretty good estimate of where the trumpet is located. But you don't experience this as music at the ear-drums *plus* an estimate of the location of the trumpeter: you just experience the music as coming from the trumpeter. And the brain uses the same information in just the same way irrespective of whether the sound waves in fact come from a trumpeter in a concert-hall or from loud-speakers in the living room.

The experience of pain might seem stony ground for a demonstration of the brain's powers of projection. The difficulty of telling the doctor 'just where it hurts' is familiar. Yet the phenomenon of 'phantom limb' pain is a dramatic example of the brain's powers of projection. A person who has lost a limb or part of a limb may go on for years feeling pain, often excruciating, localised precisely and unshakeably in the missing arm or leg. Clearly the pain cannot truly be *in* the arm, because the arm isn't there. But neural messages in the brain continue to do what they would do if there were pain in that arm, and the resulting pain experience is therefore projected onto the arm—even though other parts of the brain (the visual system, for example) clearly register the fact that there is no arm. 'Just where it hurts' is never felt to be in the brain; but that is precisely where the events (the passage of nervous impulses) that produce pain are located.

Touch also seems stony ground for our thesis. But here is what Velmans says about it, in his book *Understanding Consciousness* (p. 117):

> Notice the way this book feels hard when you press it with your fingers. The experienced hardness is subjectively located in the region of the stimulated tactile receptors at the point of contact between your fingers and the book. But the proximal neural causes of such sensations are located in the region of the somatosensory cortex. So, how does the sensation of hardness get back down to the fingers? Now press the tip of a pencil against the table on which the book sits. The table feels hard *at the point where it is pressed*. But there are no sensory organs located at the pencil tip!

In interpreting the shear force exerted on the skin by the pencil (when the pencil presses on the table), the brain habitually refers the origin of the felt resistance to the point of contact between the table and pencil tip—an everyday, illusory projection of tactile sensations beyond the surface of the skin.

## 2.3   Vision: perception versus action

But it is vision that is the queen of the senses. And the impression from this sense is utterly compelling—that we look out from our eyes, as through a perfectly clear and transparent window, on the world as it simply and really exists. It is an impression that stubbornly resists the evidence to the contrary. That evidence is contained in a vast array of visual illusions, many so familiar that they long ago entered school classrooms, museums and art galleries. These illusions demonstrate, over and over again, that the world as we see it is made according to rules imposed by the brain. Almost everybody is susceptible to them. But hardly anyone draws the necessary conclusion: that *all* our visual percepts, not just the demonstrably illusory ones, are constructed by the brain, remain inside the brain, and merely seem to form part of—are projected by the brain onto—a three-dimensional world (itself constructed by the brain) out there. I shall describe only a handful of these myriad demonstrations of the fallibility of visual perception, choosing them so as to draw out their general implications.

The first thing to make clear is that there is not just one visual system, but two (actually, more than two, but two to a first and useful approximation). They both start out with information contained in the pattern of activity in the cells of the retina caused by the light that falls there. That point of origin is what makes them both 'visual' systems. But thereafter the two systems rapidly diverge, as this information is transformed at each relay on the way up to higher levels of the nervous system, and they remain divergent up to the point at which they each, in very different ways, control behaviour. (At some stage, also, they probably converge again; but that part of the neuroscientific story is still rather unclear.) The two systems are each exceedingly complex. This is not the place to enter into that complexity (a good place to start is the excellent book by David Milner and Mel Goodale, *The Visual Brain in Action*; Fig. 2.1 presents a highly simplified diagram taken from their book). For our purposes the most important feature of the two systems is that one—call it the *perception system* (the 'ventral stream' in the figure)— underlies what we consciously see and are able to report verbally; while the other—the *action system* ('dorsal stream')—doesn't appear to be related to visual consciousness at all. It is the action system that is engaged during fast-mov ing activities carried out without the accompaniment of conscious awareness, as in the tennis example considered earlier in the chapter. As we saw in that example, the perception system comes into play only after the event, lagging fast-moving activity too late directly to influence it.

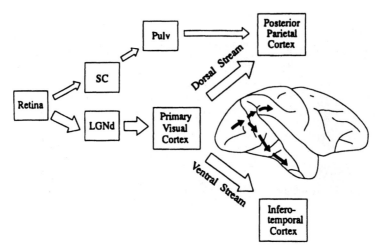

**Fig. 2.1** Schematic diagram showing major routes whereby retinal input reaches the dorsal and ventral streams. The inset shows the cortical projections on the right hemisphere of the brain of a macaque monkey. LGNd, lateral geniculate nucleus, pars dorsalis; Pulv, pulvinar nucleus; SC, superior colliculus. From Milner and Goodale (1995).

Fitting their different purposes, the two visual systems have very different properties. The action system is sensitive to rapidly changing properties of the information captured by electrochemical activity as light rays fall on the nerve cells of the retina; and it uses this information for rapid control of movements, often directed to either making or avoiding contact with the objects from which the light has been reflected. These include movements of the head and eyes, of the trunk, limbs, fingers and so on. The reason that there are, properly speaking, more than two visual systems is that the action system is made up of several subsystems, depending upon which set of movements is controlled. So, for example, movements of the eyes, most often with the goal of keeping relevant objects in central vision, are controlled by their own specialised set of brain cells, which receive visual information adapted to their own specialised needs. And so on for other sets of movements concerned with other goals, each subsystem acting as a separate 'servomechanism', along lines discussed in the next chapter.

The degree to which such visuomotor servomechanisms are isolated from one another, and their specialised role in survival, is particularly clear in species with a less complex organisation than highly evolved mammals like ourselves. Frogs, for example, have one specialised system for detecting and catching a passing fly and another for detecting and avoiding barriers in their path. If one part of the frog's brain is damaged, the animal loses its ability to 'see' flies but has no problem in 'seeing' barriers; while damage in another region of the frog brain leads to the reverse pattern of loss. Similar specialised visuomotor subsystems have been

(a)    (b)    (c)

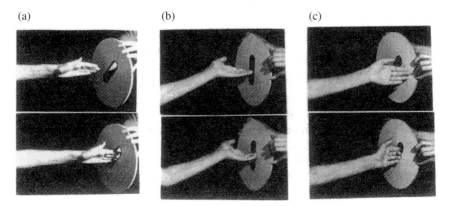

**Fig. 2.2** Illustrations of errors made by a patient with optic ataxia when reaching out to pass the hand through an oriented slot. The figure shows normal responses (a), hand-orientation errors (b), and localisation errors (c). The patient had a tumour centred in the right parietal lobe, and examples are given of her reaching respectively into the right (a) and the left (b, c) hemifield, in each case with her left hand. Single frames are shown, each taken from films made on different test trials. From Milner and Goodale (1995).

demonstrated also in monkeys and human beings. Patients with certain kinds of damage in the parietal lobes of the cerebral cortex, for example, have difficulty in correctly moving their eyes to the location of an object in space, but not in correctly grasping the object; while, if the damage is located in a different part of the same general region of the brain, the reverse is seen: a failure to grasp objects but not to move the eyes to their location ('optic ataxia'; see Fig. 2.2).

Where the action system is concerned to detect rapidly changing aspects of the visual scene, the perception system in contrast struggles to maintain visual stability. Because what we consciously see, and so can easily talk and think about, comes via the perception system, the enormity of this struggle for stability is far from obvious. Fortunately, many of the visual illusions reflect the operation of the machinery employed by the perceptual system in the struggle. In this way, they serve as a window on the perceptual system as much as one on the visual world. (This window was used particularly effectively in the early part of the twentieth century by the 'Gestalt psychologists'. I discuss their work in detail in Chapter 16. It may be helpful to read Section 16.1 before you move on.)

One of the biggest problems facing the perceptual system is that of constructing a three-dimensional world from the essentially two-dimensional array of cells in the retina that 'fire' (are active) in response to the particular pattern of light rays that fall on them. Now, if you suppose that all the perceptual system has to do is to open out on the real three-dimensional world and show us what it is like, then the overwhelmingly three-dimensional appearance of what we see comes as no surprise. But, in that case, you *should* be surprised by the capacity of the perceptual

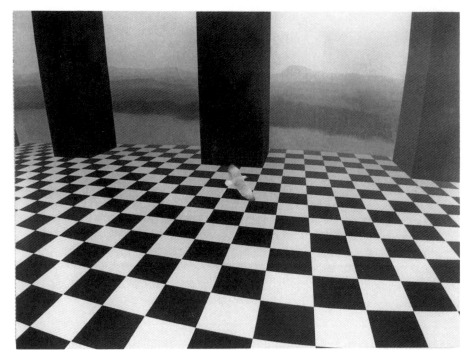

**Fig. 2.3** How two-dimensional cues can achieve quite a strong sense of depth through the use of radial perspective; painting by Peter Cresswell. From Velmans (2000).

system to achieve just the same three-dimensional effect by viewing flat surfaces—a capacity well known and thoroughly exploited since at least the time of the Renaissance, when painters discovered the laws of perspective. Figure 2.3 displays a particularly compelling recent example of this capacity. Look at this figure through a 'reduction tube' (a rolled-up piece of paper): does this not convince you that the brain constructs three-dimensional space *even when there is no three-dimensional space there*?

Notice by the way that, in asking you to look at a picture like Fig. 2.3, I can take it for granted that you will experience what nearly everyone else experiences when they view it. Philosophers sometimes endow conscious experience with an inviolable privacy, rendering it incapable of meeting the scientific requirement for replicability of empirical observations. Nothing could be further from the truth, as attested by the reliability of visual illusions, among many other phenomena.

Oddly, one doesn't normally think of this kind of painterly use of perspective as creating an 'illusion', though that is surely what it does. That term is usually reserved for particular little trick pictures invented by laboratory scientists. Several of these, too, probably depend for their effects upon the brain's attempts to create a three-dimensional world out of a two-dimensional pattern of stimulation. A

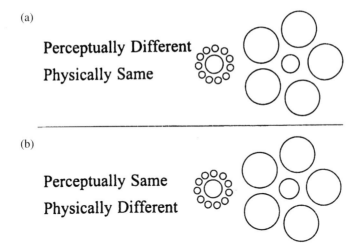

**Fig. 2.4** The 'Titchener circles' illusion. In (a) the two central discs are of the same actual size, but appear different; in (b) the disc surrounded by an annulus of large circles has been made some-what larger in size in order to appear approximately equal in size to the other central disc. From Milner and Goodale (1995).

simple example, is the 'Titchener circles' illusion. As shown in Fig. 2.4, a circle appears smaller when it is surrounded by a ring of smaller circles than when surrounded by a ring of larger circles. One hypothesis to account for this effect is that the ring of smaller circles is 'interpreted' by the brain as being further away than the ring of larger circles (since the further away an object is, the smaller is the retinal area upon which the reflected light falls). The brain also interprets each of the two central circles as belonging together with the ring of circles by which it is enclosed. If the two central circles then, as measured by a ruler, are the same size, but one is interpreted as being further away than the other, then this 'must' be bigger (to compensate for the falling off in retinal size that ought to come from being further away).

This is not to say that the rationale (convoluted but coherent) that the brain uses to produce illusions like the Titchener circles comes in the form of propositional logic. If that were the case, then understanding the logic ought to allow us to ques-tion it, to try variations on it, and so on, with consequential changes in what we perceive. But that just isn't possible. Visual illusions (like the whole of perception) are *givens*: they are constructed unconsciously and then pop, fully made, into conscious awareness. You can tell yourself (after you have applied your ruler) that the two inside circles in Fig. 2.4(a) are actually the same size; but you cannot stop yourself seeing them as being of different sizes. And this despite the fact that *the brain knows the truth all along*. It knows it, however, in another system: not in perception but in action.

This knowledge has been demonstrated in a beautiful experiment conducted in Mel Goodale's laboratory. Two thin discs were used as the central circles in displays of the kind shown in Fig. 2.4(a) and (b). Subjects were instructed to pick up the disc on the left if the two discs appeared to be of equal size (as in Fig. 2.4(b), when the discs are actually of different sizes), but to pick up the disc on the right if the two discs appeared to be of unequal size (as in Fig. 2.4(a), when they are actually the same size). The subjects were not instructed in the mysteries of Titchener circles, so they did not realise that their perceptions were illusory. It took a difference of 2 mm in the diameter of the discs for the subjects to treat them as being of equal size. In this way, then, Goodale and his colleagues were able to demonstrate and measure the extent of the perceived illusion. But, at the same time, they recorded the aperture of the subjects' grip (the distance between finger and thumb) as their hands reached for the disc. Grip aperture remained appropriate to the *actual* size of the discs—totally immune to the illusion in their perceived size.

This important experiment makes several points clear.

First, there is a remarkable degree of isolation between the action and the perceptual systems of vision. The action system takes one 'view' of the world, while the perceptual system takes another. The separation between the two systems sometimes becomes glaringly apparent in patients who have suffered brain damage. Patients with optical ataxia (as illustrated in Fig. 2.2) may nonetheless preserve the ability to make accurate verbal judgements of the location, distance and relative position of objects in the visual field. Conversely, other patients (with damage to the primary visual cortex in the occipital lobe) may suffer what Larry Weiskrantz has called 'blindsight'. They deny, verbally, seeing anything at all in that part of the visual field (the 'scotoma') that would normally be represented in the damaged region of the visual cortex. However, when tested in a variety of ways involving behaviour, e.g. pointing, or when asked just to 'guess', they show high

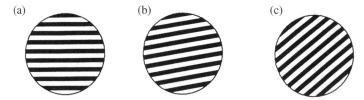

(a)     (b)     (c)

**Fig. 2.5** Stimuli used to measure orientation discrimination by a blindsight subject, D. B., in his blind field by forced-choice guessing. He was asked to guess whether a stimulus to be flashed briefly was orientated horizontally (a) or non-horizontally (c). He was virtually perfect in guessing that the grating shown in (c) was non-horizontal and that (a) was horizontal. The task was made more difficult by decreasing the angle between the horizontal and non-horizontal gratings, to measure his threshold (the limit of his ability): (b), which is $10^0$ off horizontal, was his threshold. In this task the subject reported that he saw nothing, not even the brief flash when the grating was presented. From Weiskrantz (1997).

degrees of accuracy in locating the 'unseen' object, telling the direction of orientation of a set of lines (see Fig. 2.5), or judging whether a visual stimulus is moving or stationary.

Second, both systems are able to run concurrently, each doing its own, different, job. One of the issues we shall need to consider later is how, nevertheless, the two systems are also able to communicate and cooperate with each other.

Third, the Titchener circle illusion belongs exclusively to the perceptual system, it does not affect the action of grasping. So far as I know, this is a general truth: visual illusions occur only in the perceptual system, not in the action system. It may even be a necessary truth. For what we perceive, we perceive consciously; indeed, I shall argue later that perception is the *only* form taken by conscious experience. In contrast, as shown in the residual visual capacities of blindsight patients, the visual action system proceeds without conscious awareness of the objects with which it interacts. In the absence of conscious awareness, it is difficult to comprehend what an illlusion might be. Actions can be effective or ineffective—they cannot be veridical or illusory.

## 2.4   Illusions of the will

Let's remind ourselves of the archetypal narrative structure of conscious experience which we are submitting to scrutiny. This is how the story generally goes: *I perceived* (consciously saw, heard, tasted, etc.) *this* out *there*, and so *I* then *did* (consciously formed the intention to do, and then did) *that*. In this section we move on to take a closer look at the 'I' who is allegedly the perceiving and doing subject of the narrative. The clear assumption is that this 'I' is the *conscious* self. But this assumption runs into two major problems.

First, as we have seen, for all the passion with which I might declaim that I saw the tennis ball coming over the net into the left side of the back of the court and therefore decided to run that way to meet it and give a back-handed return, that's not the way it happens. I would need to have made the decision, and indeed acted upon it, before I consciously saw the ball.

Second, there is good experimental evidence that *decisions are taken a long time before the subject becomes consciously aware of having made the decision*. In other words, the situation for the sense of agency is exactly as it is for the senses of vision and pain: consciousness occurs after the event.

This was demonstrated over two decades ago in a famous experiment by Benjamin Libet. He instructed his subjects to carry out a particular movement (a flexion of the wrist or the fingers) at a time entirely of their own choosing. The subject sat in front of a cathode ray oscilloscope displaying a spot revolving around the screen like the second hand on a clock. At the moment when the subject first consciously decided to move his wrist or finger, he noted the position of the spot, so giving the time at which this decision was made. Throughout, an

EEG (electroencephalographic) machine recorded electrical activity in the subject's brain by way of electrodes on the scalp. Now, it had long been known that, prior to the performance of any voluntary movement, the EEG shows a so-called 'readiness potential', that is, a slow negative shift. What Libet's experiment showed was that the readiness potential occurs ahead of, not only the movement, but also the first conscious experience of the intention to make the movement. And the duration of this delay before conscious awareness was not trivial: the change in the EEG occurred 350 milliseconds or more before consciousness of the intention to move. These findings (replicated recently in their essentials by Patrick Haggard and Martin Eimer) have been hotly debated over the years since Libet first reported them. This is hardly surprising, since they pose an extraordinary challenge to the deeply held intuition that one acts when and because one consciously decides to do so. But the debate has left the findings and their implication intact: the consciously experienced intention to act can occur *after* the brain already shows by its *unconscious* activity that the intention has been formed.

In retrospect, Libet's findings, flagrantly counter-intuitive as they are, should nonetheless not have caused so great a degree of scandal among the scientific and philosophical communities. For the greater part of these communities had by then abandoned Cartesian dualism. According to dualism, the stream of mental events proceeds in a medium quite separate from the stream of physical events. Communication between the two streams, according to Descartes, took place in the pineal gland, famous today rather for its production of the hormone, melatonin. Given dualism, therefore, one could have believed that the conscious wish to flex a finger might take place in advance of, or perhaps alongside, accompanying brain activity. But by the last quarter of the twentieth century, when Libet did his experiments, the weight of philosophical argument and empirical evidence had largely displaced dualism. In principle it was now generally accepted that mental events are in some way caused by activities in the brain. On that view, what *other* outcome of Libet's experiments could have been expected?

Causes must precede their effects; brain activity causes mental events; *ergo*, brain activity must precede that particular mental event that is the making of a conscious intention to do something. From this point of view, then, the only surprise in Libet's results should have lain in the duration of the delay between brain activity and conscious volition: 350 milliseconds is on any view a remarkably long time. However, Cartesian dualism is a philosophical doctrine that accords very well with the apparent facts of everyday conscious experience. For that reason, pretty well everyone still retains dualism as the default option, dominating spontaneous interpretation of the world and our place in it. So, even for the professed materialist who believes that brain activity causes mental events, first acquaintance with Libet's findings generally occasions amazement.

In fact, the delay in conscious awareness of the making of a decision fits well with the other delays we have already encountered. Consider again the tennis example. The temporal sequence of events we established earlier is: visual stimulus of ball being served → hitting of ball in the return → conscious seeing of the ball being served → conscious awareness of hitting the return. We can now expand this to read: visual stimulus of ball being served → unconscious decision about where to run, etc., in order to hit the return → hitting of the ball in return → conscious seeing of the ball being served → conscious awareness the decision about where to run, etc., → conscious awareness of hitting the return. In other words, consciousness faithfully records the correct sequence of events, but only after they are over.

This representation of a single linear sequence of behaviour passing through from unconsciousness to consciousness is, of course, greatly over-simplified. Behaviour and conscious experience are each temporally seamless. With some lag (apparently of the order of a quarter of a second), therefore, there occurs the running off of one action (or part of an action) simultaneously with the conscious recording of another that is already completed. This rather strange arrangement clearly begs the questions: how and why? We shall come back to these questions. We shall also need to consider later (see especially Chapter 19) just what it might mean for the brain to take an *unconscious* decision. We cannot just transpose our intuitive understanding of what it is like to make a conscious decision to the unconscious realm. Indeed and in general, if exactly the same things occur in and out of consciousness, that would make even more mysterious the mystery of why the brain has engineered the split between the two realms in the first place.

Everyone is very familiar with actions that run off unconsciously—that make no pretence, as it were, to dependence upon conscious volition. Some actions are so totally automatic, never having been accompanied by conscious awareness, that we don't normally deem them to be actions at all. When, for example, one rises suddenly from sitting in a chair or lying in a bed, the body makes all sorts of automatic adjustments to muscle tension, blood pressure and so on. One becomes aware of these adjustments only when they fail and you feel faint or keel over. Other actions have once been accompanied by conscious awareness but have become so routine with repeated practice that they often no longer are so accompanied. Transportation is especially replete with such examples: swimming, riding a bicycle, even driving a car. So the force of Libet's experiment does not lie in the sheer demonstration that behaviour can be governed by processes that go on outside conscious awareness. It lies, rather, in the demonstration that, even when we think we are making a conscious decision, that decision has been taken prior to our conscious awareness of it. The scandal of Libet's findings is that they show *the awareness of conscious volition to be illusory*.

Libet's findings are not the only ones to show this. There is other evidence that dissociates responsibility for action from awareness of that responsibility. This dissociation can take both possible directions: one can be responsible for an act but unaware of the responsibility; or believe one is responsible for an act which is not one's own. A dramatic example of the former case—responsibility without awareness—is the so-called 'alien hand syndrome'. After certain kinds of brain damage the patient loses the sense of ownership of the affected limb. One such report is of a woman whose 'left hand would tenaciously grope for and grasp any nearby object, pick and pull at her clothes, and even grasp her throat during sleep.… She slept with the arm tied to prevent nocturnal misbehaviour. She never denied that her left arm belonged to her, although she did refer to her limb as though it were an autonomous entity' (Banks *et al.*, 1989, p. 456). An instance of the latter case—erroneous belief in responsibility—is post-hypnotic suggestion, a phenomenon so robust that it survives exhibition on the public stage. Under hypnosis, a suggestion is made to the subject that, when the trance has ended, he will do something or other (unfurl the Stars and Stripes and wave it vigorously) in response to a signal from the hypnotist. The hypnotist duly makes the signal and the subject carries out the action—but claims the act for his own, giving all sorts of reasons for having chosen to perform it ('I saw an American mate of mine and wanted to say hallo').

So the attribution to oneself of responsibility for an act is dissociable from the responsibility itself. This dissociation raises the question: what information does a person use in making the attribution?

A neat experiment by Wegner and Wheatley (1999) begins to provide an answer to this question. They argued that you will be more likely to claim responsibility for an action if you think about it just before it occurs. To test this hypothesis they set up a task inspired by the once fashionable Ouija board. Two people (one a real subject, the other a confederate of the experimenter) placed their hands together on a computer mouse and used it jointly to move a cursor round the screen. The screen displayed pictures of about 50 small objects, e.g. a car or a swan. From time to time the two participants had to stop the movement of the cursor; and, after the stop, they were asked to rate the degree to which each was responsible for it, using a scale going from *I allowed the stop to happen* to *I intended to make the stop*. The subject also heard music and words through headphones. Some of the stops (unknown to the subject) were forced by the confederate; and sometimes the words heard through the headphones related to the picture on which the confederate was about to force a stop. The related word was presented to the subject at intervals from 30 seconds before the stop to 1 second after it. Hearing the related word before a forced stop increased the subject's rating that he intended to make the stop, but only if the word occurred 1–5 seconds in advance of the stop (not when it occurred 30 seconds in advance or 1 second after it). Even though subjects were in fact responsible for none of these stops, their ratings of responsibility at the 1- and 5-second intervals were clearly above the half-way mark. These findings clearly support the experimental hypothesis: having relevant thoughts just before an event increases your sense of responsibility for the event—even if you have done nothing to cause it.

Evidently, then, one may consciously perceive responsibility for one's actions without having it; or lack a conscious sense of the responsibility that in reality one has; and, even when one consciously has a veridical sense of responsibility, the consciousness of volition comes (as shown by Libet's experiment) after unconscious volition is already under way. More generally, the experiments discussed in this section raise the possibility—one to which we return in Chapters 17 and 18—that the central actor in the archetypal narrative, the self, is as much a construction of the brain as is the world with which the self interacts.

## Conclusions

The archetypal story of conscious experience is told like this: *I perceived* (consciously saw, heard, tasted, etc.) *this* out *there*, and so *I* then *did* (consciously formed the intention to do, and then did) *that*.

We have unpicked this story in the following ways.

1. The conscious perceiving does *not* precede the doing; rather, it follows on *after* the doing, or at best goes on in parallel with it.
2. The 'out there' of conscious experience isn't really out there at all; it's inside the head.
3. The conscious 'I' is not the true subject of the story: it is the unconscious brain.

These conclusions are not without paradox. I have committed myself in this chapter to two propositions which are, on the face of it, mutually contradictory:

(1) conscious experiences don't just represent the world out there—they *are* the world out there (leaving aside the other world—the one described by physics—also out there);
(2) conscious experiences can be illusory—indeed, illusions pertain *only* to conscious experience.

But how is it possible to judge that an experience is illusory if that experience is itself the real event? There must surely be some other means of assessing reality to come to that judgement.

This is a paradox that we shall try to resolve later (see Chapter 5). First, however, in the next chapter, we approach the Hard Problem of consciousness from another angle, by asking this question: how might the facts of conscious experience fit into current scientific understanding of the brain and behaviour?

# CHAPTER 3

# Where science and consciousness meet

The previous chapter started on the task of convincing you that there is indeed a problem of consciousness. The arguments deployed there turned mainly on matters of fact about conscious experiences. We continue on that task here, but by looking at a broader theoretical picture: how do the facts about consciousness fit into the rest of the scientific world-view?

## 3.1 Scientific reduction in biology

To get to grips with this aspect of the Hard Problem, put yourself in the position of a scientist studying the brain or behaviour. Now, science is an imperialistic pursuit. It strives continuously for a unified theory of the whole of the natural world. No sooner does it produce a theory from which one can deduce and predict empirical observations in one limited field, than it seeks to incorporate that theory into another that is wider (embracing neighbouring fields) or deeper (reduced to more elementary levels of explanation) or preferably both. In this way, for example, chemistry embraces biochemistry and is itself reduced to physics. To be sure, there are sometimes barriers to such expansion or reduction. Indeed, one of the keenest debates in the field of consciousness is whether this encompasses just such a barrier to reduction. It is therefore worth spending some time getting to understand in what such irreducibility might consist.

The best existing example of irreducibility is probably this: the processes of natural selection (and therefore those of biology) cannot be completely reduced to the laws of physics and chemistry. Importantly, however, it is not simply the case that a barrier to reduction is located at this point: there is also a principled understanding of the *nature* of the barrier.

The key argument was first clearly enunciated by Michael Polanyi. It goes as follows. The physics and chemistry upon which natural selection operates so as to maximise biological fitness are those of the DNA that makes up an individual animal's chromosomes. DNA is made up of a chain of chemical units called nucleotides or bases, of which there are four kinds: adenine (A), cytosine (C), guanine (G) or thymine (T). At each point in the double-stranded DNA helix, the laws of physics and chemistry (requiring structures to adopt the lowest energy conformation) can be satisfied *equally well in one of two ways*: A on one strand can pair with C on the other, or T can pair with G. It is precisely this physico-chemical *indifference* to what comes next that allows natural selection to work. If there were complete physico-chemical determinism of which base-pair follows which in the chain, there would be no variation—and so no possibility that biological fitness could be increased by the selection of one variant over another. In that case, the biological world would fail at the starting gun.

So far, then, from biology's being reducible to physics and chemistry, it is only because it *cannot* be so reduced that there is any biology at all. To put the same point in an equivalent, but broader, way, information (the instructions contained in a string of nucleotides as to how to make, say, a mammal) can exist only if there is a choice among alternative possibilities. Of course, those possibilities need to *respect* the laws of physics; but by definition (or they would not be possibilities) they are not fully determined by these laws. However, this failure of reductionism in no way represents a failure of scientific understanding. On the contrary: one of the triumphs of scientific enquiry is that the existence of living organisms no longer poses a mystery for which (as once appeared to be the case) it is necessary to postulate an entirely novel and special process, that of the *élan vital*.

Even in this case, then, of clear irreducibility of one science (biology) to another (physics and chemistry), there is no mystery, no gap, no lack of connection between the theories employed on each side of the divide. But, when we come to the meeting point between brain-and-behaviour and conscious experience, that is just what we find: mystery, gaps and missing connections.

The success with which biology has dealt with the one-time problem of life is often held up as the model for the way science should now approach consciousness. In considering this suggestion, it is important to bear in mind that linking biology to physics and chemistry has required two types of move. First, as we have seen, the role of natural selection and of the information content of DNA have to be understood in their own right, in a manner not fully reducible to, but not inconsistent with, the laws of physics and chemistry. Second, however, the defining properties of life (respiration, reproduction, etc.), as found in the organisms that survive natural selection, *can* themselves be reduced to specific physicochemical processes. We need to hang on to this kind of 'bifocal' perspective: physicochemical *plus* selectionist.

There is another useful way to think about the difference between the two levels of the bifocal perspective on biology. Physics and chemistry operate in such a manner that you need only the laws of these sciences, plus a set of initial conditions, to predict the way in which a system governed by them will evolve over time. The *consequences* of that evolution are not required for prediction. Biological evolution, in contrast, as governed by Darwinian natural selection, depends precisely upon the consequences of slotting *this* rather than *that* base-pair into the chain making up the genetic code for the construction of an individual organism.

Depending upon which base-pair enters the chain, the survival and reproduction of that individual will be enhanced or reduced (relative to the survival and reproduction of other individuals in which the alternative base-pair was slotted in); and, next time round, the biological world will contain correspondingly more or fewer stretches of DNA that include at that particular point in the chain the one or other pair of nucleotides. There is nothing teleological or mysterious about this process of *selection by consequences*. But there is nothing like it in unadorned physics and chemistry.

The role that selection by consequences plays at this highest layer of the laws of biology—that of natural selection—is mirrored at a series of further lower layers, like the wrapped around skins of an onion, before you reach its purely physico-chemical core. This is because natural selection has acted to produce organisms that are equipped with a huge variety of homeostatic, or 'feedback', mechanisms that serve to protect the organism's integrity and reproductive capacity against the vagaries of a constantly changing environment, so enhancing the chances of survival. The ubiquity, diversity and power of these mechanisms is reflected in the creation of a whole branch of the theory of engineering, known as 'cybernetics', to deal with them. We need not go into the details of this theory. For our purposes, its key feature is that, to understand how the theory works, we again need to take a bifocal perspective, with one level using only the laws of physics and chemistry while the other respects these laws but goes beyond them.

A system of feedback mechanisms has to be constructed from some set of components or other; and the construction of the system has to respect the particular physics and chemistry of those components. But the system also has properties (described in the mathematical equations of cybernetics) that will be the same, no matter what the components out of which it is constructed. So, in a familiar example, engineers construct thermostats in which the components are made of metal and wire. In a thermostatic system, environmental temperature is measured by a sensor of some kind. That measurement is then fed back to a central controller, and compared by the controller to a desired set point. The results of that comparison are used by the system to generate (or reduce) heat output so as to move temperature towards the set point, which changes environmental temperature, which is fed back again, and so on, optimising approximation to the set point. Household thermostats are made by engineers. But natural selection too has made thermostats, out of cells that react to changes in temperature, muscle cells, nerve cells that control the muscle cells, and so on. Now, it would be a poorly constructed thermostat that did not respect the different physical and chemical properties of these different kinds of component. But these properties are not sufficient in themselves to predict the behaviour of the system *as a thermostat*. To do that, you have to take into account the way in which the system is constructed. Conversely, it is possible to predict the behaviour of the system as a system from the equations of cybernetics. But, to predict the behaviour of a component within the system, it is necessary also to take into account the laws of physics and chemistry that are applicable to that specific type of component. And, for a complete account, both levels of explanation are required—neither can be fully reduced to the other.

Feedback of this general kind operates at every level of biology (in addition to that of natural selection itself), from the level of intracellular organelles, to the behaviour of the entire cell, to the interactions between groups of cells, to the interactions between parts of the brain, and finally to complex psychological processes in human beings. (If you wish to see just *how* complex and far-reaching this approach to human behaviour can be, take a look at Susan Hurley's introductory chapter to her edited volume, with Nick Chater, on imitation.) A particularly important level (especially for the concept of responsibility; see Chapter 19) is the guidance of learning and behaviour by reward or punishment. What is less clear, however, is whether, within this nested set of feedback systems, we need to draw any further distinctions of principle, beyond those that have already emerged in the discussion of natural selection.

There are two distinctions that may be relevant to the problem of consciousness. They both have to do with the way in which a system represents the variables that it tries to control.

The variable(s) that a feedback system controls, how that variable is measured and how such measurements are fed back to the rest of the system are key defining elements in the description of the system. In the case of a thermostat, the controlled variable is external temperature. (I consider here only the simplest case, in which the system controls a single variable; in practice, biological systems at all levels control a large number of variables simultaneously, mostly in complex interaction with each other.) Now, one can ask of such a variable: where in the system is its locus of representation? In a thermostatically controlled home heating system, it is normally relatively easy to point (literally) to this locus. Temperature may, for example, be represented in the length of a bimetallic strip that expands with heat and contracts with cold. That is the way the rest of the system receives information about how close the controlled variable is to the desired set-point. And it is precisely this—the fact that the system is designed to receive and act upon information about temperature—which allows one to talk at all of temperature as being 'represented' in the length of the bimetallic strip. On its own, the fact that the strip *does* expand with heat and contract with cold (a property it shares with many other entities) is insufficient for talk about representation.

Consider now the contrasting case of natural selection. Here, it is impossible to point to any specific locus in space or time at which survival value is computed or fed back to the chains of DNA nucleotides that survival favours or disfavours. Nor has natural selection been designed to measure or control anything. The concept of 'design' starts out as something that human engineers do. It is then reasonable (though not without conceptual risk) to extend it to what natural selection does.

A bird's wings are 'designed' (by natural selection) to keep the bird aloft. Indeed, it is almost impossible to find any other coherent way of talking about the way a bird's wings have ended up the way they are. But the process of natural selection has not itself been designed (what could have designed it?)—it just is.

We must distinguish, then, between two kinds of feedback mechanism. In the first, as in the thermostat, the controlled variable has a definite locus of representation to which the system is designed to react. In the second (natural selection), the controlled variable has no definite locus of representation and the system is not designed to react to anything. Let us call the first kind a '*servomechanism*'. That is to say, both natural selection and thermostats are 'feedback systems', but only the thermostat is a 'servomechanism'. It would seem absurd to attribute to a feedback system of the distributed kind that is natural selection a locus of conscious experience. It is not so clearly absurd, however, to make this attribution to a servomechanism, and still less so to a complex system made up of many servomechanisms. Indeed, the dominant contemporary approach to the problem of consciousness—functionalism (considered in detail in Chapter 10)—essentially does just that.

The second distinction that may be relevant to the problem of consciousness concerns the system's capacity to report the current state of the controlled variable. In the case of natural selection, nothing seems to correspond to such a 'report'. Organisms survive or do not survive, and some genes spread while others drop out; but (until human experimenters utilise methods that are quite independent of the natural selection feedback system itself), no tally is anywhere kept of either organisms or genes. Servomechanisms, by contrast, having taken a measurement of a controlled variable, must report it to the rest of the system. Otherwise, the system would be unable to take appropriate action (that is, the actions they are designed to carry out) so as to control the variable.

Servomechanisms may also report these measurements to systems other than themselves. So, for example, the mammalian brain contains a servomechanism which responds to moving stimuli in the periphery of vision by swinging the eyeballs in their sockets so that these stimuli fall into the central field of vision. Information concerning this eye-movement and the new position of the eyes is at the same time provided to other parts of the brain. These other regions use the information to cancel out what might otherwise be perceived as movement and change in spatial location on the part of other visually perceived objects. Note that all of this takes place without conscious awareness of the doings of the servomechanism (although the *consequences* of the output of the mechanism, in the form of perception of a new segment of the visual world, may be accessible to conscious awareness and report).

The difference between the diffuse feedback of natural selection and the more focussed feedback of servomechanisms is itself a product of natural selection. The process of natural selection is determined by the boundary conditions left open by the laws of physics and chemistry, by random variation, and by the interactions between organisms and their constantly changing environments. As a consequence of this process, servomechanisms come into being, because they favour survival. They do this by conferring upon organisms (at all levels of the biological world, from organelle to the whole animal) the capacity to preserve integrity of structure and function, despite changes in the environment. Selection by consequences determines natural selection; and natural selection in turn creates specialist servomechanisms that optimise selected consequences.

Now, behaviour is merely one way (albeit a very important one) in which an integrated hierarchy of servomechanisms adds to this capacity of self-preservation. At a high level in this hierarchy of feedback mechanisms is the process of learning: the acquisition, during an individual's lifetime, of patterns of behaviour that optimise rewards (which, in general—though by no means universally—favour survival) and minimise punishments (which, in general, threaten survival). Just as natural selection acts to equip individuals at conception with genes that favour survival, so learning acts to equip individuals during their lifetime with behaviour that does the same.

We do not normally suppose that the ability of servomechanisms to represent and report upon the variables they control is accompanied by conscious awareness of these variables. Yet, when we come to behaviour, this is just what we find: controlled variables (some of them, some of the time: e.g. heat, cold, pain, the pleasant taste of nutrititious food) are associated with conscious awareness. How does this association with consciousness come to take place, what kind of difference does it make to the operation of the system, is it a necessary association and, if so, why? These are ways of posing the Hard Question about consciousness, and they raise issues to which we shall return at several later points in the book (especially Chapters 7 and 18).

You may well have been bothered by the use of the word 'report' in relation to servomechanisms in the preceding paragraphs. In its normal sense, a 'report' is verbally and consciously delivered by one human being to another. Clearly, it is only in a metaphorical sense that a servomechanism can be said to report anything at all. However, my use of the word was neither a slip of the pen nor a deliberate attempt at obfuscation. For we do not know whether the difference between 'report' as used to describe what a servomechanism does and 'report' as applied to what human beings say is one that, when it comes to the problem of consciousness, *makes* a difference. If the ability of human beings to report verbally does make such a difference, in virtue of what extra ingredients does it do so? When someone says he is too hot, in what way does this differ from a thermostat equipped with a thermometer or a printout stating the same thing? This is another way of posing the Hard Question. Many theorists have proposed that consciousness requires human language. That, however, is not the position adopted here (see Chapter 6, Section 6.1).

In very general terms, then, biology makes use of two types of concept: physico-chemical laws and feedback mechanisms. The latter include both the feedback operative in natural selection, in which the controlled variables that determine survival are nowhere explicitly represented within the system; and servomechanisms, in which there is a specific locus of representation capable of reporting the values of the controlled variables to other system components and to other systems. The relationship between physicochemical laws and cybernetic mechanisms in the bifocal perspective on biology poses no deep problems. It consists in a kind of a *contract*: providing cybernetics respects the laws of physics and chemistry, its principles may be used to construct any kind of feedback system that serves a purpose. Behaviour as such does not appear to require for its explanation any principles additional to these. But we need to ask whether these same principles can account for the occurrence of the conscious experiences which (sometimes) accompany behaviour. Is this a case, like chemistry vis-à-vis physics, where complete reduction (of consciousness to the principles that govern the rest of biology) *is* possible? Or one like biology *vis-à-vis* chemistry, where reduction *isn't* possible and we know why not? If we are unable to affirm either of these positions, then we again face, now at a broad theoretical level, the Hard Problem of consciousness. In much of the rest of this book we shall be rather like a boxer, jabbing, ducking and weaving round the Hard Problem at this, its highest level of generality.

## 3.2   How does consciousness fit into neuroscience?

One of the few things we know for certain about consciousness is that, in adult human beings, it depends upon activity in the brain. The evidence for this proposition is overwhelming; we saw some examples in the previous chapter. We don't know, however, that this is a necessary connection. For example, we don't know whether consciousness could occur in a computer made of silicon chips. Nor do we know what type of activity in the brain is critical for the occurrence of consciousness. For this reason, there are as yet no answers to questions like these: What is the earliest age at which a child has conscious experiences? And do chimpanzees, or rats, or bees have such experiences? We do know, though, that not all kinds of brain activity are sufficient for consciousness. For, as we saw in the previous chapter, the brain achieves much without any accompaniment by consciousness.

These are issues to which we shall need to return. For the moment, I wish to stay at a broader level of generality. If we confine ourselves to the relationship of conscious experience to activity in the adult human brain, how would we recognise a successful scientific theory of this relationship if we had one? Such a theory would need to give answers to two questions about mechanism and two about evolution.

The mechanistic questions are:

1.  How does brain activity give rise to consciousness and the contents of conscious experience?
2.  How do consciousness and the contents of conscious experience influence behaviour?

The evolutionary questions are:

3.  How did consciousness evolve?
4.  What survival value does consciousness confer upon those organisms that possess it?

No doubt there are many other questions one could ask; but if we had a theory that could answer these four, we would have made enormous progress in integrating consciousness into scientific biology. We would also be able to give definitive answers to the more specific questions posed above: might a computer be conscious, do babies have conscious experiences, do rats? One test of a theory that purports to answer the four big questions would lie in its ability to give principled answers to these more specific questions. If it cannot give immediate answers, it must at least tell us what tests we would need to apply to computers, babies or rats to determine whether they are conscious or not. There is so far no theory that comes anywhere near this standard.

# CHAPTER 4

# Intentionality

In the last two chapters I have tried to convince you that there is indeed a Hard Problem of consciousness. In this chapter we begin to inspect this problem at a finer level of detail, by considering the nature of the gap between consciousness and brain activity. Why is it so difficult to cross?

## 4.1    The binding problem

A first difficulty facing theories of how brain activity might give rise to conscious experience lies in the sheer differences between their properties. These differences are of several kinds.

At a relatively superficial level, there are substantial differences in the temporo-spatial scales of consciousness and brain activity. The major known component of brain activity consists in the passage of electrochemical currents along and between millions ($10^{13}$ or so) of nerve cells on a millisecond time scale. There is no conceptual difficulty in relating these events in the brain to sensory input, since this similarly consists in the firing of millions of individual nerve cells specialised to respond to one or other form of physicochemical energy (light rays, sound waves, heat, mechanical pressure, specific molecules for taste and smell, and so on). Nor is there any conceptual difficulty in relating neural activity in the brain to behaviour expressed in movement. Indeed, the physiology of the neuromuscular junction, by which the brain causes muscle fibres to contract, is one of the best understood components of nervous activity. Nor, again, is there any great conceptual difficulty in understanding, at least in principle, how activity in the brain can relate sensory input to appropriate behavioural output. To achieve this understanding, one needs to take the same kind of bifocal view that we learned to adopt in the previous chapter. That is to say, one has to consider the passage of nervous impulses around the various complex and interlocking circuits of which the central nervous system is composed as falling *simultaneously* under the laws of physics and chemistry and under those of cybernetics (or 'information processing', an alternative descriptive language that can be applied to the system level of brain function). These are issues to which we shall need to return at greater length. But, as we shall see, they do not put up barriers between one part of science and another.

All of the events touched on in the previous paragraph take place on common scales of time and space. A physiologist can add up the time it takes for a sensory stimulus to activate its appropriate receptor, and for this to pass a neural message on to the central nervous system, together with the time it takes for the brain to compute an appropriate action and to cause an appropriate muscular response. In the same set of observations, a psychologist can measure the total interval between sensory input and behavioural response. These two measurements give pretty much the same answer. For a simple, unconscious sensorimotor response (for example, detection of movement at the periphery of the retina reflexly causing a movement of the eye so that the moving object now falls on the fovea—the centre—of the retina), that answer is of the order of 100 milliseconds. As to the spatial scale, all the events concerned take place in the circumscribed region provided by the brain, plus nerves in and nerves out.

However, when one looks at the temporal properties of conscious experiences, these take place on a much slower time scale. As we saw in Chapter 2, it takes about a quarter of a second (starting from sensory impact) for an event to reach conscious awareness; and this then has a duration in consciousness of upwards of a tenth of a second. As to the consciousness of a willed action, Libet's data indicate that this takes even longer—upwards of 350 milliseconds. Nonetheless, we can in the case of time at least make use of the same kind of clock. Comparison between brain activity and conscious experience with regard to their spatial scales, in contrast, is much harder, since it is not clear whether one can attribute spatial location to conscious experience at all. From one point of view, the spatial scale of consciousness is huge, since it encompasses the whole experienced world; yet, from another, a consciously experienced thought has no definite spatial location of any kind. Also, the spatial properties of conscious experience do not manifest any of the 'graininess' (millions of individual nerve cells firing away, each on a sub-millimeter scale) that is characteristic of brain activity.

There is another kind of graininess that is also characteristic of brain activity but not of conscious experience. This difference gives rise to the so-called 'binding problem'. There are (at least) two versions of the binding problem.

The first, and oldest, stems from the *multimodality* (depending on many senses) of conscious experience. We rarely if ever experience a conscious event that is isolated to just one sense. On the contrary, at any moment we are typically conscious of an integrated multimodal 'scene' (to extend this word beyond its usually purely visual meaning). We simultaneously see, hear, feel, smell, etc., a range of events or things. Sometimes each of these is a different thing for each sense (e.g. I see a chair, hear a footstep behind me, feel an itch and smell coffee); and sometimes each is a different aspect of the same thing (I see a cup, hear it chink on the saucer, feel heat on my tongue and smell coffee as I drink it from the cup). (I have settled on the vague word 'thing' in this description rather than one or other of the more technical words that philosophy has on offer, as these are all more or less burdened with conceptual baggage which I prefer to avoid.)

This 'unity of consciousness' sits uneasily next to the evidence that each of our sensory systems, all the way from sense organ (eye, ear, tongue, etc.) to brain (where there are quite different regions specialised for vision, hearing, taste, etc.), is rather strictly segregated from the others (though we shall encounter a striking exception to this rule when we consider synaesthesia in Chapter 10). This physical segregation is almost certainly important in keeping separate our experience of the different senses. For the key determinant of the specific conscious properties of each sense (that which makes visual experiences at once recognisable as different from sounds and both different from tastes, for example) appears to lie in the specific nerves stimulated and the region of the brain to which these nerve are connected. Thus, an identical electrical stimulus applied to the optic or auditory nerve produces, in the one case, a visual experience and in the other, an experience of sound. And the same is true of an identical electrical stimulus applied to those parts of the cerebral cortex to which these nerves respectively project. So the nervous system offers a good anatomical basis for our ability to distinguish clearly one sense from another. A second such basis, emphasised by Susan Hurley and Alva Noë, lies in the ability to distinguish between sensory inputs belonging to different modalities by their different responses to adjustments of the sense organs. In an obvious example (but there are many others), if I shut my eyes, visual (but not auditory or olfactory) stimuli are eliminated.

Nonetheless, all the senses *do* come together in consciousness—at any particular moment there is just one unified scene. The first binding problem is that there is as yet no known counterpart in the brain where this unification might take place. Descartes spoke of a Theatre of Consciousness. A way of expressing the first binding problem, popularised by the philosopher Dan Dennett, is to say that there is in fact no Cartesian Theatre. Actually, Dennett aims to do more with this phrase than express the binding problem, he aims to solve it. His solution is that the apparent unity of conscious experience is just that—apparent.

The second version of the binding problem is *intramodal*, pertaining, that is, to just one sense. The intramodal binding problem has come about because of the great progress that has been made in the last few decades in understanding the way in which the primate and human visual systems are put together. Very much more research has been done on vision than on all the other senses put together. So it is not yet known whether the way the other senses are organised is similar to vision, nor whether they too suffer from an intramodal binding problem. But I would be surprised if their organisation turns out to be radically different from that of vision; and there is already some evidence (in the case of audition) that the organisation is essentially the same.

We have already seen something of the intramodal binding problem for vision in Chapter 2. We discussed there the separation between the visual perception and action systems. These two systems function with a great deal of independence from one another. As we saw, one (the conscious perception system) suffers from visual illusions, the other (the unconscious action system) does not; and one can be damaged while the other is intact, leading to only one of two sets of impairments (either in grasping or in seeing objects). Yet our conscious experience lacks all knowledge of this split in the brain between two types of vision. When we both see and grasp something, and see ourselves doing the grasping, this all forms part, for consciousness, of a single scene.

Our present purpose, however, is to contrast brain activity and specifically conscious experience, so the difference *between* brain mechanisms underlying conscious and unconscious vision is of less relevance than other splits *within* the machinery that produces conscious vision. There are, in fact, a whole series of such splits. For research in which the monkey brain is experimentally damaged or the human brain is imaged in action (with magnetic resonance imaging or positron emission tomography) clearly demonstrates a state of affairs which, given normal conscious experience, is highly counter-intuitive.

Imagine that you are looking at a red kite being flown through a clear blue sky, twisting this way and that in the wind. The kite has a definite colour (red against the blue background) and location (at a certain direction, distance and height from you), a well-outlined shape, and a distinct pattern of movement, and you are able with certainty to identify it *as* a kite. All these features of your conscious experience of the kite are indissolubly bound together. No matter how hard you try, you cannot pick out for vision just the shape of the kite without simultaneously seeing its colour, motion and location; nor can you pick out for vision just its colour, motion or location. You might, at a pinch, see it as something other than a kite; though even that probably requires effort. Consciously, all these properties go together. As far as the brain is concerned, however, they do not. The visual perception system is made up of a number of separate modules, each devoted principally to the analyis of only one of these properties (see Plate 4.1). So, an area in the cerebral cortex called V4 or V8 is responsible for the allocation to the kite of its colour; another area, known as V5 or MT, is responsible for allocating its motion; a third area for recognising the kite as a particular kind of object. Damage to one of these regions deprives conscious visual perception of just that property, but not the others. Yet we cannot use that region consciously to see just one of these properties to the exclusion of the others. Conscious visual perception binds what the brain leaves asunder. This, then, is the intramodal binding problem.

These different properties of brain and conscious experience pose serious issues for any theory of how the one is linked to the other. For example, do the properties segregated in the various modules of the visual perception system come together in some other part of the brain waiting still to be discovered (a Cartesian theatre for vision)? Or does the coming together take place in conscious experience itself, with no homologous coming together in the brain?

## 4.2 Searle's model

By themselves, however, these kinds of differences between brain and consciousness do not constitute a problem radically different from others that science has
successfully overcome before. The philosopher John Searle, in a 1987 article,
points to a highly successful type of scientific theory that might work in this
context too. This ascribes to the 'micro-elements' in a system, properties from
which it is possible to deduce and predict the system's 'macro-properties'. So, for
example, the liquidity of water in bulk can be explained by the properties of the
molecules of water out of which bulk water is made up; and the solidity of a table
can be accounted for in terms of the properties of its interacting atoms. Yet if we
contemplate, not the theories that mediate these explanations, but just atoms and
molecules on the one hand and solidity and liquidity on the other, the gap between
the micro-elements and their associated macro-properties can appear so great as to
be unbridgeable. In the same way, then, it may be possible to endow the micro-
elements of neurons (nerve cells) with properties which can explain the macro-
properties of conscious experience. (This type of argument assumes, of course, that
it is indeed properties of the brain that cause conscious experience. Not everyone
accepts this assumption, by any means. But it is the common assumption of all
contemporary science and much contemporary philosophy; and I too shall take
this assumption for granted, save where it becomes necessary specifically to subject
it to scrutiny.)

The trouble with Searle's argument, however, is that it is, at least for the present,
a blank cheque. For none of the known properties of neurons (nor those of any
other elements in the nervous system, nor those of the integrated activity of
neurons, as seen for example in the electroencephalogram, or 'EEG') as yet show
sign of being able to account for the macro-properties of conscious experience.
It is therefore an act of faith to suppose that one day they will provide such an
account (just as it is an act of despair to suppose that they never will). Given the
scientific analogies proposed by Searle, it is in fact surprising that the very detailed
knowledge we already have of what neurons do has made no contribution at all to
an account of the properties of conscious experience. But there is, I think, a reason
for this. Searle's examples refer to cases in which scientists *set out* to account for the
macro-properties of matter in bulk (liquidity, solidity and the like). Accordingly,
they developed theories in which the constituents of bulk matter (molecules,
atoms and so on) were endowed with just such properties as would provide the
needed account. Once the theories passed the test of experiment, then, the question of *how* they account for the macro-properties of bulk matter could not arise.
The answer to that question was already built in at the time the theories were
constructed.

In this respect, however, nothing could be more *dis*analogous with the case of
consciousness than Searle's examples. The disanalogy has three aspects.

First, the properties with which neurons have been endowed (by theory, and then by passing the test of experiment) were never intended to account for conscious experience. They were intended to account for how physical energy input at the sensorium gives rise, after a series of transformations in the brain, to behavioural outputs. This theoretical endeavour is showing every sign of ultimate success.

Second, for the very reason that this type of theory building *without reference to consciousness* has been so successful, there is now no reason to include conscious experience in the scientific story at all. It is an embarrassment for this story that consciousness should exist at all. Existing neuroscientific theory gets on very well, thank you, without consciousness, and can in any case offer no explanation for it.

Third, given that there is a scientific story that goes seamlessly from sensory input to behavioural output *without* reference to consciousness then, when we try to add conscious experience back into the story, *we can't find anything for it to do*. Consciousness, it seems, has no causal powers, it stands outside the causal chain. How can it affect the firing of a set of neurons in the chain between input and output, if these firings have already been given a complete account in terms of the activities of other neurons that impinge upon them? And this question can be put, but not answered, at each point along the chain.

Searle's general model for a theory that would link the micro-elements of the nervous system to the macro-properties of conscious experience may one day turn out to be correct, but there is in fact no specific theory at present that fits the bill. If you hold the 'new theory' stance towards the Hard Problem of consciousness (see Chapter 1), you wait hopefully for such a theory to come along. If you are a Mysterian, you may take the view that no such theory can ever come along.

## 4.3   The intentionality of conscious experience

The kinds of difference between conscious experience and brain activity considered so far in this chapter pose serious problems for the construction of an integrated neuroscientific account of consciousness, but they do not seem permanently intractable. However, the gap between brain and consciousness looks a great deal wider when viewed from the perspective of *intentionality*: the fact that conscious experience is (almost) always about (stands for, represents) something, while activity in the brain lacks such 'aboutness'.

A central feature of virtually all the contents of consciousness (but see Chapter 18 for a major qualification in relation to the inner bodily senses) is that they are experienced *as* something or other. This is the other side of the coin that, seen from the perspective of brain organisation, constitutes the binding problem. If I see, touch and eat a banana, it would be odd to describe my experience as *seeing a patch of yellow AND seeing a curved elongated shape AND feeling a smooth surface in my hands AND smelling a sweetish odour AND tasting a sweetish taste AND feeling a warm pulpy sensation in my mouth* (though a generation of philosophers who believed in 'sense data' tried to make us talk this way). The oddness of this description is that it misses out the *intentionality* of what we perceive: namely, that what one sees, touches and eats is *a banana* and it is *as* a banana that we see, touch and eat it. Indeed, when you come to the smell and taste parts of the description, it is difficult to convey anything much about them unless you bring the missing intentionality back in, by saying that the smell and the taste are *like* those of a banana. Not only is this the way one normally experiences a banana, it is extremely difficult to experience it as anything else.

In the case of cognitive consciousness of the external world (see Chapter 1), the only major exceptions to this rule of intentionality are of a kind that proves the rule. For they consist in the consequences of certain forms of damage to the brain. These consequences are called 'agnosias'—loss of the ability to recognise an experience for what it is. Depending on the location of the damage, the agnosias can selectively affect one or other sensory modality—vision, audition, smell and so on. The neurologist Oliver Sacks, for example, graphically describes a patient with visual agnosia in his book, *The Man Who Mistook His Wife for a Hat*. The damage to this poor man's brain had the consequence that the contours of his hat and those of his wife's head had become confusible, since each had lost its normal perceived *meaning*. ('Meaning' is another way of talking about intentionality.) But in the absence of brain damage—that is, in the normal case—it is virtually impossible to experience the external world except as a continuous passage from one meaningful item to the next.

To appreciate this, try the following simple experiment. As you walk along the street, look at the number plates on the cars. Try to experience their letters and numbers as mere shapes. See whether you can prevent yourself from hearing their names (AZX 279P) in your head as you look at them. I have tried this over and over again, and I cannot do it: invariably, I hear their names whenever I look at them. I experience them *as* letters and numbers and can experience them in no other way. Other demonstrations of the sway that intentionality holds over conscious experience lie in the ambiguous figures that are the joy of the experimental psychologist. My favourite is the one that can be seen as either a duck or a rabbit (see Fig. 4.1). Note that it cannot be seen as neither, nor as both simultaneously. Furthermore, there is no time during which it is in transition from one figure to the other: one instant it is a duck and the next, a rabbit.

Now, the possession by the great majority of the contents of consciousness of the property of intentionality has been matter for the spilling of much philosophical ink. For states of the brain (which materialists tend to treat either as the causes of mental events or even as identical with them) do not, on the face of it, possess intentionality. The electrodes of the electrophysiologist encounter spikes of entirely normal electricity, and the vials of the neurochemist fill up with perfectly ordinary chemicals. We do not usually think of electricity or chemicals as standing for some-

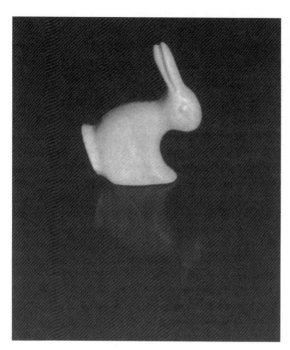

**Fig. 4.1** The duck–rabbit ambiguous picture. As the figure is rotated by 90⁰, one possible interpretation comes to be preferred over the other. From Gregory (1997).

thing, as having meaning, as being about anything but themselves. So why should we endow electricity and chemicals with these rather mysterious properties just because we find them buzzing around in the brain? Another way of putting the same point is this. The world of physics and chemistry works according to principles of causation. These principles apply perfectly well to the activities of the nervous system. One can follow without interruption the causal chain from sensory input via the brain to behavioural output. But the meaning of an event or an object does not seem—at first (see Section 4.5)—to yield to causal analysis. It appears simply to be a property inherent in the perceived event or object, without any preceding causal chain having put it there.

Arguments of this kind have been used to justify a radical conclusion: that brain states and conscious experience are incorrigibly different. Brain states have no intentionality; conscious experiences do; *ergo*, conscious experiences cannot be identical to brain states (of any kind). This argument is not so strong, however, when used against the proposition that brain states *cause* (as distinct from being identical with) conscious experiences, since of course causes can be (indeed, usually are) very different from their effects. Nonetheless, it sets up a stiff challenge to any neuroscientific theory which seriously attempts to deduce from postulates about brain states conclusions about consciousness. Somehow the theory has to deduce (to use Searle's terminology) the macro-property of intentionality from neural micro-elements that lack it.

## 4.4   Unconscious intentionality?

In Chapter 2, drawing upon the work of David Milner and Mel Goodale, we distinguished between two separate parts of the visual system: the perception system (responsible for ordinary conscious seeing) and the action system (responsible, in a largely or even entirely unconscious mode, for sensorimotor behaviour such as grasping). It is not yet known whether analogous distinctions can be made in the other senses. I shall assume that they can. Since I am about to embark on an initial sketch of a theoretical model of how brain activity becomes intentional, and since I intend this model to be generally applicable, this assumption—that there are separate perception and action systems for all the senses—is an empirical prediction from the model. The ability to make such predictions marks the border between science and philosophy; we are on the science side of the border.

As we also saw in Chapter 2, there is not one visual action system, but several. The lines of demarcation between the different action subsystems are two-fold. They are, on the one hand, anatomical: disruptions in different forms of visuomotor action follow upon damage to different parts of the brain. And, on the other, they are functional: different subsystems are dedicated to different behavioural end-points, such as moving the eyes to bring stimuli into central vision, reaching out, grasping objects. These anatomical and functional distinctions fall out together, making it reasonable to think indeed in terms of separable visuomotor subsystems.

These subsystems can all be regarded as servomechanisms, in the sense discussed in Chapter 3. There is in each case a controlled variable that the system attempts to minimise: the distance to the central fovea from a stimulus in peripheral vision; the distance between the extremity of the arm or finger and the object of reaching; the difference between grip aperture and size of the object to be grasped. These variables are defined by visual information received from the retina, together with information about movements received from the brain centres that command the movements and feedback from the muscles as they contract. Both classes of information are received and processed without accompaniment by conscious awareness. There is, so far as I can judge, only one way in which these visuomotor systems perhaps exceed the limits of straightforward application of the notion of servomechanism. This lies in the great moment-to-moment variability in the detailed parameters of the variables controlled by the subsystem ('goal variability'). So, for example, one can successfully grasp in a short space of time a great variety of objects that differ considerably in size, shape, consistency and so on. We shall return to the goal variability manifest in the brain's unconscious servomechanisms when we discuss possible contributions from conscious processing. Leaving this issue aside for the moment, however, we may reasonably consider the visual action system as consisting straightforwardly of a set of servomechanisms.

A first question to ask, then, about intentionality and meaning is whether these concepts are *already* applicable at the level of the brain's unconscious servo-mechanisms. Consider Goodale's experiment in which subjects correctly adjusted their grip aperture to the actual size of discs which, in the perceptual vision system, were subject to the Titchener illusion (see Fig. 2.4). In the absence of the demonstration that the grasping behaviour in this experiment is controlled unconsciously, the natural thing to say about it would follow the archetypal narrative of consciousness (Chapter 2). That is, the subject sees the discs *as* discs (larger, smaller or of equal size) and then reaches out to pick the appropriate one up. Should we abandon this intentional way of talking in the light of knowledge that the behaviour is in fact carried out unconsciously? If we should abandon it, then on what grounds? Because the behaviour is unconscious? Because it is based upon a simple servomechanism? Or are neither of these differences germane, and should we treat servomechanisms as possessing intentionality? If so, would this apply to all of them, down to the merest thermostat designed by human agency?

This, too, is an issue that has been much debated by philosophers. I am myself persuaded by arguments in *Mind, Meaning and Mental Disorder*, by Derek Bolton and Jonathan Hill, that it makes excellent sense to apply to the behaviour of servomechanisms the language of intentionality. Within 'functional semantics' (the term they use to describe a position similar to the one adopted here), Bolton and Hill offer the following definition of how a system can be properly said to 'interpret' a signal S as a sign of an environmental condition C: 'a system interprets a signal S as a sign of C if reception of S causes the system to respond in a way appropriate to its being the case that C' (*op. cit.*, p. 198). This definition is readily applicable to the kind of servomechanism we have been considering. One may describe, for example, the oculomotor system as responding to stimulation of peripheral retinal cells in a way that brings the fovea appropriately to bear upon the source of that stimulation. Clearly, we further need, in such an application, to explicate 'appropriateness'. But we have already outlined in principle how this explication works. The oculomotor system has been designed by natural selection to achieve just this kind of 'foveating' (bringing objects into central vision), because the ability to bring objects to central vision (where visual acuity is at its greatest) has proved conducive to the overall survival of organisms possessing an oculomotor system that works in this way.

Whether or not it is sensible to apply the language of intentionality to the activity of non-conscious servomechanisms is not, however, of primary importance for the argument pursued here. Our concern is with the problem of consciousness. It is only in order to gain a purchase upon that problem that we first need to see clearly just what non-conscious mechanisms can or cannot do. The language used to describe these non-conscious capacities is here of secondary importance. However, it would be unwise to foreclose the possibility that the capacities of non-conscious systems do not match up to the paradigmatic case of 'intentionality', 'meaning', etc., as these terms are applied to fully conscious percepts and to the words used in ordinary language to refer to these percepts. Thus it would be useful to have a separate vocabulary with which to discuss the apparently intentional capacities of non-conscious systems. In his excellent discussion of these capacities (see his 1990 paper), Stevan Harnad uses the phrase 'symbol grounding', a practice we shall follow here. So our question becomes: in what, if anything, does the symbol grounding of non-conscious systems fall short of the intentionality of conscious human beings?

What can clearly be ascribed to the visual action systems is the following. A given visual servomechanism can: (1) detect environmental inputs (in the form of changes in the activity of retinal cells) that are appropriate for the activation of its specific feedback loops; (2) activate those loops; and (3) detect successful completion of the feedback loops. In some sense at least, therefore, the system treats a given input as indicating the presence of a certain kind of environmental event and acts upon it 'appropriately'. The system is also able to report the state of its controlled variables to other visual action systems. So, for example, it might be the case that foveating a fast-moving peripheral object of vision (a fly, shall we say?) is followed by the attempt to swat the fly, requiring activation of reaching and grasping visuomotor systems. These systems do best when they receive visual information via the fovea; and this information becomes available to them as the result of the prior activation of the oculomotor system. All of this, recall (Chapter 2), is done in the absence of accompanying conscious awareness of either visual input or visuomotor actions—until these actions are over, at which time their results finally enter consciousness.

At that time, then, there is a conscious visual percept of a fly and of one's arm and hand reaching out to swat it. Does this conscious seeing of this small fast-moving object *as* a fly and *as* something to be swatted add anything of substance to the problem of intentionality, anything that needs to be explained over and above the account already offered for symbol grounding in unconscious visual action systems? Clearly, there is something of great importance added: namely, the *qualia* that make up conscious visual experience as such—*what it is like*, in Tom Nagel's well-known phrase, consciously to see something. This issue of qualia takes us to the heart of the problem of consciousness; but we don't get there properly till later. There can be no doubt that, as a rule (though not always; see Chapter 18), qualia have intentional properties. But it does not follow that the problem of intentionality, as such, becomes more intractable just because it is a system with qualia that manifests it. So it is worth continuing upon our exploration of symbol grounding and intentionality before grappling with the even harder problem posed by qualia.

There is a further important way in which visual percepts differ from the visual inputs that activate the visual action systems. The latter, as befits a system so named, are indissolubly linked to action; but conscious percepts are not. Of course, conscious percepts afford the *possibility* of action. I may contemplate a fly in consciousness for a while and then decide to swat it (or not). (I envisage here a case in which the archetypal narrative of consciousness presented in Chapter 2 has a closer fit to the reality of action than other cases that we have so far discussed.) But, for the analysis of symbol grounding that I have applied to the visuomotor systems, the mere possibility of action is not enough. For, in the case of those systems, the 'meaning' of an environmental input is grounded precisely in the action that this input causes the servomechanism to undertake. Introspectively, however, it seems pretty clear that the intentionality of a visual *percept* is not tied closely to action in this way. I may spend minutes at a time looking at a cubist painting by Picasso or Braque, seeing it now as a guitar, then as the top of a table, then as a piece of newspaper, but without these different ways of seeing being in any way tied to strumming strings, setting down plates or reading the news. This, then, is a difference that may make all the difference. For it suggests that our analysis of symbol grounding in the case of the visual action systems doesn't get off the ground (since, precisely, it is based upon action) when it is applied to the visual perception system.

Unlike the symbol grounding of unconscious action, then, the intentionality of conscious perception does not yield to analysis directly in terms of servomechanisms. However, a more indirect analysis of this kind may be applicable. The need for an analysis of *some* kind that places the burden of intentionality upon mechanisms in unconscious processing is suggested by the following consideration. The contents of consciousness are not normally constructed *in* consciousness. Rather, they spring into consciousness fully formed, and their full form includes their intentional status. For example, take another look at Fig. 4.1. You see either a rabbit-with-ears or a duck-with-a-bill. There is no conscious putting together of ears and rabbit, or of bill and duck. These animals are already formed as wholes at the time they enter your consciousness. But, if consciousness does not itself construct these intentional objects, then the construction must, by default, be achieved unconsciously. And, if that is so, then it is in *unconscious* brain processing that we must seek the mechanism of intentionality (since seeing an ambiguous figure now as a rabbit, now as a duck, is about as fully fledged an instance of intentionality as you can get).

There is in fact a volume of evidence to support this inference that unconscious processing possesses most of the hallmarks of fully-fledged intentionality. Much of this evidence has been reviewed by Max Velmans in his paper published in *Behavioral and Brain Sciences* in 1991. His examples are taken from a wide variety of behavioural and cognitive functions. Here are just two.

It has been known since the seminal work of Donald Broadbent, the founder of modern 'cognitive psychology', that one may selectively attend to verbal material presented (via headphones) to one ear while ignoring other material simultaneously presented to the other ear. Under the right experimental conditions the subject is unable to report any of the material presented to the unattended ear. This is the best experimental index currently available of non-conscious processing. (One should be wary, however, of identifying *conscious* processing with that which *is* susceptible of verbal report. That would be tantamount to deciding by *fiat* that non-verbal organisms cannot be conscious, a conclusion I reject in Section 6.1.) There is an abundance of experimental evidence, however, that the material presented to the unattended ear is nevertheless capable of influencing the interpretation of material consciously attended to in the other ear.

In one such experiment, by J. A. Groeger, subjects were asked to complete the gap in a sentence heard in the attended ear, such as 'she looked … in her fur coat' with one of two words, e.g. 'smug' or 'cosy' (Fig. 4.2). Simultaneously, the word 'snug' was presented to the unattended ear, either so that it was above or below the threshold of awareness. Presented above threshold, *snug* increased the likelihood that *smug* would be chosen as the completion word for the sentence heard in the attended ear. (The shorthand for this type of effect is that *snug* 'primed' *smug*.) When *snug* was presented to the unattended ear below the threshold of awareness, however, it primed *cosy*. There are several important inferences to be drawn from this remarkable result. First, the unconscious analysis of *snug* must have been conducted at the semantic level for it to prime *cosy* rather than *smug*. The extraction of the meaning of a word in this way is, again, one of the hallmarks of fully-fledged intentionality. Second, analysis of *snug* when this was presented above the threshold of awareness must have been dominated by the perceptual (phonetic) characteristics of the word for it to prime *smug*. Counter-intuitively, then, processing at the unconscious level appears to have been *more* intentional than processing at the conscious level. Conversely, however, the importance of the perceptual aspect of the word 'snug' for conscious processing fits well with a central feature of the approach to consciousness adopted in this book. For conscious experience is here treated as exclusively perceptual in character. Or, to put the point slightly differently and in a way that is preparatory to more extensive discussion later in the book, consciousness comes into play when function is clothed in *qualia*.

Groeger's experiment, then, is a good example of how unconscious processing can display a high degree of intentionality. A second example comes from studies of the length of time it takes to recognise a heard word.

This can be estimated by presenting to the subject for recognition successively longer fragments of a word. If the word is presented in context, that is, in a stream of normally connected speech, it takes about 200 millseconds (a fifth of a second) for accurate recogntion. That is long enough for presentation of only two phonemes (the smallest perceptible units of speech). As Velmans writes:

> Assuming a dictionary of 20,000 of American English words, knowledge of the first phoneme reduces the set of possible words to a median of 1,033, knowledge of the first two phonemes reduces the set size to a median of 87, and so on. This way, sensory analysis (a largely 'data-driven' process) contributes to word identification.

(a)

In her new fur coat she looked decidedly......

[SNUG]

Phonological prime: .... *(smug, complacent)*

Semantic prime: .... *(cosy, wealthy)*

(b)

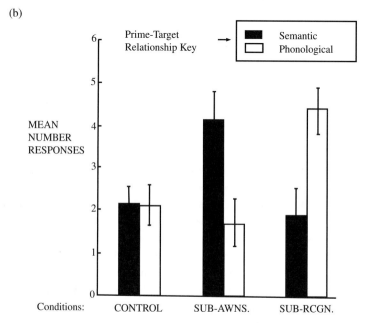

**Fig. 4.2** Groeger's (1988) experiment. (a) Example of the sentence-completion task. *Top*: the subject had to choose between one of two words to fill the gap at the end of the sentence, presented visually. *Middle*: the subject was simultaneously presented with an auditory word ('snug'); this 'prime' might be below the threshold of conscious awareness or above this threshold but below the recognition threshold. *Bottom*: the two words between which the subject had to choose contained one that was either phonologically similar to the prime ('smug' vs 'complacent') or semantically similar ('cosy' vs 'wealthy'). (b) In a control condition (*left*), with no prime presented, choices of the semantic or phonological prime were equal. When the prime was presented below the level of conscious awareness (*middle*: SUB-AWNS), choices were biased towards words semantically related to the prime. When the prime was presented above the level of awareness, but below the threshold of recognition (*right*: SUB-RCGN), choices were biased towards words phonologically related to the prime.

After two phonemes, however, a large number of possible words remain (a median of 87). Hence subjects who can identify the word on the basis of the first two phonemes must use their knowledge of the context to decide which of the remaining words is the correct one (a 'cognitively driven' process).

This highly sophisticated interaction between sensory input and cognitive analysis of the speech context is what intentionality is all about: the incoming sensory input is being heard *as* a particular word. But 200 milliseconds is too short a time (as known from other studies) for this intentional interpretation to have been accomplished by conscious processing.

It is not only in our species that unconscious intentionality can be demonstrated. A striking example lies in recent experiments from Wolf Singer's laboratory studying cats.

The experiments took as their starting point reports of human visual perception. The human subject watches two gratings, oriented e.g. at 90⁰ to each other and both moving in a direction orthogonal to the slant of the grating (see Fig. 4.3). Depending on factors such as the brightness of the intersections of the gratings or the relative width of their component bars, the subject reports one of two different percepts. In the first, 'transparent motion', the gratings are seen each to move in its respective direction, constituting two separate surfaces of which one apparently slides transparently across the other. In the second, 'pattern motion', the two gratings are combined into a single 'plaid' pattern, moving in a direction intermediate between the directions of movement of the individual grating (e.g. 45⁰ combined with 135⁰ results in perceived vertical movement). If the conditions of stimulation are changed smoothly between those that favour transparent and pattern motion, respectively, the percept at some point changes abruptly from one to the other. So the observer is perceptually categorising the stimulus as constituting two separate gratings moving in different directions *or* one plaid moving together. This clearly counts as 'intentional' perception: an almost-identical pattern of stimuli is interpreted now as one thing, now as another.

Singer presented stimuli of these kinds to cats and measured their eye-movements. These discriminated between transparent and pattern motion in just the same way as human perceptual report. He also recorded from neurons in the

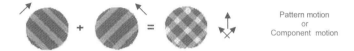

Pattern motion
or
Component motion

**Fig. 4.3** Moving gratings used to make up component motion (the two gratings are seen as sliding one over the other in the two diagonal directions) or pattern motion (they combine to be seen as a 'plaid' moving vertically). Whether component or pattern motion is perceived depends upon factors such as the brightness of the intersections of the gratings, the relative width of their component bars, etc. From Castelo-Branco *et al.* (2000).

cats' brains while they were presented with these stimuli ambiguous between transparent and pattern motion; and he was able to identify patterns of respond-ing specific to the one or other reported percept. A critical aspect of the patterns so identified is that they involved the synchronous firing of neurons widely separated in different regions of the visual cortex. Synchronous firing of this kind has been proposed as a means by which the brain solves the 'binding problem', an issue we considered above (Section 4.1) and to which we return in Chapter 15.

Singer's experiments provide impressive support for this hypothesis. Neurons in the visual system have so-called 'fields': this term denotes the region of visual space to which they are tuned to respond. In Singer's experiments, neurons in different parts of the cat's visual system fired synchronously if they each had a field that belonged to contours defining the same surface, but not if they had fields belonging to contours defining different surfaces. Now, when stimuli ambiguous between transparent and pattern motion are used, the regions of visual space which belong to the same or different surface change when the percept flips. Two points which belong together in a single surface when a plaid is seen to move ver-tically upwards no longer do so when two gratings are seen to move across one another. In agreement with this human perceptual difference, neurons in the cats' brains which fired synchronously under conditions of stimulation favour-ing a perception of pattern motion ceased to do so under conditions favouring transparent motion.

These experiments offer a powerful demonstration of intentionality in cats, and indeed in the workings of the cat's brain. But I have so far hidden from you one crucial feature of Singer's experimental set-up. His neuronal recordings were made in fully anaesthetised animals. Thus what his experiments demonstrate is *uncon-scious* intentionality in the brain of the cat. The anaesthetised state of his animals has implications also for the hypothesis that binding is accomplished by the synchronous firing of neurons across separated areas of brain. If this hypothesis is correct, it follows that binding, like intentionality, is an accomplishment of the *unconscious* brain.

## 4.5 Harnad's model for categorical representation

Unconscious processing, then, is capable of full intentionality, albeit intentionality minus qualia. What is less clear, however, is how this intentionality is achieved. Our earlier analysis, in terms of the controlled variables of a servomechanism, does not seem to fit any of the examples we have just examined: the rabbit/duck picture, Groeger's experiment, or speech perception. Can this gap between the controlled variables of a simple servomechanism and fully-fledged intentionality (minus qualia) be bridged? And can it be bridged so as to give an account of inten-tionality in unconscious processing that fits comfortably into the rest of biology and, in particular, into the physiology of the brain?

Harnad has proposed an account that seems to achieve just this. This treats intentionality as arising from the interactions between a hierarchy of three levels.

1. The first level consists of what Harnad calls 'iconic representations—analogs of the proximal stimulus on the sensory surface'. More poetically, he calls such representations 'the shadow the object casts on your receptors'. More prosaically, they are what I have been calling the controlled variables of simple servomechanisms. However we choose to name them, representations of this kind remain close to descriptions of sensory input in terms of physics and chemistry. This is the level of description with which Behaviourism was comfortable and which, in its heyday, was the only one allowed. Given just iconic representation, an organism could discriminate between inputs as being the same, different, or more or less similar, but it could not do much more than that. Identification of a stimulus as belonging to a particular category, the starting point for intentionality, would in particular be beyond its capacities. It is at Harnad's next level that such identification becomes possible.

2. Tracing the hierarchy up, then, Harnad next posits 'categorical representations' that subserve 'sorting'. It is at the transition from 1 to 2 that we go beyond the notion of the simple servomechanism that has so far served us well. But we do not leave the notion of feedback entirely behind. For level 2 depends upon the process of learning to discriminate positive and negative instances of a category, as the result of feedback received as to correct and incorrect choices. The 'sorting' of level 2 is behaviour that is learnt as a result of this feedback. If sorting is successful, the behaviour may be said to follow the rule set by the category. The 'categorical representations' of level 2 consist in connectivities between sets of neurons in the central nervous system. These connectivities change in response to the patterns relating iconic representations to behaviour to feedback. Once behaviour is successful, the connectivities may be said to represent the relevant category.

Any mystery there might have been about these processes when Harnad described them in 1990 has long since been dispelled, as they can all be discharged by so-called 'neural networks'. These are computer simulations of networks of elements (with properties based upon those of real neurons) which, initially, are randomly interconnected with one another, and with random weights attached to their ability to cause to 'fire' others with which they are connected. The 'neurons' are typically organised in several layers, of which one is an input layer (receiving, therefore, 'iconic representations'), another an output layer (producing behavioural responses) and one or more 'hidden' layers in between. Connections between 'neurons' are both within and between layers. The network is 'trained' by way of feedback as to whether a given output in response to a given input is 'correct' or 'incorrect', and this process is repeated over many trials. The network is equipped with rules according to which the weights connecting one 'neuron' to another change, depending upon whether that connection was active or not on each successful or unsuccessful trial. The general form of the rules is that weights are increased if the connection has been active on a successful trial and decreased if it has been active on an unsuccessful trial. These rules are based upon the changes known to take place in the real brain in the efficiency with which one neuron causes another to fire, depending upon increases or decreases in behavioural success (in leading to reward or punishment) that follow shortly after that particular neuronal connection has been active. In consequence of the operation of feedback and the rules for changing connectivity weights, outputs (behavioural responses) become increasingly successful. At asymptote, the final state of the connectivities between the elements in the network provides a tangible representation of the category instantiated in the regularities of the network's outputs. So, for example, neural networks have been trained in this way to recognise words or objects to high degrees of success.

3. At the third level of Harnad's hierarchy, labels are attached to the behavioural categories achieved at the second level. We are now firmly in the human species (whereas there is no reason to restrict levels 1 or 2 in this way), since the only known natural instance of such labels consists in the words or longer linguistic strings of human language. There are many who believe that consciousness is a property uniquely found in the human species and, indeed, linked indissolubly to language. As discussed later, this is not the position taken in this book. I shall therefore pay little attention here to Harnad's third level.

## 4.6 Fitting intentionality into biology

For our present purposes, then, Harnad's level 2 is critical. It is here that we move beyond simple servomechanisms and into full intentionality (identifying a stimulus *as* being an instance of Category *C*). As we saw in the previous chapter, biology as a whole manages with two classes of concept, physicochemical laws and feedback systems, these being mutually compatible but not reducible one to the other. We have also seen that Harnad's categorical representation is not mysterious (it can readily be simulated in neural networks); and that the intentionality that categorical representation underlies is not necessarily accompanied by consciousness (as in the experimental examples from Groeger's work and speech perception). One question therefore remains for this chapter. Does categorical representation, and the intentionality to which it gives rise, require any additional fundamental principles beyond those with which the rest of biology makes do?

One way of approaching this question is to pose another: in what way does the kind of system required for categorical representation differ from a simple servomechanism? Clearly, they both involve feedback. Are there qualitative differences between the types of feedback involved? They also both involve transformations ('information processing') between input and output. Do these differ qualitatively?

There is at least one potentially important difference in the way in which feedback operates in the two cases.

For a simple servomechanism the set point for the controlled variable is normally a given; or, if it changes, this is over a narrow unidimensional range. The oculomotor servomechanism, for example, is designed so as to minimise the retinal distance between the central fovea and a stimulus (especially if it is moving) initially detected in the periphery. This specification of the controlled variable is built into the oculomotor system during the normal development of the brain. These developmental pathways themselves arise, of course, as the result of Darwinian survival and evolution. Thus, feedback from the environment to the servomechanism operates only while the system is in operation, so as to indicate the effectiveness of the operation at that time; it does not participate in the specification of the system or the controlled variable themselves.

In contrast, for categorical representation, environmental feedback is itself responsible for establishing the relationships between input and output, and the corresponding states of the intervening neural networks, which come into play at the time the system operates so as to classify a stimulus $S$ as belonging to category $C$. These two processes—establishing and using the networks that mediate categorical representation—are not separated, however, in time. The system develops continuously towards asymptotic performance as it makes, and as the result of making, relevant choices. Nonetheless, we can see the same feedback (a given output being indicated as 'correct' or 'incorrect' with respect to the relevant category) as operating in two ways. In the first, it discharges the role that Darwinian survival discharges for the evolution of the oculomotor system; in the second, it operates as feedback indicating the success or failure *now* of the outcome of the networks mediating categorical representation. Now, we know that this second way in which feedback works for categorical representation can proceed in the absence of conscious awareness. Recall, for example, Groeger's experiment, described above. This showed that the word *snug*, presented below the threshold of awareness, was classified as having a meaning similar to that of *cosy*, since it biassed subsequent processing towards *cosy* rather than *smug*. It remains to be seen whether the first way in which feedback operates—so as to establish the categories—can also occur without conscious awareness. This is a matter to which we return in Chapter 8 (especially Section 8.4).

A second way in which feedback operates differently for simple servomechanisms and categorical representations, respectively, lies in its degree of generality. The variable that is controlled by a simple servomechanism is typically appropriate to that servomechanism and to nothing (or not much) else. For example, the difference between grip aperture and the size of the object to be grasped is appropriate only for the visuomotor system that mediates grasping. In strong contrast, the feedback that is used both to establish and to operate categorical representation is highly generalised. At a pre-linguistic level, this feedback is closely related to a limited number of events which have direct survival value (but a value not related to the relevant categories prior to their establishment): events such as changes in

hunger, thirst, body temperature, pain or discomfort, proximity to actual or potential sexual partners, predators, etc. These events provide feedback for the establishment of a huge variety of different categorical representations. Such 'biological
reinforcers' (rewards or punishments) are not essential for category formation. The
well-attested phenomenon of 'perceptual learning', for example, involves mere
repeated exposure to different kinds of visual patterns. Perceptual learning is then
manifest as enhanced readiness to use these patterns as the basis for rapid learning
of their association with biological reinforcers. But this role for mere stimulus
exposure in the establishment of categorical representation does not detract from
the point being made, since this too is an event of great generality. A further
important source of generalised feedback lies in social interaction. A young monkey can learn that a snake is dangerous (but a lizard is not) from observing its
mother's grimace of fear when she sees it. Human language, of course, immensely
broadens the effectiveness of social interaction. For our species, the most general
feedback for category formation comes from words meaning 'right' or 'wrong',
'correct' or 'incorrect' and so on. It is unlikely that the demarcations between
biological, social and linguistic generalised feedback are differences that, for the
problem of consciousness, make a difference. But it is possible that the generality
of feedback for categorical representations and their formation, as compared to the
narrow feedback of the simple servomechanism, does make a difference. This too
is an issue to which we return in Chapter 8.

A further way in which categorical representation differs from simple servomechanisms lies in its dimensionality. Simple servomechanisms work with a
single type of physical energy input. For the oculomotor system, for example, this
consists in electrochemical changes caused by quanta of light falling on retinal
nerve cells. Categories, in contrast, whether in perception or in language, are rarely
limited to a single sensory modality in this way. A rose, for example, is recognised
by its characteristic shape, colour, smell, its accompanying thorns that can prick
you and so on. Neural networks have no difficulty in principle in handling
such conjunctions of inputs in different modalities. However, a number of theories
of consciousness would treat the conjunction of stimuli from different modalities
as being intimately related to consciousness. For they see consciousness as the
medium in which the different senses all come together. Thus, another question which we shall for the moment (see Chapter 8) leave open is whether the
simultaneous processing of inputs across different sensory modalities requires
consciousness.

Despite these differences in the way in which the brain implements feedback in
servomechanisms and categorical representation, respectively, both fit comfortably
into the general model of theoretical biology outlined in the previous chapter. To
the laws of physics and chemistry they add, in a more or less sophisticated manner,
selection by consequences (categorical representation) plus machinery designed
to establish set points for, and to implement, controlled variables (both servo-

mechanisms and categorical representation). Thus, the same 'bifocal' perspective, shown by Polanyi to work for the interface between natural selection and physico-chemical laws (Chapter 3), works also here. We have met no further seam between biology and the physiology of brain and behaviour that might require us to pose the question: to reduce or not to reduce?

## Conclusions

We have reached two important conclusions in this chapter. First, intentionality can attach to processes that are achieved *un*consciously. Thus, it is unlikely that a deeper scrutiny of the properties of intentionality will lead *ipso facto* to a solution of the Hard Problem of consciousness. Second, the laws of physics and chemistry plus the principles of cybernetics are able in principle to accommodate, without residual mystery, intentionality and representation. These conclusions free us, therefore, to look at what consciousness *per se* brings to the party, over and above these powerful but comprehensible capacities of the unconscious brain/mind.

# CHAPTER 5

# Reality and illusion

Apuzzling question raised by the phenomena of intentionality and meaning goes as follows: 'How can a brain state, e.g. the one that is active whenever I see, hear or think of a cow (assuming there is such a brain state) represent the real object (the cow) out there in the world?'. I risked inviting this question in the previous chapter by using Harnad's term 'categorical representation'. Yet there was no need for me to run that risk. This is because, in Chapter 2, I argued that the cow perceived as being out there in the world is, in fact, not out there: it is constructed in my brain. (For the avoidance of doubt, as the lawyers say: there is also a real external, but unperceived, world that with a fair degree of certainty contains something corresponding more or less closely to the perceived cow. But the cow that human beings refer to and communicate about is the perceived one.) If that is so, questions about representation are blocked at the start. If the cow (brain state) in the head and the cow (as perceived) in the world are one and the same, then one cannot represent or stand for the other.

This conclusion seems so clear as to be almost a truism. Yet the concept of 'representation' is widely used in both scientific and philosophical discussions of these issues—so widely used, indeed, that I could not avoid it when presenting Harnad's ideas. So what stands in the way of accepting the truism? In large measure, I think, this reflects the extraordinary dominance that vision has over our other senses and, indeed, over human reasoning in general. This in itself is hardly surprising, since the brain devotes a remarkably high proportion of its overall capacity to vision. But an understanding of consciousness needs to draw upon the entirety of our experience, and this depends upon many sources other than just vision. When we consider these other sources, two points become clear that the very clarity of our visual sense obscures.

## 5.1 The unreality of the external world

The first concerns the reality of the external world perceived by our senses. When we look at an object, the impression is overwhelming that we simply have a direct window upon the world out there as it actually *is*. That, of course, does not mean the impression is correct. When we look at the sun setting in the sea, the impression that the Sun moves around the Earth is just as overwhelming. It is not surprising that it took a very long time before ordinary people accepted the Copernican view of heavenly motion: that the Earth orbits around the Sun. Nowadays, of course, that view is taken for granted by anyone with a modicum of scientific knowledge. In just the same way, I believe, most people will soon accept the counter-intuitive proposition that the external world is constructed by, and exists in, the brain.

Fortunately, this proposition is a lot less counter-intuitive when applied to senses other than vision. No-one, for example, confuses the scent of a rose with the rose. Nor do you identify the scent of the rose with the molecules that come from it to stimulate olfactory receptors in your nostrils. It is obvious that the scent of the rose is neither the rose nor the molecules, but just the impression these create in your mind. Exactly the same considerations apply to the pain you feel from a hot flame, or the music you hear in the concert hall (see Chapter 2). And vision, despite strong appearances to the contrary, is no different from these other senses.

The second point that becomes clear when you consider senses other than vision is closely related to the first. Once you abandon the notion of direct (unmediated) perception of the cow-as-it-really-is, the tempting fall-back position is to suppose that there is *both* a cow-brain-state *and* a cow-as-it-really-is, and that the former 'resembles' or 'represents' the latter. The philosophical obstacles to this line of thought are formidable and well-known. They start with one that will be immediately obvious. If the only knowledge you have of the cow is the cow-brain-state, you have no way of judging the 'resemblance' between this and any cow-as-it-really-is that might be out there. The claim that the former 'represents' the latter is therefore vacuous.

Again, the temptation to take up this fall-back position is much weaker when it is tried out for senses other than vision. The scent of a rose doesn't resemble a rose, nor is it useful to describe it as representing one. Rather, it is a *signal* of the likely presence of (among other things) the other attributes of the complex sensory construct that makes up a perceived rose—its sight, the feel of its thorns to unwary fingers and so on. And, like all signals, it is fallible. You may smell the scent of a rose when there is no other attribute of a rose around, just perfume or a woman wearing it. Under the latter circumstances, the rose scent can become a signal for the woman. And the relation between the scent and the woman is no different in principle from that between the scent and sight of the rose; the latter is merely more reliable (at least if you are in a garden or a florist's shop). Similarly, pain neither resembles the pin-prick that causes it, nor represents it; the sound of the string quartet doesn't resemble or represent the players, their instruments or the vibrations they make in the air and so on. And it makes no more sense to assert that a seen cow resembles or represents a cow-as-it-really-is. Just as for the other senses, the visual sense of the cow is *all there is to the cow that has been sighted.*

A more useful approach, I believe, is to treat all perceptual information, in whatever sensory modality, as *signals*, as we just did for the rose's scent. Signals have no need to resemble or represent what they signal. A whistle telling the gang the police are coming doesn't sound like a policeman or represent one; it is a signal, rather, for action appropriate to not getting caught. In this example, the whistle is a *conventional* signal, established by agreement between the members of the gang. It is a necessary feature of conventional signals that there is no fixed relationship between the signal and the signified. So it is natural enough that the whistle doesn't resemble a policeman. But the same holds true for perceptual signals, even though these are not capable of alteration by convention. Sensory stimuli are signals of other sensory events that they reliably (but not infallibly) precede, accompany or follow, so that one may prepare for action appropriate to these other events as needed. So the sight of a velvet dress is a signal of what you might expect if you were to touch it or pull it over your head. (This analysis of per-cepts as signals applies fairly naturally to most cases. But, as so often, music provides a counter-example. Except when it comes equipped with words, it neither signals nor represents anything at all—it just is. I take this discussion further in Section 20.2.)

Notice that these associations between signals and what they signify are all equally inside your head, constituted by patterns of connectivity between cells in various parts of the brain. So the intransigent problem (as generations of philo-sophers have found it to be) of how something in the mind can refer to (or repre-sent, or resemble) something in the external world doesn't arise. In its place we have the tractable scientific problem of how one set of neurons in the brain forms associations with another such set: in the examples just given, associations between a set that constructs the scent of a rose and one that constructs its visual appearance, or between one that constructs the visual appearance of velvet and one that constructs its feel. The same logic applies to language. The thorny philo-sophical problem of how the word 'cat' spoken or heard by you or me can refer to a creature that moves about in a world external to both of us becomes instead this tractably scientific one: how does one set of neurons (constructing the perceived cat) link up with another set of neurons (constructing the word 'cat') *in the same brain*?

Philosophical discussions of these issues have often followed John Locke in drawing a distinction between 'primary' and 'secondary' qualities. The former—principally shape, mass and motion—are held truly to be properties of an external world that is independent of the perceiver; the latter—including sound, colour, taste and smell—are accepted as being created by the observer, along lines not strongly in conflict with the position adopted here. The present position, however, treats primary qualities, too, as constructs of the perceiver's brain. The only access we have to an external reality that is independent of perception (other than by way of our *unconscious* cybernetically controlled transactions with that reality) is through the kind of rational enquiry which culminates in natural science. None-theless, the distinction between primary and secondary qualities has an interesting echo in the facts of biology. For there is a second sense, besides the one analysed above, in which secondary qualities often, but primary qualities rarely, act as signals.

Natural selection has frequently evolved mechanisms that depend for their contribution to fitness upon the passage of signals either from one member of a species to another or between members of different species. Most of these use as the signalling medium one or other of the secondary qualities. Examples abound. Within a species, these often depend upon sexual selection: the bright patterns of the peacock's tail, the red rump of a female monkey in heat or the songs of the birds are well-known examples. Between species, the sweet scents and bright colours of flowers act as powerful attractants to the insects that pollinate them. Closer to home, the reds and oranges of ripe fruit tell primates, including ourselves, when they are best to eat. This example (considered in greater detail in the next chapter) is particularly instructive. It involves a striking process of co-evolution. The fruit benefits from being taken and eaten by monkeys, because in so doing the monkeys scatter their seed. The monkeys benefit by way of an improved diet. But, for this arrangement to work it was necessary, not only for the fruit to evolve the appropriate pigmented surfaces, but for the monkeys to evolve a whole new sensory modality—trichromatic colour vision. That is why you and I can see so many colours today.

So, far from the colours of fruit having always been out there waiting to be seen, it was their co-evolution with the colour vision of monkeys that created the poss-ibility of their being seen at all. Nor is this an isolated example. The scents and colours of flowers depend in just the same way upon co-evolution of appro-priate sensory systems in the pollinating insect species, as beautifully described by Richard Dawkins in his book, *Climbing Mount Improbable*. Just how often such processes have occurred it is impossible to say. But as an interesting exercise in time travel, imagine visiting planet Earth before biology began, stripped of plants, trees, insects or other animals. There would have been precious little around in the way of even potentialities for creating experiences of colour, odour or taste, and not much for sound either, other than wind, thunder or the occasional falling rock. For, on today's Earth, most of what goes on in these modalities consists of the passage of signals from one plant or animal to another.

Let us, then, follow our own counsel (Chapter 2) and dispense with the biggest illusion of all: that the perceived world is external to our brains (while—once more, for the avoidance of doubt—accepting that there is some real world or other that *is* external to our brains). And let us dispense too with all further talk of representation.

That, of course, still leaves open a big question: how can brain states endow the percepts to which they give rise (or, possibly, to which they are identical) with an intentionality that is evidently not possessed by the micro-elements that make up the nervous system? In the previous chapter we made good progress in providing an answer to this question. In so doing, we narrowed the ground upon which to look for aspects of intentionality that are specific to conscious processing. There remain just a few features which, in that chapter, we were unable to find in unconscious processing that possesses intentionality. These are: (1) feedback used to establish (as well as implement) the controlled variables of a servomechanism; (2) feedback provided by generalised reinforcers (biological, social or linguistic), as distinct from feedback limited to a variable appropriate to a single servo-mechanism; and (3) information processing and feedback specified in multimodal rather than unimodal terms. In Chapter 8 we shall ask whether these features provide any useful clues as to the specific functions of conscious processing.

## 5.2  The paradox of illusion

First, however, we must return to some unfinished business. Part of the evidence for the conclusion that the perceived world is created by the brain and resides there lies in the phenomena of illusions. But, as noted at the end of Chapter 2, this then faces us with a paradox: how is it possible to judge that an experience is illusory if that experience is itself the real event?

The solution to this paradox rests in that very multiplicity of sensory and perceptual systems which has given rise to most of the other puzzles we have been struggling to resolve. The fact that the perceived world is created by the brain does not mean that there is not also a real world out there—this is not an essay in Berkeleyan idealism. There *is* a real world, but we do not directly perceive it. We do, however, interact with the real world, continuously, actively and *unconsciously*. It is in the fruits of these interactions that the test of illusion lies. Even these interactions, however, do not put us directly in touch with the real world. They, too, are mediated by partial information at sensory surfaces integrated in their own fashion by partial systems in the brain.

It is the *conscious* perceptual systems that are subject to illusion. One cannot even sensibly speak of an 'illusion' in unconscious sensory processing (error yes, but illusion no). The conscious perceptual systems present to us a world outside that appears to carry a guarantee of its own authenticity. When that authenticity is challenged by other evidence, the experiencing subject may come to the conclusion that he is indeed faced with an illusion. Yet the illusion itself persists (see, for example, Fig. 2.4). Thus, one can argue to oneself that one is experiencing an illusion, but one cannot argue the illusory experience away. Indeed, it is this failure of knowledge or thought to eliminate illusions that allows art and entertainment to make such excellent use of them. Everyone knows that the depiction of motion (a galloping horse, a rushing train) on film is actually a series of still frames. You can even freeze the frames at will on your home video. And no-one believes that a painting really displays a three-dimensional world, no matter how skilful the painter (see Fig. 2.3, for example). Yet this knowledge—fortunately for our enjoyment—does not in any way weaken the illusion.

There are, however, some circumstances in which illusory perceptual experiences can be corrected. The nature of these circumstances may provide a resolution of the paradox that consciousness constructs its own reality and yet recognises, on occasion, that it suffers from illusion.

A series of classic experiments (reviewed by Susan Hurley in her penetrating book, *Consciousness in Action*, pp. 285 and 346 *et seq.*) has studied what happens to visual perception when people wear various kinds of distorting lenses or prisms. These perform transformations like left-right or up-down reversals on the retinal image. Initially, the viewer's perceptual experience—disturbingly—follows the reversal. Strictly speaking, this is not an illusion of the kind we have considered so far, since its source lies, not in something done by the brain alone, but by an experimenter who interferes with the normal input to the brain. Nonetheless, what follows is highly instructive. For eventually—after many days or weeks spent continuously wearing the prisms—the subject adapts and comes to see the world again in its normal orientation.

The requirement for this adaptation appears to consist in extensive practice *interacting* with the distorted visual environment. A subject wearing left-right reversing goggles, for example, was instructed, over and over again, to do things like pick up a book 'on the right with your left hand and place it on the right-hand chair' (an experiment by James Taylor). Another subject actually rode a bicycle while wearing distorting goggles (an experiment by Ivo Kohler). Now, these sensorimotor interactions are of course the province of those same visuomotor action systems that we considered in Chapter 2. And these, as we saw, operate in the absence of conscious awareness. Thus, the 'reality' that (eventually) corrects illusory experience in the *conscious* perceptual visual system is provided by the activities of the *unconscious* visual action systems. There is too little empirical evidence, however, to be sure that this conclusion can be generalised to all circumstances and all sensory modalities.

Where, then, does this leave 'reality'? What is the real external world or *ding an sich* (Immanuel Kant's 'thing in itself') that lies beyond the constructions of the conscious mind?

Undoubtedly our best approximation to the *ding an sich* is provided by the theories and discoveries of natural science. However, the sensorimotor servomechanisms, of which the visuomotor action systems constitute a prime example, are necessarily also closely linked to outside reality. But that link consists only in changes caused in sensory receptors by the various forms of physical energy for which these are specialised: quanta of light on the retina, air vibrations on the ear drums, molecules of various kinds on the olfactory mucosa and so on. And even these forms of physical energy are not directly sensed. They are subject to various kinds of complex transformation at the energy-receptor interface; and they are further altered by the operations of the very servomechanisms that they activate. Worse, neither before nor after these transformations are they available to consciousness (except by way of scientific analysis).

What *is* available to consciousness is only its own construction of a world based upon the activities of unconscious mechanisms and, as we have just seen, corrigible (sometimes and to some extent) by them. Corrections of this kind, however, are not often needed. For the most part, conscious perception is a sufficiently good guide to the real world outside that we can use it to navigate through it with considerable success. (It is doubtful that this would be true if we did not also have our unconscious sensory systems to rely upon; but I know of no experimental means to test that proposition.) For the good fit between conscious experience and outside reality, the idealist philosopher Berkeley called in God. In this more materialist age, it is Evolution that we must thank.

We have not yet, however, reached the heart of the Hard Problem of consciousness. We do so in the next chapter.

# CHAPTER 6

# Enter qualia

The thrust of the argument so far has been in two directions, which may at times have seemed mutually contradictory. For, on the one hand, I have been striving to convince you that conscious experience constitutes a Hard Problem for the natural sciences. At the same time, however, I have been trying to reduce progressively the extent of that problem by showing just how much can be achieved by a brain acting unconsciously. These unconscious achievements, moreover, can be analysed in a manner fully compatible with general biological principles. So, for example, in Chapter 4 we were able to analyse (unconscious) intentionality in just such a manner. But it is now time to come to the heart of the problem of consciousness: *qualia*.

'Qualia' is the plural of 'quale'. The word is used to refer to the distinctive qualitative features of conscious experience: features such as the redness of a red rose or the outline of a tree against the sky; the sound made by a violin playing a high 'C', the sounds of words in a language you understand, or speech sounds in a language you don't understand (and in which, therefore, you probably cannot even distinguish the separate words); the feel of a piece of velvet; the smell of Chanel Number 5; the taste of an Espresso coffee; the warmth of the sun upon your skin or the cold of a piece of steel; the tiredness in your limbs after a long walk; the shudder in your arm and the 'smack' of the racket when you hit a tennis ball; the pain of toothache; the bodily sensations of fear or hunger; itches and tickles; an imagined banana; the green after-image you experience after gazing too long at a red patch of colour; the thought 'I wonder if it's going to rain?', heard (if you are like me) as a string of speech sounds inside your head; a melody sung by someone else, sung by you, or running inside your head; the contents of your dream (if you remember it) last night; and, if you happen to experience them, hallucinations.

I could go on adding to this list indefinitely, but by now you probably have a pretty good idea of what I mean. Unless, that is, you are a *zombie*. This is a philosophical invention intended to cover the possibility that there may exist beings which act just like humankind but do not experience any qualia. It is a stark illustration of our lack of understanding of the functions of consciousness that no-one is at present sure whether zombies could or could not exist in reality. That is to say, we do not have a theory from which it can be deduced what kinds (if any) of information processing or behaviour could or could not be executed in the absence of qualia.

I doubt that I can add to your understanding of qualia by offering you an extended definition, or by entering into the long and tortuous philosophical debates that centre upon their existence or nature. But I may be able to help by giving you some negative instances. The processes by which you breathe, walk, ride a bicycle, hit a tennis ball, withdraw your finger from a hot surface, produce a sentence, comprehend sentences spoken by others, read a page of prose, generate thoughts—these processes of *action* are all discharged without the aid of qualia. To be sure, they are *accompanied* by qualia. But these do not directly reflect the *processes* of action. Qualia appear, rather, to reflect the consequences of, or triggers to, action: you feel (or hear, see…) your chest heaving as a result of your breathing, the wobble of the bicycle you ride, the pain due to contact with the hot surface from which your finger retracts, the sounds of the words you utter, read or think.

Thus, in terms of the concepts developed in Chapter 4, qualia reflect *variables controlled by servomechanisms*, not the processes by which a servomechanism controls them. Or, to summarise in more familiar psychological terms, qualia are perceptual. I intend this summary in a very strong sense. Qualia are *exclusively* perceptual[1]. Furthermore, the Hard Problem of consciousness lies *exclusively* in the existence of qualia. As we have seen in the last few chapters, it is possible to use types of explanation familiar from other branches of biology to account for sensory detection, sensorimotor action and the extraction of meaningful (intentional) categories grounded in the activities of such sensorimotor feedback mechanisms. It remains to account *only* for qualia. Success on that front would solve the Hard Problem.

This is not a treatise in philosophy (though I hope well enough informed by it to avoid the more egregious forms of philosophical error). The success we seek lies within empirical science. For it to be attained, we would need to know of qualia (in terms that link up effectively with the rest of natural science):

1.  *What* are they?
2.  *How* does the brain produce them?
3.  *Why* does the brain produce them (given that it can perform so many complex operations, even to the level of intentionality, without them)?

---

[1]   A warning about terminology. 'Perception' is typically used in philosophy to refer to *successful* or *veridical* perception, that is, to cases in which there is a real something out there in the world and this is what is being perceived. This terminology does not work for the constructivist position adopted in this book, identifying as it does a perceived-cow with the cow-in-the-world. In any case, it is commonplace within neuroscience and psychology to describe as 'perceptual' also experiences such as hallucinations, to which on any account nothing corresponds in the external world and so there is no possibility of 'successful' perception. In this book, therefore, 'perception' is used to cover all sensory experience, whether veridical or not.

4. What do they *do*?
5. How did they *evolve*?
6. What *survival value* do they confer?
7. Is it *only brains* that can produce them?

No theory at present comes anywhere near answering all of these questions, nor even any one of them satisfactorily. An answer to Question 7 will almost certainly have to wait upon answers to the others. This is because, in the absence of a general theory of consciousness, there are no behavioural tests by which we can distinguish whether a computer, a robot or a Martian possesses qualia. Questions 1–3 are likely to prove the hardest of all. Questions 4–6 go together: if we knew what qualia permit an organism to do that otherwise it cannot, then the survival value of this function is likely to be obvious.

We have to start somewhere, and the fourth question in the list looks a little more tractable than the rest. This is not because it is clear what additional functions (behavioural or cognitive) qualia bring to the party, but rather because (as we have already seen repeatedly) the experimental evidence indicates that the brain can do an awful lot without them. That eliminates a lot of possibilities that common sense otherwise finds very appealing. We don't, for example, need qualia in order to act swiftly, to act voluntarily, to sense stimuli across the gamut of our sensory modalities, to extract meaningful categories from stimuli, to react emotionally, to solve problems, to learn or to remember. (Some of the items in this list have been discussed already; we shall come to others later; and all of them are to be found in Max Velmans' 1991 article in *The Brain and Behavioral Sciences*.)

So what do qualia do? What do they do, moreover, that could have conferred upon them sufficient survival value for them to have evolved? A possible answer to these questions is suggested by the lateness of conscious awareness, discussed in Chapter 2 (see Section 2.1). Before setting out this answer (in Chapters 7 and 8), however, we need in this chapter to enter into two necessary digressions: one on animal consciousness, and the other on epiphenomenalism.

## 6.1 Consciousness in animals?

To recapitulate: we become conscious of events only after we have had time to respond to them behaviourally and, often, have already done so. This rule applies even to one's own volitions, as Libet's famous experiments show (Section 2.4): the brain decides and then we become aware of its decision. This pattern severely restricts the range of possible uses to which qualia might be put. They clearly are not essential for what one might call 'on-line' behaviour: the kind of rapid reaction that saves you from a traffic accident these days and saved our ancestors from the lion's maw in earlier times. From the evolutionary point of view, that rules out a great deal of behaviour that contributes rather directly to survival.

A large chunk of the survival value that remains lies in the winning of a mate. And indeed there are theorists who believe that sexual selection has played a determining role in the evolution of the human species. According to this line of thought, just as a peahen requires an especially fancy tail on a peacock before she will mate with him, so a woman requires of her man high intelligence or a good singing voice. In this way, one might account for the rapid development of intelligence and artistic talent in recent human evolution. That may be so, but it does little to help with the evolution of qualia. In the first place, there is no evidence that intelligence depends upon qualia. A better case can be made out for song, and for all the arts; indeed, these appear to depend rather specially upon the impact made by qualia (see Section 9.2). But, while qualia may be essential for artistic experience, the notion that artistic experience provides the survival value for consciousness, as sometimes suggested, is too fanciful to be taken seriously.

A powerful reason for rejecting this line of thought is that it almost certainly entails a restriction of qualia to the human species. I have indicated before, my aversion to a restriction of this nature. It is time to justify the aversion.

We don't as yet know why or how qualia are linked to particular forms of brain function and behaviour; but we do know that they are so linked, reliably and systematically. If I touch a hot surface and rapidly withdraw my hand, it is certain that I shall also feel pain (even though it comes too late to affect the withdrawal). That certainty applies also to nearly everyone else (apart from a few individuals who lack normal pain sensation). If we are given an opiate analgesic, such as morphine, and the experiment is repeated, we shall almost certainly all report that our sensation of pain is reduced (and withdraw our hands a little less quickly). We cannot ask a rat or a mouse if it feels pain, but we can observe its speed of withdrawal from a hot surface. Rodents respond to opiates just as human beings do. They do so because their brains contain the same receptors for opiates, and the same endogenous opiates that act upon these receptors, as does the human brain. We *could* maintain that, nonetheless, only human beings experience pain, just as one could maintain the Ptolemaic view of the Heavens despite the observations made by Copernicus. But it just isn't parsimonious to do so, especially since observations like these can readily be multiplied many times over.

I will give here just one more example. It draws upon the phenomenon of binocular rivalry. A stereoscope is an instrument that presents one image to one eye and a different image simultaneously to the other ('dichoptic presentation'). When you look through it, the brain normally attempts to fuse the two images into a single percept. But if the pairs of images differ too much (see Plate 6.1a–d, for some examples), fusion is not possible. What you consciously see under these conditions is now one of the images and now the other. The alternation between the two images is largely automatic, little influenced by deliberate effort to see the one or the other. Depending on the characteristics of the stimuli, one (e.g. the brighter or more sharply outlined) may be seen for a greater proportion of the time than the other, but transitions between the two continue.

All this can be determined by having a human observer report what he is sees. But exactly the same results are obtained if you substitute for the human observer a monkey. The animal has previously been trained, with identical stimuli presented to both eyes, to obtain a favourite fruit juice by pressing one lever when it sees one of the two stereoscopic images (e.g. the starburst pattern shown in Plate 6.2) and to press another when it sees the other (the face). When it is then tested under conditions of binocular rivalry, it 'reports' (by pressing the levers) perceptual domi-nance, now of the starburst, now of the face. Furthermore, the frequency with which the monkey reports one or other of the two stimuli depends upon exactly the same stimulus characteristics as does human report (Plate 6.1e–g).

We are dealing with the probabilistic world of empirical science, not the cer-tainties of mathematics or the desired certainties of philosophy. So these elegant observations, due to Nikos Logothetis, *could* be interpreted in a way which avoided attributing to monkeys in the binocular rivalry experiment the same kind of switching between two consciously perceived visual percepts that human beings report under identical conditions. But scientific parsimony requires us wherever possible to attribute identical observations to identical mechanisms. Neither in the human nor in the monkey binocular rivalry experiment does the pattern of stimu-lation on the retinae of the two eyes change when the report (e.g. of starburst or face) changes. In the human case, we know that what is reported is a change in the consciously perceived percept. It is parsimonious to suppose that this is true also of the monkey.

It is known, moreover, from research with human subjects that the deter-mination of which of the rivalrous stimuli is, at any given moment, consciously perceived is made at a relatively central point in the stream of visual processing, after area V1, the primary visual cortex (see Plate 4.1). Further experiments from Logothetis' laboratory lead to the same conclusion with regard to the monkey. He recorded from individual neurons at several points in the visual system in the monkey brain during the binocular rivalry experiment. Cells were observed whose firing pattern correlated with the stimulus currently being reported as 'seen' by the monkey, that is, they discharged vigorously when the monkey reported the starburst but not when it reported the face, or *vice versa*. The proportion of such cells rose as they were recorded in successively higher reaches of the visual sys-tem (Fig. 6.1). Furthermore, these cells were all binocular, that is, driven by signals from either eye. Thus binocular rivalry does not reflect a simple switching mechan-ism between the eyes (as is clear also from perceptual experiments with human subjects; see Plate 6.1c). Rather, there is somehow a moment-by-moment selection for perception of one of two percepts (starburst or face) which the brain has already fully constructed. In the human being, this selection is for *conscious* perception; it is almost perverse therefore to suppose that, in the monkey, it is not.

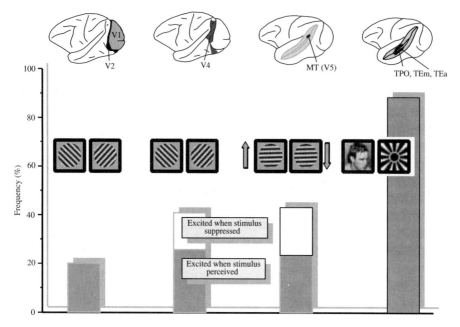

**Fig. 6.1** Distribution of perception-related activity in binocular rivalry experiments (Plates 6.1 and 6.2) in monkey visual cortex. The higher in the visual system (going from V1/V2, on the left of the figure, to regions in the inferotemporal cortex on the right), the greater the frequency of perception-related neural responses. From Logothetis (1998).

A further inference from Logothetis' experiments concerns intentionality, reinforcing the conclusions we drew in Chapter 4 (Section 4.4; see the discussion of Wolf Singer's experiments). Recall that, throughout the binocular rivalry experiment, the pattern of stimulation on the retina is constant. Yet the monkey sometimes reports the starburst and sometimes the face. This is just the kind of phenomenon that philosophers include in their concept of intentionality: that is to say, a constant input from the world outside is interpreted *as* this or *as* that. So the monkey (and, indeed, the neurons in the monkey's brain from which Logothetis recorded) displays intentionality, just as do Singer's cats and the neurons in their brains.

Any Ptolemaic neuroscience that attempted to interpret these results without attributing to the monkey qualia (of starbursts or faces) and intentionality (the capacity to see an identical pattern of stimulation as one or other of these percepts) would be strained indeed. So I conclude, from this and the other examples considered above and in Chapter 4, that animals have qualia and intentionality. I also conclude that experiments like those of Logothetis and Singer are well on the way to finding the neural mechanisms that underlie intentionality. I would like to be able to add that they are on the way to discovering the neural basis of qualia:

but that is a higher hurdle that we shall attempt to clear later (see especially Chapter 13).

## 6.2    Epiphenomenalism

Animals then—at least, the mammals to which we have confined this brief discussion—have qualia. That rules out a large number of false leads. We need not take seriously suggestions that consciousness began with the Greeks or requires human language or that its survival value (by way of sexual selection) lies in its contribution to specifically human intelligence or artistic sensitivity.

But we are still left with the puzzle of finding a function for conscious experience, one moreover that has sufficient behavioural power to have mediated its Darwinian selection. We failed to find it in the kind of rapid on-line behaviour needed to avoid a predator (which takes place too fast for consciousness to come into it); and it is unlikely that the female rat, cat or even monkey picks her mate for the quality of his conscious life. So where does that leave us?

We should leave no stone unturned. Thus we shall have to take seriously even the possibility that consciousness actually has *no* real function: that it is an epiphenomenon. I confess that I find this solution deeply unattractive. But it has been proposed by some eminent thinkers.

An *epiphenomenon* is, as it were, only half involved in causality: it is caused but has no further causal effects of its own. An analogy (a version of one first proposed by Thomas Huxley) may make the concept clearer. Steam in a steam-powered locomotive plays a causal role in driving the train's wheels. But suppose that excess steam blown off through the funnel comes out sounding like the melody of 'She'll be Coming Round the Mountain When She Comes'. This melody plays no part in powering the train, though it is caused by the same events that do power it. In the same way, epiphenomenalists suppose that conscious experiences are caused by the same brain processes that drive behaviour, but do not themselves add to the causal effects of those processes.

The epiphenomenalist position may be taken to an extreme at which it denies *all* causal effects to consciousness. In that case, there is a trivial way in which it is so clearly wrong that it is difficult to see how anyone could ever espouse it. To begin with, books about the problem of consciousness could not be written if conscious experiences had no causal effects, for their production is one such effect. (Philosophers have speculated that zombies with no conscious experience might nonetheless develop the behavioural capacities that allow them to write such books. I shall, however, ignore this bizarre speculation.) More generally, neither language nor artistic creation, at least as we know them, would be possible without qualia (I leave till Section 9.2 justification of this point).

But there remains a serious core to the epiphenomenalist position, which cannot be dismissed so lightly. This concerns the role played by qualia in the brain processes which, at any given moment, appear simultaneously to give rise to them and to discharge other functions. So, to revert to the example of competitive tennis (Chapter 2), when Venus Williams sees her sister Serena's serve only after she has returned it, what role does this perception play in her return stroke (fully accounted for, as it is, by the brain's unconscious sensorimotor functions)? From this point of view (that of the 'ongoing causal efficacy', if any, of conscious experience; see Section 9.3), the epiphenomenalist position looks much more tempting. The steam engine analogy is useful in relating the extreme and core epiphenomenalist positions. If a train does happen to whistle 'She'll be Coming Round the Mountain' as it passes by, this is likely to occasion comment and maybe make you too whistle. So the melody has causal effects. But it is very unlikely to contribute to the powering of the train.

Steven Harnad, in a paper published in 2002, has put the epiphenomenalist argument particularly forcefully, within an evolutionary context. Whatever conscious experiences are, they appear to constitute a rather significant addition to the rest of the biological stable. Ever since Darwin, a standard response to a significant piece of biology has been to ask: what is its survival value? And, indeed, that is just what this section is asking of consciousness. Now, survival value is enhanced if a characteristic increases the chances of an individual's (1) staying alive and/or (2) producing more offspring. So let us suppose that the brain is affected by a series of genetic mutations that change its functions and enhance survival value; and let us also suppose that these mutations lead at the same time to some new form of conscious experience. The increase in survival value requires changes in behaviour (the individual might run faster to escape a predator, mate more successfully, etc.). These changes (argues Harnad) can be fully accounted for by the brain processes, and their output in behaviour, to which the new mutations give rise. Therefore, the accompanying conscious experiences do not contribute *in their own right* to the enhanced survival value: they just come along for the ride.

A concrete example may make this point clearer. Most mammals do not possess full trichromatic colour vision. Accepting, as argued above, that sub-primate mammals (at least) have qualia, they must see the world with much less variety of colours than do most human beings, or even entirely in shades of black, white and grey (as we do at night). Trichromatic colour vision evolved in the mammalian line at the primate level (though very rich forms of colour vision have separately evolved in other lines, including, for example, birds and bees). Its evolution in primates depended upon the addition to the retina of new types of cell, sorting light according to wavelength in the red/green part of the spectrum, and new modules to the visual system specialised for colour vision. These developments provided monkeys with the ability to respond differentially to differently coloured surfaces, e.g. to pick out ripe red fruit from a background of green foliage and so improve their diet. These developments are all explicable—and perhaps even *fully* explicable—within our standard understanding of biology, physiology and behaviour. There is no need to add into this explanation any mention of qualia. Yet, given the close evolutionary relationship between the human and other primate species, it is likely that the development of colour vision in monkeys was accompanied by the development of the same qualia of red, green, orange, yellow, etc., by which it is accompanied in us. What *additional* survival value did these qualia bring to the party? If they brought none, as Harnad argues, they are epiphenomena.

It might seem that the difficulty that is leading us up the epiphenomenalist path is purely empirical. Surely, if we wait a bit and do a bit more research, someone will come up with a survival function for consciousness. Indeed, in the next chapter I shall propose just such a function. However, the problem goes deeper than this. Pretty well everyone now takes it for granted that conscious experiences result from brain activity. Dualism—the notion that consciousness occupies a separate 'psychic' realm—is moribund. So, whenever a function is discovered or proposed for consciousness, the assumption is that there are brain processes that cause (or even, on a widely accepted view, are identical with) the accompanying conscious experiences. Those same brain processes participate in the seemingly closed world of natural science. They are caused by other processes in the brain (and by related input received via the sense organs from the environment) and they lead to further brain processes (and, by way of output to muscles and glands, to behaviour). There seems to be nowhere in this chain that might allow for an extra contribution from conscious experience. And, if there were a gap in the chain, no-one has proposed a way in which conscious experience could contribute to its filling in a manner compatible with the way in which the rest of the chain operates. So this is not merely an empirical difficulty, it is also a conceptual one. That is why it is part of the Hard Problem.

We seem to be faced, then, with hard choices between cherished assumptions.

If we go with epiphenomenalism, we have to abandon the natural-science approach in general and natural selection in particular. In general, there is no room in the standard scientific world-view for a class of entities that stands aside from full causal interaction with other classes. And, in particular, no other significant biological phenomenon stands outside the framework of natural selection.

If we require that conscious experiences should fully participate in causal interactions with other biological phenomena (and, in particular, with brain processes and behaviour), we have to abandon the assumption that brain function and behaviour will yield to a full explanation within the framework of existing neuroscientific and psychological concepts. Worse, this line of thought risks leading back to a dualism whose rejection is widely seen as a major conquest in contemporary discussions of consciousness. The conceptual revolution needed to accommodate such a return to dualism would be seismic.

Faced with this dilemma, I can do little more at present than state a preference. If conscious experiences are epiphenomena, like the melody whistled by the steam engine, there is not much more, scientifically speaking, to say about them. So to adopt epiphenomenalism is a way of giving up on the Hard Problem. But it is too early to give up. Science has only committed itself to serious consideration of the problem within the last couple of decades. To find causal powers for conscious events will not be easy. But the search should be continued. And, if it leads us back to dualism, so be it.

The situation may not, however, be so dire. Searle's model, outlined in Section 4.2, offers a potential way out of the dilemma. This treats conscious experience as a 'macro-property' that depends entirely on the properties of the 'micro-elements' (nerve cells, etc.) that make up the brain, in the same way that the solidity of an object depends upon the physical properties of the interacting atoms that compose it. Solidity does not have *separate* causal properties over and above these atomic-level properties. But the varying degrees of solidity possessed by tables and packets of butter have very distinct causal effects when you attempt to place a cup of hot tea upon them. It may be that consciousness will eventually be shown to relate to the properties of interacting brain cells in much the same way that solidity relates to interacting atoms. In that case, we would have a conceptually coherent way out of the epiphenomenalist trap. But recall that Searle's model is at present a blank cheque. No-one has yet come up with a theory of how the properties of brain cells might give rise to those of consciousness.

# CHAPTER 7

# A survival value for consciousness?

Any account of the survival value of conscious experience must respect its lateness relative to the behaviour it accompanies, as described in Section 2.1. Most existing proposals as to the functions of consciousness ignore this constraint. In consequence, they posit in this role functions which, on the evidence, are discharged unconsciously—before consciousness comes into play. I shall therefore not consider such proposals here. Instead I concentrate on a proposal of my own, published in an article in *The Behavioral and Brain Sciences* in 1995, which explicitly takes the lateness of conscious experience as its point of departure.

According to this account, the principal function discharged by conscious experience is that of a 'late error detector'. This account explains the purpose that is served by having conscious experience occur after on-line behaviour has already taken place. But we also need an account of just what the brain is doing during the period (some hundreds of milliseconds) while it is constructing the contents of consciousness. My 1995 hypothesis dealt with this aspect of the problem by proposing that the brain acts as a comparator system, predicting what should be happening next on a moment-to-moment basis and detecting departures from prediction. This hypothesis still seems to me to be on the right lines. But I now think that it needs supplementation. In particular, we need also to take into account the manner in which the perceptual world constructed by consciousness differs from the sensorimotor interactions discharged by the unconscious brain. In this chapter, therefore, I outline the hypothesis from three points of view. I first present the proposed function of conscious experience—late error detection. I then outline the comparator mechanism required to discharge this function. Finally, I situate the comparator mechanism in the broader perspective provided by a general theory of the nature of conscious perception, as distinct from unconscious sensory detection.

## 7.1 Late error detection

Given the conclusion that animals such as rats or cats, like human beings, have a conscious life, as I concluded in Chapter 6, we need to seek a survival value for consciousness that is commensurately basic and phylogenetically ancient. We cannot find this survival value in the immediacy of on-line behaviour, because consciousness comes too late. But it comes only one or two hundreds of milliseconds late. When it does come, it seems to be particularly concerned with novelty or error: the unexpected has an especially privileged chance of 'gaining access' to consciousness, as the mysterious phrase has it. So the proposal is that consciousness acts as a late error detector.

Here are two examples of what I mean.

The first concerns pain. Pain is in many ways the quintessential conscious experience, uncluttered by representation of entities in the outside world (other than the location, e.g. in a limb, to which the pain is referred) or by conceptual complexity. When it occurs, and especially if it is intense, it dominates experience to the exclusion of all other contents of consciousness. It has a primitive urgency and simplicity that make it feel, phylogenetically speaking, ancient, as indeed is the physiology that underlies it (see Chapter 18). Yet it shares with other qualia a key characteristic. It comes too late: the hand is withdrawn from the flame long before the pain is felt. So pain does not serve the purpose of on-line withdrawal from the source of potential damage. That is achieved unconsciously. An alternative is that pain serves to cause the individual to rehearse the action that led to it. In other words: your hand goes too close to a flame, you withdraw it (unconsciously), *you then feel the pain and, in consequence, you review the action* that just led you to approach the flame too close and too incautiously. The evolutionary benefit of this process would lie in the decreased likelihood that you will commit the same error next time round (with a consequent increase in your chances of survival). This is the process I term 'late error detection'.

For the second example, let's go back to our game of tennis. Serena Williams has just received Venus' serve and tried to hit it back (all unconsciously achieved), but this time she misses the ball. Along lines discussed in Chapter 2, this is all 'replayed' in consciousness after the event. We can now see this replay, however, as serving a purpose. It allows Serena to consider what she did wrong and (if necessary and possible) to take steps not to commit the same error next time round. We did not evolve to play tennis; but the same mechanism of late error detection that allowed our ancestors to perfect their skills in avoiding flames or predators can now be put to more enjoyable uses.

The temptation at this point is to throw our hats up in the air: we did it! We found a survival value for consciousness, one moreover that fits the temporal facts. But beware. Notice the phrase I set in italics two paragraphs up. This gives to consciousness a causal role. It is *in consequence* of the pain that you review your action. Well, yes, of course: that's exactly how it feels, doesn't it? That is why, in books like this one, it is so easy—and so frequently done—to first state the Hard Problem and then quietly slip it back under the carpet. But, when we try this on, there is likely to be a Stevan Harnad who will—quite rightly—drag it out again. For we don't at present understand how conscious experience, whether or not seemingly equipped with the right kind of survival value, can have causal effects in its own right, as distinct from those of the brain processes it accompanies. This is a central feature of the Hard Problem. So I shall avoid the temptation to slip it back under the carpet, but rather leave it dangling for now in the air.

## 7.2   The comparator system

A system can detect error only if it has an expectation of what the correct state of affairs should be like. This formulation in no way implies the explicit, consciously experienced, kind of expectation that human beings are able to express in language. Mechanistically implemented systems able to predict and to compare outcomes with prediction are commonplace. Consider, for example, the way in which a guided missile extrapolates the trajectory of a moving target and alters its own course accordingly so as to minimise the distance between them. Indeed, prediction (the desired set-point) and comparison with prediction (feedback) are essential features of all negative feedback servomechanisms. There are many biological examples of such 'comparator systems'. Reaching out to grasp an object, as studied for example in Goodale's experiment illustrated in Fig. 2.4, requires continuous comparison between the position of the object reached for, the position the reaching limb has so far attained, the object's size in relation to current grip aperture, and so on. So there is nothing remarkable in postulating that the entry of novel aspects of the environment 'into' consciousness results from the operation of such a comparator system. Note that the operation of the system must itself be unconscious. We usually become aware that an element in our environment is novel or unexpected at precisely the same moment that we become aware of it at all. So the element's novelty must be computed prior to our becoming conscious of it.

Most of the brain's comparator systems—and there are many—are encapsulated. That is, they serve just one limited function, as in the reach-and-grasp example. The comparator system I have proposed for consciousness, however, has a much more general scope of activity. This is an inevitable consequence of the broad-ranging multimodality of conscious experience. Our conscious awareness is 'grabbed' by whatever is most unexpected at any moment, be this visual, auditory, olfactory and so on (or any combination of these and the other senses). The comparator that funnels this diversity of novel elements into consciousness must correspondingly be all-embracing. I have tried to capture the information processing capabilities that such a system requires in the sketch shown in Fig. 7.1. I have also made some suggestions as to the particular regions of the brain which discharge its functions. For the moment, we give these only scant attention (but see Chapter 14).

To understand the workings of the system depicted in Fig. 7.1, we need first to quantise time—that is to think in terms of successive discrete moments. Call such a

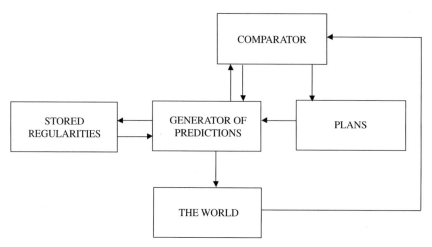

**Fig. 7.1** The kinds of information processing required for the successful functioning of the comparator system (for details see text). From Gray and McNaughton (2000).

moment *t* and the following one *t*+1. The duration of a moment is of the order of a tenth of a second (one hundred milliseconds). This duration is derived from certain of the physiological characteristics of the neural mechanisms postulated as discharging the comparator function. The overall function of the system is then: in the light of information available to it at time *t*, to predict what the perceived world should be like at time *t*+1; and then to compare the actual state of the world at time *t*+1 to this prediction so as to detect 'match' (the world is as it is predicted to be) or 'mismatch' (it isn't). In greater detail, the operations of the system are as follows.

1.  At time *t* the system takes in information describing the current state of the world, as this has been received and analysed (unconsciously) by the sensory systems of the brain. These systems principally occupy sensory regions in the back of the brain's neocortex, and regions in the middle of the brain called the thalamus. To have a useful label, therefore, I shall refer to them as 'thalamocortical sensory systems'. Now, as we saw in Chapter 4, this unconscious sensory analysis can proceed up to the level of intentionality. Thus, even though at this stage nothing has yet entered consciousness, we can envisage the results of sensory analysis as consisting in representations of what are capable of becoming fully conscious, multimodal percepts: e.g. in warm sunshine a scented red rose is swaying in the breeze as a bird sings in a near-by tree (elaborate on this as you will).

2.  The system also receives information concerning the brain's own 'motor programs' or 'plans'. Only by taking account what you are going to do next can the brain predict what you will next perceive.

3.  The system in addition has access to information held in memory stores. These are based on past regularities in the subject's history from which associations have been extracted and learned. These regularities, for example, may take the

form of predictive relations between events (e.g. flashes of lightning followed by claps of thunder) or between behaviour and events (e.g. pressing a switch turns on the light).

4. By putting these sources of information together the system can predict what the state of the world should be like at time $t+1$. Expressed in language, the prediction would run something like this: 'when I was last in a state of the world similar to the one I am in now, and in that situation I did what I am doing now, then the world next took on the following appearances'. Except, of course, that the prediction is actually formulated in the firing of neurons across many systems in the brain (*which* systems is a matter we shall come to later in the book).

5. The next step is to compare this prediction of how the world should appear at $t+1$ to the sensory analysis computed (still unconsciously) by the thalamocortical systems (as defined in point 1). This process of comparison will reveal elements of agreement ('match') between the predicted and actual states of affairs and elements of disagreement ('mismatch'). Mismatches may take the form of predicted elements that fail to appear (you press the switch but the light does not come on) or unpredicted elements that do appear (the light comes on all by itself).

6. We now finally come to the point at which some of what the brain has been unconsciously analysing finally enters consciousness. This is the central feature of the hypothesis I am proposing. A great array of experimental data shows that, at any moment, we are consciously aware of only a fragment of the complete sensory information which the brain has taken through to a pretty complete, but unconscious, analysis. The fragment that enters consciousness, so the hypothesis holds, consists in a subset of the outputs of the comparator system. This subset is made up of elements which are either (a) unexpected or (b) provide salient feedback for ongoing motor programs.

It is not my intention in this book to present a thorough exposition of a complex theory (see the second edition, 2000, of my book, with Neil McNaughton, *The Neuropsychology of Anxiety*). So I hope this brief outline of the 'comparator' hypothesis of the contents of consciousness will serve its purpose. It does need supplementation, however, to avoid some likely misunderstandings.

First, the quantisation of time does not imply that conscious experience should be jerky, like a video played slowly enough that each frame becomes separately visible. (Any such implication would, of course, be flagrantly in conflict with the experienced continuity of consciousness.) At any given time, the brain 'enters' into consciousness the results of the last comparison-plus-selection process while *simultaneously* preparing the prediction for the next one. So every moment is, in terms of the above exposition, both $t$ and $t+1$. Unconscious and conscious processing proceed in parallel, with the unconscious always in advance. Furthermore, there is a minimum duration for a conscious experience, and within this duration temporal order is blurred. That duration is of the order of a tenth of a second, about the same as the time which the comparator takes to make each successive comparison.

Furthermore, most of the contents of consciousness remain the same moment by moment. This is presumably because the furniture of the real external world, which constrains the constructs of consciousness into appropriate perceptual approximation, also remains largely the same from moment to moment. According to the comparator hypothesis (and in agreement with much evidence), we become consciously aware principally of those elements in this background or 'context' that either change or are of particular importance to us (given what we are trying to achieve) at that moment. The stability of the context (to the extent that it is consciously perceived, for much of it never enters consciousness at all) contributes to the continuity of conscious experience, seamlessly unifying each successive moment.

Additional smoothing of a process which, as described above, may appear to run the risk of jerkiness lies in the type of decision made by the comparator. This is not simply a binary choice between match and mismatch. Rather, the comparator produces a list of all the elements submitted to the comparison process, each annotated according to its degree of match/mismatch (the degree, in other words, to which the element matches in detail the prediction that has been made for it). Elements then enter consciousness depending on this degree of mismatch and can consequently be perceived as utterly, slightly, not at all unexpected and so on. What finally enters consciousness, then, is a nuanced set of elements among which some stand out as commanding particular attention because of the extent of their departure from expectation. In addition, other elements command attention because, although they are just as expected, they are important for ongoing motor programs: that is, in terms used earlier in this book, they act as controlled variables in respect of the operation of one or other of the brain's currently activated servo-mechanisms.

## 7.3   The nature of conscious perception

We shall have more to say later about the proposal that the contents of consciousness consist in outputs from a comparator system. However, before pursuing this proposal further, we need to situate it in a broader context. The contents of consciousness are perceptual. Yet so far we have considered them only under the limited aspect of their degree of novelty or unexpectedness. What is the nature of the more general perceptual functions that they discharge? And how, if at all, do these differ from the sensory detection discharged by unconscious sensorimotor servomechanisms?

A likely answer to this question relates directly to the differences in the temporal properties of conscious and unconscious sensory processing, respectively, with which we are already familiar. As I have emphasised, the time-base of conscious experience is slower than that of unconscious sensory processing. For visually-guided grasping or striking to be performed successfully, especially if the object to be grasped or struck is moving rapidly (as when a cat pounces on a bird or a tennis player returns a fast serve), the visual information defining the location of the object and the distance and trajectory still to be traversed must be updated on a time scale of at most tens of milliseconds. The brain is very good at operating on this fast time scale. But, when it comes to conscious perception, in any sensory modality, it chooses to operate much more slowly, on a scale of one or more hundreds of milliseconds for each conscious 'moment' or 'scene'. Until now, we have treated the lateness of conscious experience largely as a limitation that has to be accommodated by any analysis of what consciousness can or cannot do. But I now wish to consider this fact from a more positive point of view. What function is achieved by having consciousness operate in such a leisurely manner?

The comparator hypothesis goes some way to proposing such a function. The computational effort required by a comparator system (Fig. 7.1) must take time. And, indeed, the unit adopted for the quantisation of time in the comparator circuitry (*c.* 100 milliseconds) is based upon considerations of that kind applied to both the computations themselves and the neural machinery postulated as discharging them. But recall that most of the operations of the comparator are performed unconsciously. It is only when all the work is done that the list of annotated comparisons ('a clap of thunder, unexpected'; 'darkening of the sky, not much different from a moment ago') enters consciousness. The final entry into consciousness of such an annotated list does not seem, on its own, sufficient to account for the slow sweep of conscious experience.

The extra ingredient, until now missing from our account, has been elegantly expressed by the visual scientist, Semir Zeki. As he writes (about colour vision), the brain must 'reconstruct the constant properties of surfaces from the information reaching it which, itself, is never constant' (Zeki, 1993, pp. 233–4). This reconstruction of (relatively) constant percepts from ever-changing sensory inputs is the main business to which conscious experience appears to be directed. Testimony to the success with which the reconstruction is achieved lies in the extraordinary difficulty we have in distinguishing it from the real world 'out there', for which it serves in fact only as a model. And, to return to the comparator function, it is only against such a background of smoothed out ephemeral change that it is possible to detect *important* change in the model of the real world. Otherwise, everything would be in flux and all of equal importance.

How does conscious perception achieve this transmutation of the ever-changing into the constant? There are two ways of putting this question. The first asks for an account of the detailed machinery by which the brain performs the relevant computations. This is (a very difficult) Easy Question. We shall deal with it now, by way of one detailed example, that of colour vision. The second question asks for an account of the contribution specifically of conscious experience to the making of the transmutation. That is part of the Hard Question, and we shall save it till the next chapter.

The cells of the retina are activated by the quanta of light (photons) that they absorb. These trigger the cell to transmit a signal further up the visual system. Like other such signals in the nervous system, this consists in successive waves of electrochemical activity ('action potentials' or 'spikes') that pass down the fibre (the 'axon') connecting one cell to another. The intensity of discharge of the cell is reflected in a frequency code—the 'firing rate' or number of spikes per second. If all cells in the retina responded equally to photons independently of their wavelength, the visual world would lack all colour. This indeed is what happens with some individuals who lack the genetic machinery that specifies differential cellular reactions to different wavelengths of light. That machinery consists in the possession by cells ('cones') in the fovea (the central region of the retina) of one or other of three different 'visual pigments'. The absorption spectra of these pigments have maximal sensitivity, respectively, at short (S; violet), middle (M; green) or long (L; yellow-red) wavelengths, as depicted in Plate 7.1b. These spectra overlap considerably and, particularly in the case of the M and L pigments, lie quite close to each other. So the distinction the retina makes between different wavelengths of light is not categorical. Nor, in any case, does incident light come neatly separated into S, M or L categories. Rather, except under special circumstances not normally found outside a laboratory, the eye is continuously bathed in light of all wavelengths. So S, M and L cones are normally all activated simultaneously by incident light. However, their firing rates do depend upon the wavelength of the light. Other things being equal, a shift in wavelength from the violet through the green to the red end of the spectrum is reflected in changes in the firing rates of S, M and L cones that follow the shapes of their absorption curves (Plate 7.1). But these rates do not signal colour, nor even wavelength. The firing rate in a given cell is a signal only of the intensity of the light that falls upon it, that is, of the total number of photons captured by the cell. The wavelength of any particular photon, and its relation to the absorption spectrum of a given cone, affect only the probability that the photon will be absorbed by the cone. But the resulting firing rate carries no information about what that wavelength was.

The aim of the game of colour vision is to extract information about the wavelengths of light preferentially reflected from surfaces. Any given uniform surface reflects specific proportions of the light incident upon it at each wavelength, and this property of 'reflectance' is (relatively) permanent. It would provide useful information, therefore, if the nervous system were able to measure reflectances. And, indeed, it turns out that the property to which perceived colour most closely relates is surface reflectance. However, a first problem for the nervous system in obtaining this information is that, as we have just seen, it receives no signals from retinal cells that are unambiguously related to wavelength. A second problem is that the mixture of wavelengths of light reflected by surfaces changes in different conditions of illumination. To quote again from Zeki (*op. cit.* pp. 227–8):

If, for example, one were to view an orange or banana in a room lit by tungsten light, and then in a room lit by fluorescent light and then, successively, in daylight on a cloudy day and on a sunny day, and at dawn and at dusk, one would find that the orange will continue to look orange in colour and the banana will continue to look yellow. There may be some changes in the shade of yellow and orange, but the colour will remain the same. Yet, if one were to measure the wavelength composition of the light reflected from these surfaces in these different conditions, one will find profound variations. In natural viewing conditions there is thus no prespecified wavelength composition, or code, that leads to a particular colour and to that colour alone. Indeed, if the colours of objects changed with every change in the illumination in which they are viewed, then colour will lose its significance as a biological signalling mechanism since the object could not then be faithfully recognised by its colour any more.

Consider then three retinal cones, each containing a different pigment (S, M or L), upon which light is reflected from the same uniform surface. The brain can, and does, compare the intensity with which each of these cones fires and can thus compute the ratios between these firing rates. But these ratios are functions of two unknown variables: the wavelength composition of the incident light and the reflectance of the surface. It is therefore indeterminate from the ratios whether, say, the S cone is firing fastest because the incident light lies at the violet end of the spectrum, or because the surface has a relatively high reflectance for short-wave light; and the equivalent arguments hold true also for the firing rates of the M and L cones. From this, we can infer that it is impossible for the brain to determine the reflectance of a *single* surface. Experimentally, this indeed turns out to be the case. Take the design illustrated in Plate 7.2, known as a 'Mondrian' after Piet Mondrian, the Dutch artist who popularised this kind of abstract painting. It consists of an arrangement of rectangles or more complex polygons, each differently and uniformly coloured. Now, if one of these polygons (e.g. the green one picked out in the right-hand panel of Plate 7.2) is viewed in isolation through a small aperture, illuminated with light of mixed wavelength composition, it is seen as white or grey, depending upon the intensity of illumination, irrespective of the colour (reflectance) of the surface. So, the rectangle may be red, green, blue, yellow or whatever, but the viewer will report it always as white.

However, a further computation is able to resolve this ambiguity. This computation requires a comparison between, on the one hand, the ratios with which, one surface causes S, M and L cones to fire and, on the other, the same ratios arising from light reflected by other surfaces. These 'ratios of ratios' are capable of ordering surfaces according to their relative reflectances in the short-, middle- and long-wave portions of the visible spectrum. It is *this* ordering that the brain perceives as the colours of surfaces. Experimentally, this is demonstrated by having the viewer first report the colour of the rectangle marked by a circle in Plate 7.2 when it is viewed in isolation as above, and then widening the aperture so that it encompasses also other rectangles surrounding it. With this widening of view, the rectangle that appeared white is at once seen as green (or red, or blue, etc.), despite the fact that the light it reflects is in no way altered by the change in viewing conditions. The computation, of course, is not performed consciously—the change of perceived colour (so far as conscious awareness is concerned) just happens. As with all conscious experience, it is only the final perceptual result—a white or a green rectangle—of which one is aware.

These experiments—pioneered by Edwin Land—provide a clear demonstration that colour is not, as such, an inherent property of a surface. When it is isolated in the aperture viewing condition, a rectangle appears white; when the same rectangle, illuminated in an identical manner, is seen surrounded by other rectangles in the Mondrian design, it takes on a colour. The colour is determined by the taking of ratios (across rectangles) of ratios (across differently pigmented cones) of neuronal firing rates. But there *is* an inherent property of surfaces to which colour, when fully computed by the taking of ratios of ratios, corresponds: the surface's reflectance (across all wavelengths of light, but as estimated by the relative activity induced only in S, M and L cones).

Now, surface reflectance is a property of the real world out there. Kant called this real world the *ding an sich*, and believed it to be unknowable. The position adopted here agrees with Kant, in taking the perceived world to be quite different from the *ding an sich*. But it holds that, to a very considerable degree, we can obtain knowledge of the *ding an sich*, and this in two ways. First, the perceptual world as constructed by the brain is in many ways a faithful guide to (some) semi-permanent properties of the *ding an sich*. In the example considered here, colour is a good guide to surface reflectance; and surface reflectance is itself a good guide to certain objects of supreme biological importance. Second, the development of natural science, based upon rational thought applied to conscious perception, is able to elucidate the properties of the *ding an sich* to a degree that far surpasses the modelling capacities of unaided perception. Surface reflectance is an excellent case in point.

The main purpose of this discussion of colour vision has been to illustrate how conscious perception constructs an approximate model of aspects of the real world on a time-base longer than the rapidly changing visual inputs to which the visual action systems (grasping, reaching, etc.) are best adapted. The specifics of the wavelength composition of light incident upon, and reflected from, objects are in constant and rapid flux. Those specifics combine with the absorption spectra of cones to produce a further pattern of rapid flux in the firing rates of retinal cells. The brain's colour vision system uses these specifics to model (by the taking of ratios of ratios) the more enduring properties of surface reflectance. Having used them, it discards them—necessarily so, since the specifics of the flux are actively incompatible with the enduring qualities that colour vision strives to model. So we are aware of colours (*created* by the brain and *related* to reflecting surfaces in the external world, but *not* part of those surfaces), but we are not aware of the moment-by-moment changes in the wavelength composition of the light that actually impact upon the retina.

I have chosen colour vision as my example, since perceptual modelling of the world has been particularly clearly worked out in this modality. However, it seems generally to be true that conscious perception fulfills this role: that of constructing a model of aspects of the real world which are likely to be biologically useful and informative on a time-scale that is longer than the time-scale of unconscious sensorimotor action. (For want of a better word, I shall call this time-scale and model 'semi-permanent' or 'relatively enduring'.) This hypothesis should provide significant purchase for the empirical testing of the theory of conscious experience to which these arguments are leading.

Note, however, that, in normal human terms, the semi-permanent time-scale of conscious perception is still very short. The time-scale of rapid unconscious sensori-motor action is measured in tens of milliseconds; that of conscious perception in hundreds. But once something has been identified as enduring for hundreds of milliseconds, the chances are that it will last for minutes, days or even in some cases years. So it is with the reflectance of surfaces.

## 7.4   The evolution of colour vision

A further advantage of the example of colour vision is that we have a pretty good idea of how it evolved. It is possible, indeed, to infer something about the particular surfaces whose reflectance took on a biological role of sufficient significance to drive the evolution of colour vision.

As previously noted, human colour vision is 'trichromatic': that is, it is based upon three photopigments contained in different retinal cones. Astonishingly, it has been estimated that, using just these three starting points, we are potentially able to distinguish more than two million colours. Trichromacy first appeared in the human line of ancestry about 30 million years ago, with the evolution of the Old World primates. Most mammals are 'dichromats', that is, they possess just two classes of cone photopigments, as illustrated in Plate 7.1a. Human beings maintain this phylogenetically old system, but have added the more recently evolved Old World primate system (right-hand side of Plate 7.3). The older system (which contrasts activity in S cones with that in a mixture of M and L cones; see the left-hand side of Plate 7.3) is maximally discriminative of colours over the violet to yellow region of the visible spectrum. The newer system (which contrasts activity in L and M cones; right-hand side of Plate 7.3) is maximally discriminative over the red to blue region (Plate 7.1). The newer system thus conferred on Old World monkeys the capacity to make sharper distinctions between red, orange and yellow objects. What were these objects?

Old World monkeys eat fruit, and plenty of it; in many species well over 50% of the diet comes in this form. The fruits they eat have certain typical characteristics:

they tend to weigh about 5–50 g, to contain small seeds, and to be yellow, orange or red in colour when they are ripe. In the absence of trichromatic vision, they are very difficult to distinguish against the foliage of the forest background, as illustrated in Plate 7.4. Similarly, tender young leaves of a reddish colour are another preferred food. It is plausible, therefore, that the key survival value that drove the evolution of trichromatic colour vision in Old World monkeys lay in the new dietary opportunities it afforded. But this was probably not a one-way evolutionary street. A good case has been made, by John Mollon in particular, that the plants upon which these monkeys feed use the monkeys as a major route by which to disperse their seeds and so increase the survival of their own genes. This is because the monkeys excrete the seeds at a considerable distance from the plant where they found the fruit. So there has been co-evolution of the plants and the monkeys: the plants evolved fruit that was discriminable by and attractive to the monkeys, just as the monkeys evolved a new perceptual system, that of colour vision, by which they were able to locate the fruit.

Now, I am in great danger of leading you to suppose, in virtue of the argument I have been pursuing, that this evolutionary story is about the *conscious* perception of coloured fruit. There is, of course, no need to suppose this at all. Colour is like all other features of the visual world, in that a human observer can discriminate between, say, red and orange (by pressing a button on the left when he sees red, and a button on the right when he sees orange) faster than the time it takes for the consciously available percept of these colours to form. Similarly, the phenomenon of 'blindsight' (see Fig. 2.5) applies also to colour vision. Thus, Alan Cowey and Petra Stoerig have demonstrated that, in patients with damage to the visual system and who deny conscious perception of colours, the ability to discriminate between visual stimuli differing in wavelength of light nonetheless persists; and they have demonstrated similar effects in monkeys. So it is a mistake to infer that an Old World monkey, using his newly evolved trichromacy to pick out a ripe red berry, required the conscious percept of the berry or its redness to do so. The distinction between the visual perception and visual action systems is not straightforwardly that the former necessarily involves conscious percepts and the latter unconscious sensory detection. The distinction is more subtle. The rapidly changing visual information upon which sensorimotor action is based is (so far as I can tell) never available to conscious awareness. However, the information that gives rise to percepts is available *both* consciously *and* unconsciously, with the latter preceding the former. So, colour (as distinct from mere wavelength discrimination) is a construct of visual perception and capable of entering consciousness. But, like all other percepts, it is first constructed by the unconscious brain; and it is capable of exerting behavioural effects while remaining at that unconscious level. The question that therefore remains—a key part of the Hard Problem—concerns whether and, if so, how percepts can exert behavioural, and therefore causal, effects when they *do* enter consciousness and *in virtue of* that entry into consciousness.

## Conclusions

Three ideas have been sketched in this chapter: (1) that conscious perception aids Darwinian survival by providing a means for late error detection; (2) that a central component of the machinery that achieves late error detection is a general-purpose comparator system; and (3) that perception constructs a model of the semi-permanent properties of the real world on a time-base slower than that at which sensorimotor action systems function. These ideas will be further developed and integrated in the next chapter, where I present the main lines of a general theory of the survival value of conscious experience.

# CHAPTER 8

# Creeping up on the hard problem

We have spent a long time circling round the Hard Problem of consciousness. Let's see how close we've got.

My intentions in this chapter are, first, to set out a series of starting assumptions that any theory of consciousness will need either to make or to choose between; and second, to sketch a (partial) theory based upon these assumptions.

## 8.1 The assumptions

For the most part the assumptions (A1–A9, below) have been justified in earlier chapters.

### A1 The scope of conscious experience

The whole of the perceived world, extending to its most substantial features (solidity, three-dimensional extension, etc.), is a construct of the brain. There must be a good fit between this constructed model and the real external world 'out there', otherwise our efforts to interact with the real world would not be the spectacular success that they are. There must also be a good fit between the constructs of the world made by each and every other human brain, otherwise we would not agree as often as we do in our modes of interacting with the world. Nonetheless, the only direct contact we have with the real external world is by way of our unconscious sensorimotor action systems.

### A2 Perception models enduring features of the world

We took colour vision as a relatively well-understood example of this aspect of perception. To recapitulate, the wavelength composition of light falling on the retina is in constant flux. For the purposes of colour vision, this flux represents the only portion of the real external world with which the brain is in direct contact. The brain has no direct contact with the surfaces from which light is reflected. Yet, by way of a highly complex set of transformations and computations, it is able to model important and relatively enduring features of objects, namely, the reflectances of their surfaces. Knowledge of these surface reflectances provides biologically useful information, which aids survival. The modelling takes the form of experienced colours (plus the unconscious brain processes that cause the entry of these qualia into consciousness and either cause or constitute them). Generalising from this example, I assume that all perception has this characteristic of modelling relatively enduring features of the external world.

## A3   Survival value

Whatever consciousness is, it is too important to be a mere accidental by-product of other biological forces. A strong reason to suppose that conscious experience has survival value is this. It is only by appealing to evolutionary selection pressures that we can explain the good fit that exists between our perception of the world and our actions in dealing with it, or between my perceptions and yours. Biological characteristics that are not under strong selection pressure show random drift, which would be expected to destroy the fit. I assume, therefore, that consciousness has a survival value *in its own right*. That rules out epiphenomenalism, but leaves us with the problem of identifying the causal effects of consciousness *in its own right*.

## A4   The necessity of consciousness

A corollary of the assumption that consciousness confers survival value and has been the subject of natural selection is that it was perhaps a *necessary* evolutionary development. The brain is capable of a myriad wonderful things without deploying consciousness. Had it been able, without evolving consciousness, to add to its repertoire whatever it is that conscious processing additionally renders possible, then it is likely that it would have done so. So I assume that consciousness was the easiest and perhaps the only way to extend the brain's repertoire, at least at that point in biological evolution.

## A5   Animal consciousness

Relative to the development of our species, conscious experience is phylogenetically old. I do not know how old. Indeed, one of the benefits we would look to in a successful theory is an objective index of whether or not a given species has conscious experience. But we can, I believe, safely assume that mammals possess conscious experiences. That rules out as the survival value of consciousness anything exclusively human. Language, for example, cannot be necessary for conscious experience. The reverse, however, may be true: it may be that language (and other functions) could not have evolved in the absence of conscious experience.

## A6   Qualia

The contents of conscious experience are purely and entirely perceptual. This does not imply that they consist in what the philosophers call 'sense-data': as-yet uninterpreted sensory fragments awaiting integration into a meaningful or 'intentional' whole. On the contrary, the contents of consciousness are almost always (but see Chapter 18) intentional, that is, interpreted as having meaning.

### A7    Qualia are constructed by the unconscious brain

This point may seem obvious, since it is (almost) universally accepted that conscious experiences are products of the brain; and, apart from these constructs themselves, the brain's activities remain unconscious. It is nonetheless worth emphasising. It is commonly supposed that conscious experience is in some sense voluntary. Nothing could be further from the truth. Percepts just happen: they 'pop in' to consciousness automatically and involuntarily. We can choose not to turn our eyes towards a red apple or to keep them shut. But if the apple is in our field of view (and if we are paying attention) we cannot choose not to see it. Even in the case of ambiguous percepts, like the one in Fig. 4.1, the 'flip' between conscious perception of the one (a duck) or the other (a rabbit) happens automatically, with little influence from conscious deliberation.

### A8    Conscious experience is selective

The brain carries out a huge variety of processes, most of them highly complex and many of them simultaneously. We are consciously aware of only a tiny, highly selected subset of these processes. Unavailability for conscious experience takes two forms.

(a) There are processes of which one is never aware. This is the obverse of Assumption 6: we are never aware of the processing of the brain except when this eventuates in percepts. We are unaware, for example, of how we undertake actions, other than by way of percepts of the goals to which the actions are directed.

(b) Within the perceptual realm in which conscious experience is possible, it is restricted to only a small part of what might be consciously experienced at that time.

One can distinguish between these two kinds of unconscious processing by calling the former 'unconscious' and the latter 'preconscious'. These considerations greatly weaken hypotheses, proposed for example by Daniel Dennett, Marcel Kinsbourne and Susan Greenfield, according to which the neural activities of which one becomes conscious may be located anywhere in the brain, determined solely by the spread and intensity of one centre of activity relative to others (see Chapter 11).

### A9    Conscious experience comes too late to affect on-line processing and action

This is more than an assumption: it is supported by a large array of experimental evidence, which Max Velmans reviewed in 1991 (see Chapter 2). Libet's experiments show that this lateness applies also to the experience of oneself making a decision. The decision is made by the unconscious brain and enters conscious awareness only after the event.

Given these assumptions, let's see what kind of a theory we can build on them. Some of its elements have been introduced in earlier chapters, others are new.

## 8.2   Late error detection vs change blindness

The survival value of conscious experience lies in the provision of a mechanism to take a second look (one or two hundreds of milliseconds after on-line behavioural responding becomes possible) at something which, in the immediacy of action, has just gone wrong. This wrongness can take the form of an error in a motor program, or simply a departure from the expected state of the environment: something unexpected happens, or something that should have happened does not. The error signal can be specific (this particular subgoal in a motor program has not been reached, or this particular element in the environment has undergone unexpected change); or it can be highly generalised, as in the case of pain. (The distinction between these two types of error signal is pursued in greater detail in Chapter 18.) Pain, indeed, may reflect a very early stage in the evolution of the error detection mechanism, providing as it does an undifferentiated and universal signal of important (potentially tissue-damaging) error.

For the detection of error and change there must be a prediction of the expected state of affairs without error or change. Given that the errors that enter conscious experience cross all modalities, the comparator must be similarly multimodal. Given the intentionality of much of conscious experience, the comparator must work at a level at which perceptual systems have been able to construct (if they are needed) fully interpreted percepts, e.g. of objects. Given that conscious experiences are automatic and involuntary and that there is no awareness of the process by which they enter consciousness, the operations of the comparator system and the detection of error must be conducted preconsciously.

Indeed, there is evidence for a complementary assertion: that conscious perception is itself (as distinct from the preconscious processes by which the contents of consciousness are constructed) extraordinarily *insensitive* to departure from expectation. This assertion is supported by a series of experiments on 'change blindness'. Change blindness has been demonstrated across a diversity of situations, ranging from the stripped down experimental laboratory to the complexity of everyday life.

Many of the laboratory experiments have focussed on what happens during saccades. These rapid movements of the eyes jump from one part of the visual field to another, with each saccade lasting about a tenth of a second (depending on the exact distance the eyes travel). Their purpose is to bring to bear central vision (with its higher density of receptors per degree of visual angle) upon successive parts of

(a)

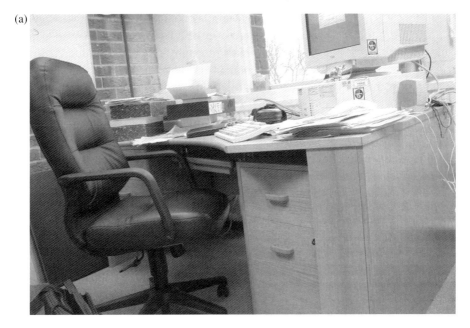

(b)

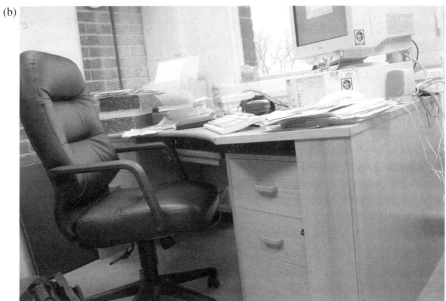

**Fig. 8.1** A pair of photographs, kindly provided by Professor Tom Trościanko, of the kind used by Blackmore *et al.* (1995) to study change blindness. For explanation, see text.

the visual field. Saccades occur several times a second, for the most part without our being aware of them or aware that vision is completely interrupted during their occurrence. In the experiments on change blindness, the onset of a saccade is used to trigger a change in the visual display that the subject is viewing, so as to ask the question: does the subject notice the change? The answer is that, even with very gross changes, the subject surprisingly often notices nothing. Susan Blackmore and her colleagues, for example, changed pictures like the one in Fig. 8.1a to pictures like the one in Fig. 8.1b, in which the black box file on the desk disappears. All the subject had to do was report whether the pictures were the same or different. Over a series of similar pictures, some of which changed and others did not, subjects correctly reported change only 55% of the time. This did not differ significantly from the 50% 'correct' that would be expected from totally random responding. More recent experiments show that change blindness is not necessarily linked to saccades as such. It seems, rather, that any interruption to visual processing, e.g. a simple white, blank field flashed up for a tenth of a second while the change is made, can achieve the same effect.

An even more dramatic example of change blindness comes from a naturalistic study carried out by Simons and Levin. The method they used was so clever that

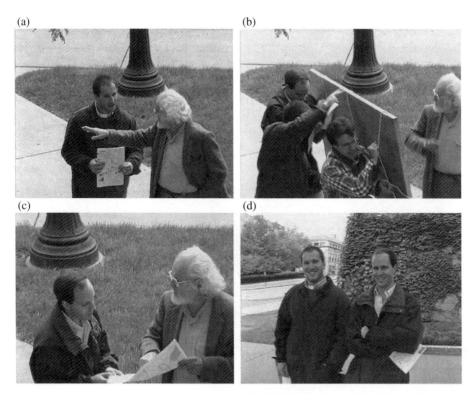

**Fig. 8.2** Simons and Levin's (1998) naturalistic study of change blindness. (a) A first experimenter (*left*) approaches an unwitting subject and asks for directions. (b) The two experimenters swap places behind the interposed door. (c) The second experimenter carries on the conversation with the subject. (d) The two experimenters side-by-side.

it deserves to be set out in detail. The experiment was conducted on the campus of Cornell University.

> An experimenter carrying a campus map asked unsuspecting pedestrians for directions to a nearby building (Fig. 8.2a). Pedestrians had a clear view of the experimenter starting from a distance of approximately 20 metres as they walked down a sidewalk. After the experimenter and pedestrian had been talking for 10–15 seconds, two other experimenters carrying a door rudely passed between them (Fig. 8.2b). As the door passed, the first experimenter grabbed the back of the door, and the experimenter who had been carrying that part of the door stayed behind and continued to ask for directions (Fig. 8.2c). The door blocked the pedestrian's view for approximately 1 second (Fig. 8.2b). From the subject's perspective, the door briefly occluded his or her conversation partner, and when it was gone a different person was revealed. As the door passed, subjects typically made eye contact with the second experimenter before continuing to give directions. The entire interaction took 2–5 minutes. The two experimenters wore different clothing and differed in height by approximately 5 cm (Fig. 8.2d). Their voices were also clearly distinguishable.

At the end of the interaction, the second experimenter asked subjects if they had noticed anything unusual and, if they did not mention the switch in their conversation partner, they were directly asked, 'Did you notice that I'm not the same person who approached you to ask for directions?'. Only 7 out of 15 subjects had noticed the change. This small proportion was reduced still further in a second experiment. This aimed to test the hypothesis that, the more subjects perceived their conversation partners as belonging to the same group as themselves, the greater would be the attention paid to their individual characteristics. In the first experiment the conversation partners had looked and dressed like the students they accosted. In the second, they dressed up like building workers. Despite the marked differences between the two fake building workers (Fig. 8.3), now only 4 out of 12 subjects noticed the switch between them.

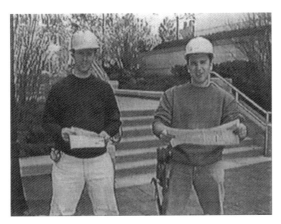

**Fig. 8.3** Simon and Levin's (1998) second experiment, in which the two experimenters were dressed as construction workers.

Both on the short time scale of a saccade, then, and the long time scale of normal social interaction, conscious perception is extraordinarily insensitive to quite gross change. How do these observations fit with the notion that consciousness discharges the function of a late error detector? And how do they fit with other observations demonstrating that novel, unusual or unexpected events have privileged access to conscious awareness (see, for example, the description of 'visual pop-out' in Section 10.5)?

The opposition between these two sets of data is more apparent than real, once due credit is given to the activities of the unconscious brain. As noted at the beginning of this section, the workings of the comparator system are conducted unconsciously. It is as a result of this unconscious processing that novel, unusual or unpredicted events are detected and entered into conscious awareness. For its part, conscious perception is concerned with the construction of a model of the relatively enduring features of the external world, an assumption already made and developed further in the next section. The construction of enduring features requires, precisely, the smoothing out of fluctuations in moment-to-moment sensory detection. So the medium of conscious perception is not the one in which one expects to find great sensitivity to change. This does not matter, so long as unconscious mechanisms are able to detect change and to alert the conscious system as and when required. The conscious system is then able to evaluate these alerts within the framework afforded by its construction of the more enduring features of the world.

Given these considerations, the change blindness experiments can be understood as follows. They are so designed as to prevent the *unconscious* detection of change. It is known, for example, that during saccades, visual input is suppressed. Similarly, it is likely that the one-second period during which vision of the conversation partner was blocked by the door in the Simons and Levin experiment (see Fig. 8.2b) would be sufficiently long to prevent operation of the unconscious detection of change in the pattern of visual input before and after the interruption. Thus, detection of change in both experiments would be dependent only upon conscious processing.

## 8.3  The nature of perception

As noted above, the central function of the perceptual systems is that of constructing a model of the relatively enduring features (relative, that is, to the rapid flux of physical energy at sensory receptor surfaces) of the external world. This model is naïvely experienced as actually *being* the external world. The perceptual model provides the 'medium' in which the comparator system reports expectations, error and change. Perception retains the sensory origin of the sources of information it uses to construct the model. Thus, we are aware not only of the visual or auditory or tactile aspects of say a cat, but also of these aspects as *being* visual, auditory or tactile. However, perception puts the different modalities together to make a single percept, of *Felix* sitting in my lap and purring while I stroke it. This putting together of modalities can be illusory. So, for example, a skilled ventriloquist takes advantage of this mechanism when he 'throws' his voice: his lips don't move, the puppet's lips do, and the audience therefore (automatically and without conscious inference) 'binds' the ventriloquist's voice to the puppet. Thus, the thrust of conscious perception is towards the construction of relatively enduring sources of multiple sensory information—'objects'.

The objects so constructed are located within a definite spatial and temporal framework. These frameworks are as much constructed by the brain as are the perceptual objects situated in them. Indeed, as clearly articulated by Immanuel Kant, space and time as constructed and contributed by the perceiving subject are necessary preconditions for the perception of anything else.

Space for the action systems is egocentric, that is to say, its metric is in co-ordinates of direction and distance from parts of the body. That is all that is needed to guide, say, a grasp or a kick. But space for the perceptual systems is also allocentric, that is, it utilises a map in which the relationships between locations of objects can be specified independently of the location of the observing subject, who himself has a location on the same map. Conscious experience is almost always (but see Chapter 18) situated in such a three-dimensional allocentric spatial framework. Conversely, utilisation of that framework appears to depend intimately upon conscious processing. This is so even in the case of the kind of rapid action that is paradigmatic of unconscious processing. When I ski fast down a slope full of 'moguls' (as skiers call bumps), the movements of my body and limbs are controlled without conscious awareness. However, I consciously scrutinise the positions of the moguls on the slope and *seem* to use the results of the scrutiny to plan my next turn. But I say 'seem' advisedly. We saw in Chapter 2 how misleading one's conscious intuitions can be. I don't know of any experimental work that could determine the accuracy of these intuitions concerning the special role that conscious processing may play in the strategic use of allocentric space (in my example, so as to navigate an array of moguls spatially distributed on a ski slope). But that is not to say that such an experiment could not be done.

The brain uses different regions for the construction of egocentric and allocentric space. This will be an important clue when we come (in Chapters 14 and 15) to ask about the functions of specific brain regions in the construction of conscious experience. Vision plays an important role in the construction of three-dimensional allocentric space, as we saw in Chapter 2 (consider, for example, Fig. 2.3). But other sensory modalities, such as sound and the vestibular sense of balance, also contribute to this construction. This multimodal spatial frame is used to guide the conjunction of modality-specific qualia into their combination as a unifed object. For example, in the ventriloquist's illusion, the auditory percept of the voice is subjectively displaced to join in space the visual percept of the puppet's moving lips.

Objects are situated also in a temporal framework. This can be used to separate one moment from another or to bind them together. Both these operations can give rise to illusion, as well-illustrated in the perception of motion. Anyone who has visited a discotheque with good strobe lighting has seen frantically moving dancers freeze-framed into successive stationary appearances. Conversely, if two spatially separated lights are switched on so that just after one has gone out the other comes on, then (depending on the intervals and distances between the lights) what is seen is a single light moving between the two points. The perception of movement in cinema or video films (in which, of course, nothing actually moves) depends upon this so-called 'phi' phenomenon. The temporal framework constructed by the brain is thus used to parse objects and events into successive moments, and to aid in their identification as 'the same' and 'different' across such moments.

## 8.4  Remediating error

By definition, a late error detection mechanism operates only after the error has been made (though this point is qualified below). However, late error detection permits changes to be made to action plans so as to adapt them more successfully to similar situations in the future. The theory contains several postulates concerning these changes and the way in which they are made. The central notion behind the postulates is that the brain is able to use conscious processing so as to modify the set-points of variables controlled by unconscious servomechanisms. (This, of course, still begs the question—part of the Hard Problem—of how conscious processing can achieve this, or indeed anything else.) There are different cases of this general principle.

### (a)  Juxtaposition of controlled variables

We have conceived of unconscious action systems as consisting in more or less complex instances of servomechanisms, each acting so as to control one or perhaps a few variables (Section 3.1). There is only a limited degree of communication between servomechanisms as to the states of their several sets of controlled variables. In contrast, entry into conscious perception seems to be particularly privileged for events in which there is a need to conjoin controlled variables of different kinds. Especially important in this respect are occasions on which the function of a servomechanism controlling a variable of one modality leads to error in relation to another servomechanism operating in a different modality. Under these conditions, conscious perception appears to serve as a medium in which multimodally conflicting information can be juxtaposed, permitting resolution of the conflict. The psychologist Bernard Baars calls this kind of process a 'global workspace': consciousness, in his view, permits the 'broadcasting' of the otherwise encapsulated contents of each servomechanism, so that they may be compared one to another. Although the view advocated here differs in important respects from that of Baars (see Chapter 11), his terminology is apt.

Consider the following example, taken from personal experience. I am a keen skier. I own my own skis and I am very familiar with them. One day I marched out from lunch looking towards the slopes to which I was headed. I had stuck my skis into the snow and, as I reached them, I hefted them up in my left hand without looking at them. After I had taken two or three more paces I experienced something like a little blue light blinking (literally) at me in the corner of my left eye. I turned my head to see what this light was, to discover that the skis were not after all mine. These skis had a small piece of blue decoration on the bindings, which mine did not. This was what my comparator system, acting unconsciously, had picked up as a discrepancy from the input that would be expected to enter my peripheral vision had I hefted up my skis and ski bindings (which, notice, I would have been completely unable to describe had I been asked to do so a moment before). So, the action servomechanism had failed to detect any discrepancy in the size or weight of the hefted skis; but the visual system had picked up a blue colour where no blue should have been. The resulting 'popping' of blue into my conscious awareness (automatically and involuntarily) permitted me to juxtapose the outputs from these different modalities, each with its separate servomechanism, and so revise the motor program that had picked up the wrong skis.

### (b) Contextual disambiguation of action programs

The type of case described in (a) is a one-off correction of a motor program that has gone wrong. A different type of case is one in which it becomes necessary to distinguish between two (or more) motor programs, both of which are right but under different circumstances. It is in this type of case that the spatial framework, into which conscious experience of the external world is slotted, comes into its own. For the spatial context provided by this framework can serve to select between such conflicting programs.

Consider, for example, an animal that forages for food at a distance from its burrow. The route by which it returns to the burrow must differ considerably, depending upon the point to which its foraging has taken it. From a given location, it must start with a turn left (rather than right) or must head for a particular landmark (rather than move further away from that landmark and towards a different one). Without an allocentric spatial map, there would be well-nigh insuperable problems in learning each different motor program to get the animal home from each different point in its environment and in keeping these programs separate from each other. In any case, this is not the way mammals (at least) do it. If they did, they could not find their way home to their burrow from a new location without learning by trial and error the new route required. In contrast to this laborious scenario, there is a wealth of evidence, much of it gained with the laboratory rat, demonstrating that, once an animal has learned to navigate to a base from a small number of locations, it can at once navigate there from others, so long as the relationships between major landmarks remain the same. The construction of such enduring landmarks, as well as the spatial framework that defines their interrelationships, according to the theory being developed here, forms part of the business of conscious perception.

The same basic machinery can be deployed to disambiguate the correct motor program under conditions other than purely spatial. For example, a street-wise urban rat may frequently visit a particular garbage can in search of food. But the motor program that takes the rat to the garbage needs to be overridden if there is an odour of cat in the air. Juxtaposition of these different circumstances so as to acquire the appropriate contextual 'tagging' that permits the rat both, today, to get food and tomorrow (when the cat is around) to avoid predation—these are functions, on the present theory, to which conscious perception makes a critical contribution.

### (c)    Addition of new controlled variables

I have frequently emphasised the fact that highly skilled, complex motor action programs (competition tennis, for example) run too fast for conscious processing to play any part. However, it can be objected that, when these skills are first learned, conscious awareness of the requirements of the new action pattern plays an important role in the learning. This objection is probably correct. But we need an understanding of the exact role played by conscious awareness in such early learning. An important aspect seems to lie in the identification of key variables for feedback and their desired set-points. Here are some personal examples (most readers will no doubt be able to supply others of their own).

One of the things a skier needs to learn is to keep his skis close together. Looking down at the skis to see how far they are apart is not a good idea, as you need to watch where you are going. But one day I noticed that when my skis are close to each other they make a little clattering sound as from time to time the edges touch. So that sound took on the role for me of a feedback signal (a controlled variable) that I can use to check that I am skiing the way I want to. Once the signal is established, by this conscious route, it can be used by the brain unconsciously. Indeed, if it is to be of any use once the motor program starts running off fast, it *must* be used unconsciously. A well-known ploy to put a skilled opponent off his game is to tell him to pay close conscious attention to whatever it is that he is doing. Conversely, one's best performance (and here dancing is as good an example as any sport) most often comes when you are least consciously aware of what is guiding your movements.

A good sports instructor often draws the novice's attention to feedback of this kind. When I was trying to master getting my weight into the right place after a parallel turn, my ski instructor taught the class to bend down and touch the back of one ski-boot while standing otherwise still with a straight back. Notice, he said, the feeling in the side of your waist when you do this. Sure enough, I get just that feeling if I make a good turn on a bumpy slope, so I am able to use this as feedback to monitor how well I am skiing. Often extra sources of feedback of this kind play a valuable role even though, after initial learning, they are not available for direct use. My ability to dive greatly improved one summer at a pool where I could always see my reflection in the water. Until that time I never had any idea at all what my body was doing between launch and an often painful arrival in the water. Now I was able to use my reflection to keep my body straight. That summer's learning transferred to other conditions lacking reflection to guide the dive. Presumably, feedback from vision had enabled establishment of the correct settings for other feedback signals (from muscles, stretch receptors, etc.), which my unconscious servomechanisms had before been unable to get right.

Notice that this discussion, like the earlier discussion of servomechanisms in Chapter 3, assumes that behavioural output is designed to produce sensory input. The more common picture supposes just the reverse: that sensory inputs produce behavioural outputs (as enshrined in the archetypal narrative of consciousness considered in Chapter 2). It is past time to justify this assumption more explicitly. To do so briefly I draw upon a telling experiment by Franz Mechsner and his colleagues at the Max Planck Institute in Munich (for a much more detailed account, see Hurley's book, *Consciousness in Action*).

When people spontaneously move both hands there is a well-known tendency towards mirror symmetry—moving the hands towards and away from each other, for example. Traditionally, such 'bimanual symmetry' has been attributed to factors on the output side, e.g. a tendency simultaneously to activate homologous muscles in the two limbs. The Munich group used the test of bimanual symmetry illustrated in Fig. 8.4. The standard form of the test is shown in Fig. 8.4a and b. The subject finds it much easier to move the two index fingers successively towards and away from each other (mirror symmetry) than successively in the same (parallel) directions. In this standard form of the test one cannot separate between the possible contributions of output (motoric) or input (sensory) factors, respectively, since they both operate in the same direction. However, the test shown in Fig. 8.4e and f discriminates between the two types of factor by having the subject hold one palm up and the other down. Now, if co-activation of homologous muscles (or any other motoric variable) is responsible for the preference for bimanual mirror symmetry, then it should be easier for the subject to move the fingers in a parallel than in a symmetric manner. The results of the experiment were just the opposite: it remained easier to move the fingers successively towards and away from each other. Thus the tendency towards bimanual mirror symmetry rests upon a sensory not a motoric basis. The sense concerned is not necessarily visual, since the same results were obtained when viewing of the fingers was prevented. Under these

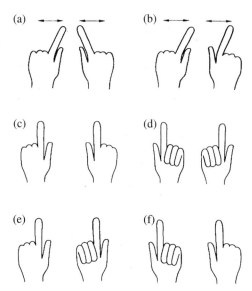

**Fig. 8.4** Instructed, synchronous finger oscillation patterns and hand positions. (a) Symmetrical movement. (b) Parallel movement. (c, d) Congruous position with both palms up or both palms down. (e, f) Incongruous positions with one palm up and the other palm down. From Mechsner *et al.* (2001).

conditions sensory feedback was presumably provided by way of the sense of proprioception (feelings arising in muscle and joint receptors as the fingers move).

A second experiment in the same report reinforces the conclusion from the first. In this experiment the subject was asked to perform an action that is under normal conditions virtually impossible: to turn two crank handles in a ratio of 4:3 turns of the one to turns of the other. But this task was easy to perform if the two crank handles were attached by gears to visible flags which, when the cranks were turned in the 4:3 ratio, moved at the same speed (Fig. 8.5). This bimanual pattern of movement, like others, was easier if the flags were moved in mirror symmetry than if they were turned 'in parallel', i.e. so that they both turned in the same direction at the same time.

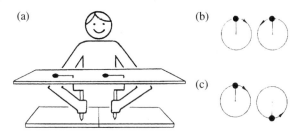

**Fig. 8.5** Instructed synchronous circling of flags. (a) Apparatus. The participant circles two visible flags using his or her hidden hands. The left flag moves coincidentally with the left hand, whereas the right flag moves according to a well-defined angle and/or frequency transformation with regard to the right hand (see text). (b) Symmetry, that is, $0^0$ relative angle. (c) Antiphase, that is, $180^0$ relative angle. From Mechsner *et al.* (2001).

In summary, the most important determinant of motor action patterns lies in the sensory controlled variables (feedback) to which the pattern is directed. Conscious perception of feedback signals may aid in the establishment of the motor pattern during early learning. However, once the action pattern is fast and fluent, conscious perception of feedback no longer plays a determinant role (although unconscious detection of sensory feedback continues to do so).

### (d)   Modification of the value of reinforcers

The most generalised forms of feedback lie in the rewards and punishments ('reinforcers') that motivate learning and the performance of learned actions. Anthony Dickinson and Bernard Balleine report an ingenious experiment, which suggests that change in the value of reinforcers may rely, at least in part, upon conscious perception.

Their experiment was performed with thirsty laboratory rats. These were first taught two actions for two different types of reward: to press a lever for sucrose and to pull a chain for saline. (As in all such laboratory experiments everything was in fact 'counterbalanced', half of the subjects getting the reverse assignment of action to type of reward. In this way, any special influence of lever-pressing over chain-pulling or sucrose over saline is controlled out of the results.) Then, after a session of this kind, the rat was made to feel sick (by injection of an emetic drug, lithium chloride). Now, it has been known for some time that this sequence of taste (sucrose or saline) followed by sickness produces a conditioned malaise to the taste when the animal next encounters it. This is known as a 'conditioned taste aversion', 'conditioning' being the general term for the process, originally studied by Ivan Pavlov, by which animals form associations between events that follow each other in time. (Much the same often happens to people who experience sickness during radiation therapy. They may find that food which they ate over that period later makes them feel sick.) Earlier work had also shown that, not surprisingly, rats will cease to work (by pressing levers, pulling chains, or the like) for a one-time reward which has come to be associated with sickness.

Dickinson and Balleine had already demonstrated that this loss of the motivation to work for a reward becomes manifest only if, after the initial conditioning session, the rat is allowed (in a 're-exposure session') to drink the once-rewarding fluid. So, for example, suppose the rat has learnt to press a lever for sucrose and to pull a chain for saline, and has then been made sick after ingesting both these substances. If it is now allowed to drink the sucrose (but not the saline) and is then once more given the opportunity to press a lever and pull a chain, it shows a reduced tendency only to press the lever—chain-pulling continues unabated. It is as though the rat needs to discover that, when it drinks the sucrose, it no longer tastes so good (or even induces nausea) before it can use that information to devalue the reward of sucrose (and so to give up on lever-pressing).

The anthropomorphic language I am applying here to the rat is no accident. Dickinson explicitly draws a parallel between these observations and an incident in his own life. He first tasted water melon on a summer holiday in Italy and thought it great stuff. Unfortunately, however, just after eating the water melon, and for reasons that had nothing to do with this innocuous fruit, he fell violently sick. Next day he once more came across a water melon and bit gleefully into it—only to find that he at once inexplicably (except that we can now explain it as a conditioned taste aversion) felt extremely sick. The rats in his experiments, he believes, similarly don't know that sucrose will make them ill until they try it.

On the basis of these experiments Dickinson and Balleine propose the hypothesis that the function of conscious experience is to act as an interface at which emotional reactions (in the example, a conditioned taste aversion to the hitherto pleasant sucrose solution) can interact with a cognitive and behavioural action program (performing the action of lever-pressing to obtain sucrose). To test the possible role of specifically conscious perception of the conditioned taste aversion, they carried out a final experiment in the series. In this experiment, during the critical re-exposure session (when the rats drink sucrose for the first time after the sickness induced by lithium), half of them are given a drug, ondansetron, which in human beings acts as an anti-emetic. Sure enough, when once more given the opportunity to press a lever for sucrose, the ones that had been re-exposed to sucrose plus ondansetron carried on pressing merrily, as though they expected the sucrose to be just as tasty as ever.

From these experiments we may infer (at increasing levels of abstraction and risk) that: (1) in the re-exposure session, the specific bodily reaction that teaches the rat to devalue the once rewarding sucrose is reverse peristalsis (since this is blocked by ondansetron); (2) the blockade of reverse peristalsis by ondansetron is accompanied by a loss of the conscious perception of nausea (since this is what happens in human beings given ondansetron); (3) if (2) is correct, then (reinforcing our earlier conclusions) rats share conscious percepts with human beings; (4) conscious perception of the changed value of a reinforcer plays a critical role in the resetting of the servo-mechanism that directs behaviour to the gaining of that reinforcer. As noted, Dickinson and Balleine wish then to draw the still more general inference that the key function of conscious experience is to provide a medium in which emotional reactions can influence such goal-directed behaviour. My own inference is broader still: that the phenomenon demonstrated by Dickinson and Balleine is a further instance of the general role of conscious perception in permitting change in the variables controlled by unconscious servomechanisms.

## Conclusions

In sum, I propose that a key function of consciousness is to permit, in the simulated 'real world' medium of perceptual experience, the juxtaposition and comparison of variables controlled by different unconscious servomechanisms, especially when these are in different sensory modalities; and the modification of their set-points in the light of a wider array of information than any single servomechanism has at its command. Note that this is a version of 'global workspace' theory, considered—and criticised—in Chapter 11 below. Note also that such theories provide a *functionalist* account of consciousness: they assume that a solution to the Hard Problem should consist in a description of specific information processing functions which require conscious experience for their discharge. This assumption has not been justified. Worse, in Chapter 10, I provide evidence that it is false. Here, then, lies a nodal point of tension in the argument developed in this book. Its resolution comes later.

# CHAPTER 9

# Epiphenomenalism revisited

The last chapter was profligate in suggesting that consciousness *does* various things. But many thinkers do not accept the possibility that consciousness is the kind of thing that can do anything at all (see the earlier discussion of epiphenomenalism in Section 6.2). So anyone who claims causality for consciousness has to offer at least some kind of explanation of how this might be achieved. It is time I grasped this nettle.

I referred in Section 7.3 to consciousness as a 'medium'. I shall here explain what I mean by this term. The explanation risks raising a host of anti-Cartesian demons. But this too is a nettle that must be grasped. Let's start by recapitulating some of the major points that have gone before. I shall state them as though they were fact, but they are of course for the most part hypotheses.

## 9.1 Causality and consciousness

As outlined in Chapter 6, conscious experience serves three linked functions.

(1) it contains a model of the relatively enduring features of the external world; and the model is experienced as though it *is* the external world;
(2) within the framework afforded by this model, features that are particularly relevant to ongoing motor programs or which depart from expectation are monitored and emphasised;
(3) within the framework of the model, the controlled variables and set-points of the brain's unconscious servomechanisms can be juxtaposed, combined and modified; in this way, error can be corrected.

Points (2) and (3) together constitute the 'late error detection' that gives consciousness its initial (phylogenetically speaking) survival value. The model of the external world (point 1) provides an essential medium in which late error detection can operate.

These three functions, then, are what conscious experience is *for*. But note that I have formulated points (1)–(3) without saying explicitly that consciousness *does* anything. That is because most, and perhaps all, of the doing lies with *unconscious* mechanisms. Unconscious mechanisms are responsible for (1), the construction of the model of the external world that enters consciousness; and this unconscious construction proceeds even to the point at which meaning and intentionality are invested in objects or events (see Section 4.4). Unconscious mechanisms are responsible also for (2), the comparator process that either ticks off a motor program as 'going according to plan' or detects novelty and error. That leaves only (3), the correction of error by modification of the activities of unconscious servo-mechanisms. Whether this is achieved in conscious or unconscious processing is an open empirical issue deserving experimental investigation. Given the assumption that error correction often requires the juxtaposition of controlled variables in different sensory modalities, there is a potentially important overlap between this issue and the 'binding problem' (Section 4.1). In that case, the issue becomes this: does the binding of features across different submodalities (e.g. colour and motion in vision) or different modalities (e.g. vision and audition) take place unconsciously or within consciousness or both? This is almost certainly a tractable problem, experimentally speaking.

If the unconscious brain does all or at least most of the work, what use does it make of conscious experience? To this question I give an old answer: that *consciousness acts as a medium of display.*

This answer today risks provoking a great yawn and a standard objection—of infinite regress. If there is a display, there has to be an observer of the display; and, if the observer of the display has to use conscious experience to witness it, then who acts as the next observer observing this display (and so on *ad infinitum*)? But, to quote from the philosopher Jerry Fodor (*The Language of Thought*, p. 189): 'This is a bad argument. It assumes, quite without justification, that if recovering information from the external environment requires having an image, recovering information from an image must require having an image too. But why should we assume that?' In any case, the objection misses the point made here. The medium of consciousness is used by the *unconscious* brain, not by a second conscious entity.

Before pursuing this line of argument further, let's grasp the other nettle: how can conscious experience have causal effects in a world whose causality is otherwise provided by processes that fit the laws of physics and chemistry? We are supposing that conscious experience acts as a medium for the display of (a constructed model of) the external world; that the unconscious brain reports in this medium the detection of 'late' error; and that the medium of conscious experience plays a role in the correction of the error. In order to discharge these functions, in what causal interactions must consciousness engage?

The first way of answering this question turns on the causal powers of the unconscious brain. For it is the unconscious brain which causes conscious experience. Nowadays, this postulate is uncontentious. It is taken for granted by scientists and philosophers alike that consciousness is a product of the brain. In fact, though, despite the consensus, this direction of causality, brain-to-consciousness, poses as thorny a problem as its converse, consciousness-to-brain, but one that I shall leave aside till later chapters. Here we concentrate on the complementary, scandalous (because it threatens us with dualism), possibility: that conscious experience causally affects the unconscious brain.

Analogies are dangerous tools, especially in relation to consciousness. Nonetheless, I find this one useful. Suppose I am in St Marks Square in Venice and have sufficient artistic talent (this is a counterfactual example!) to make a passable sketch of it. Later, I use the sketch as an aid to recall St Marks. Thus the sketch expands my capacity to remember—a causal effect. But the sketch clearly doesn't have this causal effect in its own right. The sketch is made by the brain (via hands controlling a paint brush) and later used by the brain. All the causal *mechanisms* lie in the brain. Still, any full description of the causal chain that leads to my recall of St Marks, must include an account of the role played by the sketch.

The nature of the causal role played by the sketch in this example is unproblematic. But can the analogy be properly applied where it is needed, that is, to my initial conscious perception of St Marks? Let's see.

Like my sketch, the visual percept of St Marks is constructed by my (unconscious) brain. Like the sketch, the percept expands the powers of my brain. Blindsight (see Section 2.3) occurs in the absence of conscious vision; but it is very limited in scope. It does not permit, for example, appreciation of the full three-dimensional lay-out of the square, its colours, its symmetry and so on. A person with only blindsight could not navigate from one side of the square to the other. So conscious vision involves *something* that has causal effects: the seeing person acts in and on the world in ways that, without it, are impossible. (This inference is not totally safe, however: the damage in a blindsight patient impairs unconscious as well as conscious visual processing.) Just how does conscious vision exert these causal effects? The sketch analogy suggests that conscious perception, like the sketch of St Marks, deploys no causal mechanisms of its own. The percept is there, like the sketch, merely as a display, one used by the unconscious brain.

This suggestion, however, begs the further question: how does the unconscious brain *inspect* the display? Before contemplating possible answers to this question, recall that there are not two things to inspect: not St Marks *and* my percept of St Marks. My percept of St Marks *is* St Marks—that's all (for me at the time of inspection) there is. And this percept is in my brain, made up of activity in whatever circuits have been activated in its construction, in the visual cortex and the other parts of the brain with which the visual cortex interacts.

There are two main ways in which one can answer the question: how does the unconscious brain inspect the display?

The first relies on direct routes to the rest of the brain from the neural circuitry and activity responsible for the construction of the display. Such routes are abundant and increasingly well-documented, and communication along them is unproblematic. The relevant information can be passed on in the usual way—by the passage of electrochemical signals along neural pathways. So, on this account, the display of conscious perception (like the sketch of St Marks) does have causal *effects* (as, given both introspective and experimental evidence, seems to be the case), but these do not require the attribution to consciousness of additional causal *mechanisms* over and above those possessed by the well-understood electrochemical activity of the brain.

Seductive as this solution to the problem is, it begs a further question. If the brain activity responsible for the construction of conscious percepts can communicate its constructs directly to the rest of the brain, why does the brain bother to construct the conscious percept at all? On this line of argument the conscious display has no additional effects of its own, over and above those of the brain activities upon which it rests. In other words, if we go down this route, we wind up on the epiphenomenalist horn of the dilemma. The conscious display is like the melody played by the steam escaping from the steam engine: it does no work, just adds metaphysical spice to life.

If epiphenomenalism is not to your taste, you have to give the conscious perceptual display some real work of its own to do. This implies that the unconscious brain in some way *inspects the display itself* and utilises the results of the inspection. Now, introspectively, that is of course just the way it seems. If I am in St Marks Square and aim to visit the cathedral, I locate it in conscious vision and walk towards it. The major qualification we need place upon this view from naïve introspection is that the perceived square through which I navigate is not 'out there', where it seems to be, but (along with the perceived body doing the navigating) inside my brain. In today's world of virtual reality machines, this assertion may seem less outrageous than it once did. For, if you are immersed in such a machine, using a joy-stick to navigate around a visually and tactually perceived environment, that environment can feel uncannily like 'the real world'. In this case, of course, you know that it isn't 'real', but entirely constructed by the computer controlling the show, in collusion with your brain. On this analogy, the 'real world' is similarly a virtual reality show, constructed in consciousness by the brain, and through which the unconscious brain navigates. This line of thought does justice to the facts of introspection, while perhaps offering a model for eventual theoretical development.

But we have learnt by now not to trust introspection unless it can be supported by other means. And this line of argument is taking us dangerously close to the other horn of the dilemma: dualism. For it suggests the following sequence:

(1) the unconscious brain constructs a display in a medium, that of conscious perception, fundamentally different from its usual medium of electrochemical activity in and between nerve cells;
(2) it inspects the conscious constructed display;
(3) it uses the results of the display to change the workings of its usual electrochemical medium.

Nonetheless, besides accounting for the effects of the conscious perceptual display in action, this sequence would also give natural selection something to work on in the evolution of conscious experience. For selection would now be, not just of brain circuits, but of brain circuits *and* the conscious experience to which they give rise. So this solution to the problem preserves overall scientific causation and ropes consciousness into the Darwinian corral along with the rest of biology. These would be major gains, even at the potential price of dualism.

Is there any way of escaping from the epiphenomenalist trap without falling into the dualist pit? Most of the solutions on offer, I fear, are verbal only. Chief among them are various forms of 'dual aspect' theory.

These state, roughly, that the brain activity that makes conscious experience happen and the conscious experience itself are, despite all appearance to the contrary, identical. They just happen to be observed in different ways. A brain scientist observes one aspect, electrochemical events in nerves, etc., from the 'third-person point of view'; while the experiencing subject observes the identical events, but from a different 'first-person point of view'. Theories of this kind have been elaborated in great detail, most recently by Max Velmans in his book, *Understanding Consciousness*. They are often buttressed by case studies from the history of science in which two apparently distinct entities have been shown in fact to be identical. Familiar examples are the identiification of both the Morning and Evening Star with the one planet, Venus; the unification of electricity and magnetism into a single theory of electromagnetism; or the realisation that those white puffy things in the sky called clouds are identical to the massed droplets of water encountered if we move right into them. But there is a major difference between such examples and the problem of consciousness. In each example, there is a detailed account of just how it is that the apparently different entities are identical, and of just how their two different manifestations arise and relate to one another. Perhaps we shall one day have such a theory for the relations between brain activity and conscious experience. But we don't have it yet. So the dual aspect notion at present expresses no more than a pious hope. It is an understandable hope, one that I share. If dual aspect theory were correct, it would escape both epiphenomenalism and dualism. But, as Hamlet says of the hawk and the hand-saw, I can tell the difference between a hope and a theory.

## 9.2   Language, science, aesthetics

The determined epiphenomenalist seeks to deny that conscious perception has causal effects in its own right (as distinct from the brain activities that give rise to conscious perception). Such a denial is not too difficult for the case of simply seeing something, for example, St Marks Square. There are, however, more complex human activities in which the causal role played by conscious perception is much harder to deny. These include language, science and aesthetic appreciation.

What we sense unconsciously activates appropriate servomechanisms but provides no purchase for language, since literally we cannot speak of it. We can speak only about the world as it is constructed in conscious perception. Correspondingly, the grain of language is set almost entirely at the level of the semi-permanent features of the world modelled in conscious perception. Thus conscious perception appears to be an essential precondition of human language: it provides the entities to which words refer. Here, then, is a massive causal effect attributable to conscious perception.

The sketch analogy seems to apply well to the case of language. A perceived rose (not the rose *ding an sich*, whatever that may be) provides a causal basis for speech about roses. There must, then, be causal interactions between (1) the brain circuitry whose activity is responsible for the construction of the percept of a rose and (2) the circuitry whose activity instantiates the linguistically expressed concept, 'rose'. Such interactions are likely to play a particularly important developmental role in the establishment of the concept on the back of the percept; and they probably continue to play an important role whenever the concept is used. So, at first glance, the epiphenomenalist argument rehearsed above for simple visual perception appears to be valid for language too. That is, speech about roses is based entirely upon direct links between circuits of types (1) and (2); and the conscious perception, as such, of the rose (or for that matter of the word 'rose') plays no causal role above and beyond the activity of the neural circuits which give rise to it.

However, language is based, not only upon features of the external world as modelled in one's own perception, but also upon consensus between different users of the same language. If there were no consensus, there could be no language. For the consensus to be possible, there needs to be a common set of referents. No individual can speak about events picked up only by unconscious sensory detection; *a fortiori* there can be no publicly agreed set of such events. (It is irrelevant to this conclusion that the very recent development of an empirical science of behaviour is able to demonstrate the unconscious detection of events, and so make these available for public discourse. Discourse of this kind is parasitic on the preceding existence of language.) These considerations give rise to a seemingly paradoxical conclusion. Despite the fact that the external world is constructed in each brain separately, *conscious perception is the only route by which a common set of referents can be created*. As argued earlier, evolution has ensured that the contents of conscious perception provide good guides to the real external world and are closely similar in most members of the same species. It is this similarity of perception under similar circumstances which permits establishment of the shared corpus of referents to which utterances refer. Furthermore, the consensus *cannot* be based upon the activities that underlie, in each perceiver's brain, the construction of the perceptual world, since these activities are of course *not* shared between brains (except via the conscious percept itself). Thus, for language to be possible, conscious percepts must do real causal work over and above the brain activities that give rise to them.

This is a very important conclusion. But note that it does *not* entail that the on-line production or comprehension of speech is a conscious process; we have indeed seen earlier that this is not so. Thus the case of language resembles the case of learning motor skills (considered above), in that conscious percepts play a critical role in the establishment of the parameters of feedback but not necessarily in the execution of the program once it has been learned. This resemblance is not surprising, since language is itself a motor program, albeit the most complex one in the human repertoire. Part of this complexity lies in the fact that there are two quite separate classes of feedback that need to be established and coordinated. The first is the one that this section has been mainly addressing: feedback (including from other language users) concerning those items within conscious perception to which language refers. The second consists in feedback (acoustic and articulatory) indicating that the correct words have been spoken or heard.

In the previous section we found grounds only of scientific or philosophical taste to justify the rejection of epiphenomenalism. The argument from language offers stronger, empirical, grounds for this rejection. Notice however that it holds only if one first abandons the naïve realist view that we directly perceive the external world out there. Given direct perception, the consensus of referents between language users might be based upon the real furniture of the real world. But, as we have seen, the scientific evidence overwhelmingly supports the view that the apparently real world to which language refers is constructed separately in each brain.

The same general argument applies also to the construction of scientific knowledge. Even though most of the contents of this knowledge refer, not to features of the conscious perceptual world, but to entities (wavelength of light, vibrations in the air, etc.) that activate unconscious sensory detection mechanisms, it is only by way of publicly replicable experiment that the corpus of scientific knowledge is built up. Such public replicability relies upon the results of conscious perception communicated from one member to the other of the scientific community in linguistic form.

Aesthetics provides a very different angle from which to attack epiphenomenalism. Consider the appreciation of beauty in any of its forms. This invariably involves contemplation of the constructs of conscious perception: the sight of the sunset or a painting by Titian; the sound of a nightingale, a song or a string quartet; the smell of a rose; the words of a poem heard in your head. Typical of all these instances is that they involve no action. You *can* point to the sunset or talk about it, but you don't need to do this or anything else in order to appreciate its beauty. It is sufficient—indeed usually optimal—just to sit and look at it. The unconscious action systems of the brain are best left still. But strip the aesthetic experience of its conscious content and there is nothing left. Sometimes, it is true, its hovering presence can be felt before you become aware of the qualia in which the full experience comes clothed. So, for example, I sometimes sense only the melodic shape, without words, of a line of poetry struggling to enter my conscious awareness (like the 'tip of the tongue' phenomenon with which everyone is familiar, when a word struggles to fill a semantic gap in the stream of discourse). But this type of experience demonstrates only that, like everything else in consciousness, the qualia that give us aesthetic pleasure are the products of the unconscious brain. For the aesthetic pleasure itself, it is a *sine qua non* that there should be consciously experienced qualia: without conscious perception there is no beauty. Here, then, is another massive causal effect attributable to conscious perception.

'Beauty is in the eye of the beholder'—this common saying is normally taken to mean that we each have different reactions to the same thing (sunset, sonata, scent or sonnet) in the real world. But the saying is true also on a much deeper level. Each of these objects of beauty is a construct of the brain. It is the brain that makes, not just the sunset's beauty, but the sunset. And it is the brain that then contemplates the sunset it has created. I find it hard even to give sense to the notion that this act of contemplation is directed at the neural activity that gives rise to the percept of the sunset rather than to the perceived sunset.

## 9.3   Ongoing causal efficacy for consciousness?

Language, science and the appreciation of artistic beauty constitute in this way major causal consequences of the existence of conscious experience. But they fall short of demonstrating that conscious experiences play a causal role in *the functioning of the brain that produces them at the time they are so produced*—what one might call 'ongoing causal efficacy'. Given the lateness of conscious experience, coupled with the abundant evidence that such experience is always the outcome of a prior chain of unconscious brain processes (see Chapter 2), the lack of evidence for ongoing causal efficacy of consciousness in the brain is perhaps not surprising. But it *is* worrying. For it leaves open the possibility that, insofar as it is linked to ongoing brain activity, conscious experience is indeed a mere epiphenomenon. Its causal effects may be exerted in the same way as those exerted by my sketch of St Marks: as an external *aide-mémoire*. The brain can achieve many things, given the *aide-mémoire*, that it could not do otherwise; but the *aide-mémoire* itself is causally inactive. The case may be the same for the seeming ongoing causal efficacy of conscious experience.

There are, however, a few pieces of experimental evidence that suggest (but no stronger word is possible) true ongoing causal efficacy for conscious experience. Here are three examples.

First, consider a seminal experiment reported in 1980 by the Cambridge psychologist, Tony Marcel. This turns on the abundance in English, as in other languages, of 'polysemous' words—words with more than one meaning. To make sense of such words we rely upon their context. No-one, for example, is likely to mistake Shakespeare's 'bank for love to lie and play on' (*The Winter's Tale*) as a place to cash a cheque.

Marcel presented his subjects with a series of three words, of which the final one might be a real word or a string of letters looking like a word but not in fact composing one. The subjects had to press a button as fast as possible to indicate whether the third word was real or not—a so-called 'lexical decision' task. Marcel asked whether the speed with which subjects reached this decision on trials when the third word was in fact real would be affected by the semantic relationships holding between the words in the series. The fastest decision times occurred when all three words were semantically related as part of a common network, as in *HAND–PALM–WRIST*. (This kind of influence of one meaning, usually but not necessarily packaged in a word, on another that follows is known as 'semantic priming'.) However, by placing a polysemous word in the middle, Marcel was able to arrange that the first two words and the last two were related, but not the first and third. An example would be: *TREE–PALM–WRIST*. The decision that *WRIST* was a real word under these conditions was slowed down compared to a control condition in which all three words were unrelated (*TREE–RACE–WRIST*). This result implies that, in the sequence *TREE–PALM–WRIST*, the primed meaning of 'palm' ('a kind of tree') inhibited its meaning as 'a part of the hand', so delaying recognition of 'wrist' as a meaningful word.

These were Marcel's results when all three words were clearly visible. In a further condition, however, he used the same triplets of words but with the one in the middle masked so that it was not consciously seen. Priming still occurred, but now it took a different form. Compared to the control condition in which all three words were unrelated, decision times were faster when the second word primed the third, irrespective of the semantic relationship between the first and second words. So 'wrist' was recognised as a word faster in strings of both the form *HAND–PALM(masked)–WRIST* and the form *TREE–PALM(masked)–WRIST*.

A comparison between Marcel's results in the two conditions (the middle word in the series masked *versus* unmasked) suggests a clear role for conscious processing in the determination of semantic context. When it is masked from conscious perception, the middle word in the triplet ('palm') is analysed in both its meanings (as a tree and as part of the hand), irrespective of what has gone before. Both of these meanings are then available to prime the third word ('wrist') as required. Conscious perception of the middle word changes this pattern. Priming is now restricted by the meaning of the previously seen word, 'tree', so that 'palm' is interpreted *only* as 'a kind of tree', not as 'a part of the hand'. Note that the meaning of 'palm' as 'a part of the hand' does not merely fail to get accessed, it is actively inhibited, since decision times to series of the form *TREE–PALM–WRIST* were actually slower than to three unrelated words. So conscious perception appears to extend the duration of context (this now plays over three items, not just two) and to narrow it (one meaning of the polysemous word is picked out at the expense of the other). The former effect—extension of duration—has also been demonstrated in other experiments on semantic priming. Greenwald and his colleagues, for example, have shown that the effects of a masked semantic prime are confined to a brief window of time (around 60–100 milliseconds), whereas those of an unmasked prime extend for up to 400 milliseconds.

As a second example, consider again Groeger's experiment (Fig. 4.2). This demonstrated that the choice between the words 'smug' and 'cosy' (to fill the gap in 'she looked ... in her fur coat') was primed differently by prior auditory presentation of the word 'snug', depending on whether 'snug' was above or below the threshold for conscious perception. Below the threshold, priming followed the semantic route, favouring 'cosy' over 'smug'; above the threshold, it followed the phonetic route, favouring 'smug' over 'cosy'. The most natural interpretation of this result is that it was the conscious perception of the phonetics—the qualia—of 'snug' which *caused* this latter effect.

There is, however, a perhaps always unavoidable weakness in these arguments, one which Stevan Harnad would be quick to point out. There must be different neural events taking place when Marcel masks or leaves unmasked the central word in his triplets, or when Groeger's 'snug' is consciously heard or not. So the different types of priming observed in these cases may arise directly from these differences in neural activity, with the accompanying conscious experience playing no causal role of its own. There is, however, one further line of experimentation that—just possibly—may allow us to take the argument further. Like a number of other points made in this book, it turns on the phenomenon of synaesthesia (for a detailed account of this fascinating condition, see Chapter 10).

Jason Mattingley, Anna Rich and their colleagues in Melbourne, Australia, studied a group of 'colour-grapheme' synaesthetes, who experience colours when they see single letters or digits ('graphemes'). Their experiments are based upon the well-known phenomenon of 'Stroop' interference (named for the psychologist who discovered it). In a common version of this type of experiment you are asked to name, as fast as possible, the colour in which either a string of *X*s or the name of a colour is presented to you. If the colour name differs from the 'ink' colour (e.g. the word 'red' printed in green), your naming speed will be reliably slowed down. This is the Stroop effect. Mattingley's group demonstrated just such an effect when their colour-grapheme synaesthetes were shown letters or digits in different ink colours and asked to name the colour. If this was incongruent with the synaesthetic colour triggered by the grapheme, they took longer to name the physical colour in which it was displayed. (This is one among many recent demonstrations that the experiences synaesthetes report are real and have observable effects upon behaviour.) In a further experiment the synaesthetes were presented with a black-and-white display of a grapheme followed by a patch of colour. Their task now was simply to name the colour. Colour naming was again slowed down if the synaesthetic colour triggered by the grapheme was incongruent with that of the colour patch.

This variant on the standard Stroop paradigm permitted the introduction of a further twist: the priming grapheme could now be presented in a manner that blocked it out from conscious perception. This was achieved by very brief presentation (for just 28 or 56 milliseconds) followed by a visual mask. This manoeuvre eliminated the Stroop interference observed when the grapheme was consciously perceived.

Now this result might seem trivial. What else do you expect when the interfering grapheme is not consciously seen? However, results obtained by the Canadian psychologist, Philip Merikle, suggest that blockade by masking of the synaesthetic Stroop effect may be anything but trivial. Merikle has reported a series of experiments closely analogous to Mattingley's, but with non-synaesthetes. The subjects were shown a colour name followed by a patch of colour that they had to name as fast as possible. The expected Stroop effect was obtained: colour naming was slowed down when the colour name was incongruent with the colour of the patch. Remarkably, however, when the same experiment was carried out with the colour word not consciously perceptible (it was presented for 33 milliseconds, followed by a mask), the Stroop effect was still obtained. So Mattingley's Stroop effect primed by synaesthetically-induced colours differs from Merikle's with non-synaesthetes primed by colour names: the former does not survive removal of the priming stimulus from conscious perception, the latter does.

This difference is intriguing. It suggests, contrary to epiphenomenalism, that synaesthetically induced colours *require* conscious experience if they are to affect behaviour—bringing us perilously close to dualism (Fig. 9.1). But the strength of the argument is weakened by depending upon a contrast between two different experiments using two different groups of subjects. A more powerful design would be one in which, within a single experimental paradigm, the same subjects show both a standard Stroop effect and one that is synaesthetically induced. We are currently planning an experiment of this kind. If we are able to show that masking affects the two kinds of Stroop effect differently, as suggested by joint consideration of the Mattingley and Merikle results, this might offer a way to put the effects of the specifically conscious perception of synaesthetic priming stimuli under closer experimental scrutiny. In this way we might be able to bring epiphenomalist claims into the laboratory—and that would be triumph enough. For the while, that is the best I can offer. The case against epiphenomenalism is not water-tight by a long way; but it is getting stronger. So, for the rest of this book, I shall assume that consciousness plays a full causal role in the natural world. The question is: how?

## 9.4 The evolution and ontogeny of consciousness

Conscious experience is clearly related in some fashion to the brain. If we said this about any other aspect of brain function, we would expect it to have evolved

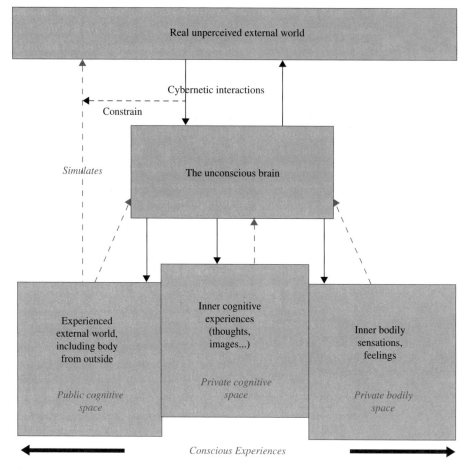

**Fig. 9.1** Perilous proximity to dualism. A modification to Fig. 1.1 (dashed lines going back up to 'the unconscious brain') to illustrate the possibility that conscious experience might have causal effects on the activities of the unconscious brain *in its own right* (that is, over and above any effects of the neural activity that gives rise to the conscious experience).

(during phylogeny); and we would expect (given sufficient time, work and ingenuity) to trace the course of its evolution. We would also expect it to develop during an individual's lifetime (ontogeny). The brain does not start life with the capacity to control walking or do mathematics—these functions develop as the brain matures and as it learns about its environment (though such learning plays a much greater part in the achievement of mathematics than of walking). These, then, are questions that it is reasonable to pose also in the case of consciousness. But is there any relevant evidence with which to answer them?

The short answer is 'No'—though it is perverse to say so, given that whole books (including Euan MacPhail's *The Evolution of Consciousness* and Merlin Donald's

*A Mind So Rare*) have been devoted to the topic. The trouble is that all such discussions make entirely arbitrary assumptions about what kind of behaviour does or does not entail the underpinning of conscious experience. And, as we have seen, behaviour is notorious in *not* itself providing a reliable index of the occurrence of conscious experience. This is the case even when the behaving individual is alive, adult and human—how much worse, then, when one tries to infer the conscious underpinnings of behaviour in other species, especially when these are no longer even extant. The ontogeny of conscious experience is not much easier to tackle, even if one confines oneself to the human species, and for the same reasons. A mother is normally in no doubt that a cry of pain is a reliable sign that her infant is consciously experiencing pain; but many scientists and philosophers have grave doubts on the score. (So grave, indeed, that some of the more radical opponents of experiments with animals reckon that it would be ethically sounder to work with human infants—a curious opinion that I do not share.) Resolving these disparate views is unlikely to be possible until we have a clearer idea of the mechanisms by which the brain creates qualia. Then we could perhaps get a grip on the ontogeny of conscious experience by enquiring when these mechanisms become functional, and a similar grip on its phylogeny by enquiring when they evolved.

The line of argument pursued in the previous section may, however, offer an unexpected purchase upon the ontogenetic issues. Consider in this context Peter Hobson's careful observations (described in his book, *The Cradle of Thought*) of joint attention in mother–child dyads. Here is how Hobson describes a relevant instance—one that will be familiar to any mother (*loc. cit.*, pp. 107–8). His description refers to the 'triangle of joint attention' reproduced here as Fig. 9.2.

> We can apply the triangle to the case of a twelve-month-old who is confronted with a disquieting object. A new toy suddenly pronounces 'I am a robot!'. The child is looking at the toy (the world), and now she feels both interested and afraid. She looks to her mother, who is standing nearby. The mother is looking at the robot with amused surprise. Noting her daughter's anxiety, she might also show faint pretend-anxiety. This would make it easier for the child to link in with her state, and at the same time to modify her own feelings. In the case we are considering, the

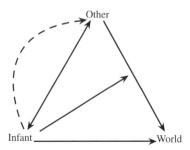

**Fig. 9.2** Hobson's (2002) triangle of joint attention (see text for explanation).

infant perceives the mother's attitude to be directed towards the toy. The mother may look reassuringly at her baby, but by her alternating looks between her baby and the toy it is clear to any observer (including the baby) that she is giving her baby reassurance *about* the toy. In this way the baby relates to her mother's way of relating to the toy—the arrow that bisects the triangle—and comes to modify her own feelings towards the toy. Her anxiety turns not to fear but to curiosity; her hesitation turns not to retreat but to timid exploration. She has been moved by the attitude of her mother to construe the world differently.

Hobson himself draws many fascinating inferences from this kind of mother–child interaction. But the one I want now to draw differs from any of them. For this inference, the key feature of the episode is that the interaction depends upon mother and daughter's both recognising an object in the external world—the toy robot. If we had retained an analysis of the external world in which *it is really out there*, this fact would tell us little about consciousness. For interactions between a world really out there and behaviour directed towards it can be accomplished *unconsciously*. Indeed, that is just what happens when visual action systems discharge their normal cybernetic functions. But there are two substantial planks in our overall argument which, taken together, lead now to a different analysis. The first is that the consciously perceived world is *not* really out there at all—it is constructed by each and everyone's brain. The second is that communication between two individuals requires reference to just such conscious percepts constructed in the brains of each of them—for reference to *unconscious* stimuli is simply impossible (Section 9.2). On these two planks we can rest the conclusion that, when mother and daughter communicate about the toy robot in Hobson's vignette, they must each have a conscious percept of the toy. (That their communication is accomplished without fully-fledged language does not affect the argument.)

From observations such as these, then (provided they are interpreted within an appropriate theoretical framework), we may infer that the one-year-old child in Hobson's vignette has reached a stage of development that permits conscious perception. Interestingly, at 8 months of age children do not yet show this capacity for shared attention to perceived objects (Hobson, *loc. cit.*, p. 64). Does this mean they lack conscious perception? *This* inference would be illegitimate. While it seems reasonable to infer conscious perception from certain kinds of behaviour, one cannot infer from the absence of that behaviour to the absence of perception. This difficulty in arriving at negative conclusions is, of course, a general feature of scientific inference. But, in case you are in any doubt as to its application to consciousness, consider the impossibility of inferring the absence of conscious experience in a motionless, sleeping adult who may be in the middle of a dream. Nonetheless, despite this limitation, it is progress to be able to make a reasonably tight inference to the presence of conscious experience in a one-year-old child.

## Conclusions

The Hard Problem of consciousness can be stripped down to one (still Hard) but double-edged question: *how does the unconscious brain create and inspect the display medium (qualia) of conscious perception?* I call this one question rather than two because I suspect (but cannot demonstrate) that any scientifically acceptable account of how the brain creates qualia will at the same time constitute an account of how it inspects them. St-Marks-as-virtual-reality, as discussed above, *may* offer a model of how this could be achieved. What is certain is that the first half of the question, 'how does the brain create qualia?', is enough to keep science going for a long time to come. So, for the rest of the book, this is the half we shall concentrate upon.

# CHAPTER 10

# Scrutinising functionalism

We concluded the previous chapter by asking the question: *how does the unconscious brain create and inspect the display medium of conscious perception?* If the argument so far is correct, the Hard Problem of consciousness can be reduced to just this question. In this chapter we start on the exploration of some possible ways to answer it.

## 10.1  Foreclosures

In the search for useful answers, getting the question right is half the battle. The way I have formulated the Hard Problem has already foreclosed some options. Some of the foreclosures were made explicit earlier, but they should be borne in mind.

First, like any formulation of the Hard Problem, this one presupposes that there *is* such a thing as conscious experience, and that it can be picked out (in some way or another) as being different from either behaviour or brain activity. I have not spent much time justifying this assumption, since the contrary view—that there is really no such thing as consciousness—is unlikely to find favour among most readers. Are we not familiar enough with our own conscious experiences?

But it is worth putting on record that some Radical Behaviourists (an endangered but living species) do not accept the reality of conscious experience. They treat subjective accounts of experience as fundamentally misguided, and replace them with statements about behaviour. Once, in a heated argument with one such, Howard Rachlin, I came up triumphantly with an example which, surely, would convince him that some conscious experiences just don't translate into behavioural terms. Suppose, I asked, you come into a room and see two individuals both sitting motionless in arm-chairs; a gramophone is playing a Mozart string quartet; one of the two individuals is listening to the music, but the other is deaf: how can you describe the difference between what is going on in these two individuals without reference to the subjective experience of the one listening to Mozart? Quick as a flash, Howard answered as follows: the one who isn't deaf has a whole lot of behavioural patterns which will include, when he is later asked, making verbal statements about Mozart and string quartets. That is how 'listening to music' is translated into behavioural terms. Since then I have given up all attempt to convince Radical Behaviourists that conscious experience is independently real.

Second, again like any formulation of the Hard Problem, this one supposes that such a *problem* exists. As we saw in Chapter 1, not everyone agrees with this. A majority of working scientists, in particular, take the view that the problem of consciousness will be solved in the same general way as the problem of life was solved. That is to say, there will be solutions to each of the separate aspects that today appear to make up the Hard Problem, and these solutions will require no more than the detail of experimental discovery plus standard biological explanation. If this point of view is correct, then it will be sufficient to discover more and more about the detailed brain mechanisms that underlie conscious perception, and all will then fall into place.

Let me be clear that, if this should prove to be the case, I shall applaud. I have no desire—as do those whom Dan Dennett aptly christened the New Mysterians—for consciousness to remain mysterious; and, if there is a solution to be found within normal science, so much the better. But there are strong reasons to doubt that this will be so.

Chapter 3 described the contract that biology made with physics and chemistry: biological explanation will respect their laws, provided these allow selection by consequences (in natural selection and in the feedback mechanisms designed by natural selection). That contract works well enough over the rest of biology, but seems to break down for the special medium of conscious perception. It is not selection by consequences where the difficulty principally lies. If one could sort the physics out, there doesn't seem to be an insuperable problem in finding causal effects for conscious perception to produce. Though these are much more restricted than appears to introspection, they still provide enough purchase for natural selection to work. As to servomechanisms, we identified in Section 8.4 a range of ways in which conscious perception is likely to increase their scope and efficiency. To be sure, acceptance of these causal effects for consciousness *per se* means that we are also foreclosing on epiphenomenalism; but we found good reason to do this in Chapter 9.

The problem, rather, lies in the physics and chemistry. It isn't that conscious experience doesn't obey their laws, it is rather that they don't seem to apply to it at all. None of the usual measurements make any sense. You cannot speak of the position, mass, momentum, acceleration, energy, etc., of qualia, let alone measure them. And the fact that you *can* apply all these concepts to the brain and the brain's components doesn't help, once you decide (as we did when we killed off epiphenomenalism) that conscious experience is capable of having causal effects over and above those of its underlying neural activities.

This, by the way, is not a problem just for psychology and neuroscience. Physics aims to give a complete and completely unified account of the entire universe. Thus it cannot rest easy with a set of natural phenomena, such as those of conscious experience, which resist physical measurement and explanation. So either consciousness must be made to fit contemporary physics or physics itself must change to accommodate consciousness. Some physicists, like Roger Penrose (whose theory we consider in Chapter 16), advocate just that.

The scientific stakes, therefore, are high—so high, in fact, that I shall not yet foreclose on the possibility that there will after all be a 'normal science' account of consciousness. The most promising contemporary attempt to construct such an account flies under the banner of 'functionalism'—a doctrine that this chapter therefore submits to close scrutiny.

Now, the single fact about consciousness of which we can be most certain is that it is in some way connected to the activity of the human brain. So the brain is a good place to start in seeking possible solutions to the Hard Problem. The trouble is that there are many different ways in which to think about the brain; and, depending on the way you choose, you arrive at quite different types of solution.

For the brain is:

(1) a system which
(2) interacts with an environment
(3) and is made up of physicochemical components;
(4) these components are biological cells,
(5) more specifically, neural cells.

Depending upon which of (1)–(5) you think comprise the critical conditions for consciousness, you can end up with wildly divergent hypotheses. Functionalism takes (1) and/or (2) as its starting point.

## 10.2   Conscious computers?

Suppose the only thing that matters for the making of conscious experience is the nature of the system, irrespective of the components of which it is made. Then, if you make a system that has functions identical to those of the human brain but make it out of different components (silicon chips, for example), the system will have conscious experience. In its extreme form, this line of thought leads to the supposition that computers which merely *simulate* functions identical to those of the human brain would experience consciousness.

The famous Turing test encapsulates this supposition. You face two closed doors through which you feed a series of test questions. Printed answers to your questions are slipped back under the doors. The answers coming from the door to your left are as convincing as those from the door to your right. No matter how complicated you make the questions, how demanding of what you take to be intelligence or emotion or social skills or aesthetic appreciation or any other human attribute, you cannot distinguish between the quality of the answers from left and right. You then open the doors: on the left, you see a human being typing the answers into a computer console and, on the right, just a computer producing the answers itself.

The computer has just passed the Turing test. If you regard this test as valid, then you must concede that the computer has all the functions of the human brain— including that of being conscious. (Strictly speaking, Turing introduced his test as one of intelligent behaviour; but the general form of the argument can be, and frequently is, applied to consciousness.)

No computer has yet passed the Turing test. But this has not prevented the notion that a sufficiently sophisticated computer would develop consciousness from gaining wide currency, not only in science fiction, but also among philosophers and scientists, especially those working on 'artificial intelligence'. This field is devoted to making computers as clever as they can get. There are already well-known demonstrations that they can be very clever indeed—clever enough to beat Grand Masters at chess, for example. However, there are convincing theoretical arguments that make it unlikely that, no matter how clever they become, computers will ever develop consciousness.

These arguments turn on the distinction, most familiar in the context of ordinary language, between syntax and semantics: that is, between the rules that govern the ways in which strings of symbols can be put together (syntax) and the meanings to be attached to the strings (semantics). If you have ever learned Latin, you know how to take the stem of a verb and conjugate it (*am-o, am-as, am-at* and so on). You can do this without any idea of what the verb means, or even if the stem doesn't exist at all. That's syntax without semantics. And that, critically, is what computers do: they conjugate strings of symbols without any knowledge of the meanings of the strings.

In most computers, the strings take the form of a series of interconnecting switches, each of which at any one time can be either open or closed. The two possible positions of the switches can be regarded as *0*s (closed) and *1*s (open), and so the positions of a series of switches can be used to represent numbers in the binary arithmetic that most children nowadays learn at school. This is the way the computer's 'machine code' works. Higher-order computer languages merely provide ways of manipulating the machine code in a manner less laborious than that required to specify each and every change in switch position. So all that computers do is to transform one set of switch positions into another. The sets of positions are enormously complex and the switching takes place at a very great speed. Nonetheless, that's all there is. The interpretation of the series of switch positions— even at their most basic level as *0*s and *1*s—is carried out, not by the computer, but by the human beings who build, program and use it.

This line of argument may appear to contradict a common way of describing computers, namely, that they are systems for the processing of 'information'. But this is something of a weasel word. In its everyday sense, 'information' is information *about* something, it conveys meaning. But I have just asserted that computers cannot on their own compute meaning. The information they process is interpreted by human beings; for the computer itself, it is *un*interpreted information.

The reason that, nonetheless, it is common to apply the language of information processing to computers is that the word 'information' has a second, technical, sense within the mathematical theory of 'information' or 'communication'. Consider again a series of computer switches in open or closed positions, or their equivalent as a string of 0s and 1s. Let's say the string is just four units long. At each position in the string, there are just two possibilities: 0 or 1. Across all four positions, there are therefore $2^4 = 16$ possibilities. If you have no further knowledge of the switch settings, your total 'uncertainty' is quantified as these 16 possibilities, expressed in 'bits', that is, powers of the base 2. So, here, the uncertainty is 4 bits ($16 = 2^4$). You are given 'information' in the sense of mathematical communication theory to the extent that you are able to reduce this uncertainty. To know all the actual switch settings is to reduce uncertainty completely, so you would gain 4 bits of information. It is in this sense, and this sense only, that computers, properly speaking, transmit information: as switch positions are set, the uncertainty as to what possible strings the settings *might* form is reduced. This, by the way, is exactly the same sense in which a chain of nucleotides constituting a stretch of DNA can be said to transmit information. And, just as DNA is ignorant of the proteins for which it is 'coding', so a computer is ignorant of what its switch settings stand for.

To dramatise the distinction between syntax and semantics, John Searle (in his 1980 paper published in *Behavioral and Brain Sciences*) used an analogy, which has since become famous as the 'Chinese Room'. Again imagine the two doors set up for the Turing test. You feed into each door a series of Chinese words written in Chinese pictograms. Out from behind the doors come their English equivalents, written in normal Latin script. The outputs from the two doors are equally accurate. You then open up the doors. Behind one is a bilingual speaker of Chinese and English who knows what the words in both languages mean; he is performing a normal task of translation. Behind the other is, this time, not a computer but another human being. This person speaks neither Chinese nor English. But he has a look-up table: two long columns with Chinese pictograms on one side and equivalent English words on the other. So he just looks up the pictogram he receives and sends back its English equivalent—without the least understanding of what the words *mean*. Computers are like the second person.

Searle's analogy has led to intense, sometimes ferocious, debate. For my part, I find the argument totally convincing. Conscious experiences are nearly always 'intentional' (Chapter 4). What we perceive is perceived, immediately and automatically, as this or that meaningful entity. In Fig. 10.1, for example, you see either a vase or two profiles facing one another. You cannot see both of these percepts at once; and it is extremely difficult to see the figure as a series of lines that form nothing particular, neither vase nor profiles. Given these assumptions, then, the argument is simple. Conscious experiences are imbued with meaning; computers cannot (without human interpretation) compute meaning; therefore, computers cannot be conscious.

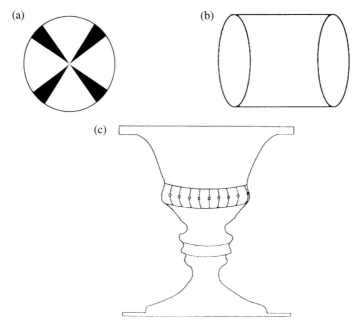

**Fig. 10.1** Kinds of ambiguities: (a) figure-ground switching (or object and space swapping); (b) depth flipping; (c) object changing. From Gregory (1997).

But beware. Whatever the force and clarity of this argument, this has not prevented many eminent thinkers from continuing to believe the opposite: that, with increasing complexity of the processing they perform, the day will come when computers develop consciousness. Our further discussion here, however, will take it as established that this can never happen.

## 10.3   Conscious robots?

Computers are systems for the processing of information, in the technical sense of this word. So, for that matter, are brains. Rather than multiple series of switch positions, the brain employs multiple series of 'spikes' (passages of electochemical currents along and between neurons) to determine which, out of a very large number of possibilities, will be the actual total state of neuronal events at any one time. In the previous section we have seen that a system of this kind is incapable on its own of generating meaning, and therefore incapable of having conscious experience. We can accept this conclusion without contradiction for computers, but clearly not for brains, since we know that brains do have conscious experiences. So what do we need to add to an information-processing system for it to cross the barrier between syntax and semantics?

Computers don't interact directly with their environment (except in the trivial sense of the human environment that programs them and interprets their output). But robots do. Might such interactions be sufficient to endow a robot, made out of silicon chips, tin cans or anything else, with the capacity to interpret in a meaningful way its own informational states?

Let us return to the Chinese room, but this time apply its lessons to a robot rather than a computer. We can readily see the difference between the modes of operation of the two people in the Chinese room, the one doing normal translation, the other using a look-up table. But is this a difference that matters? Maybe, behaviourists might argue, 'meaning' is as fictional a concept as is (for them) consciousness itself.

Suppose all there is to understanding the meaning of a 'stimulus' (whether it be a word, object, faces or anything else) is simply to have a repertoire of behavioural responses appropriate to all the different circumstances in which you might encounter it. Then the difference between the two people in the Chinese room is that the one who understands Chinese and English has a very large and varied behavioural repertoire (depending on environmental circumstances, the sentences in which the words are embedded, and so on) for responding to Chinese words, whereas the other one has a very limited repertoire (that of picking out correspondences between pictograms and words in the same row of the look-up table). On this analysis, they can both give a 'meaning' to a Chinese pictogram, but in the one case it is very broad and in the other, very narrow. Or, to put the same point in the behaviourist manner, neither can truly be said to give a meaning to a Chinese pictogram, because 'meaning' is in both cases a misleading abstraction from the real facts of behavioural dispositions.

Robots differ from computers in that they are endowed with just such behavioural dispositions. The dispositions may be built in at the time the robot is constructed. More interestingly, they can also be acquired by learning, which is the way that human beings acquire most of their behavioural dispositions. So, if this behaviourist analysis of meaning is correct, the language of meaning may perhaps be applied to robotic behaviour as appropriately as to the human kind. This, indeed, is a step we have already taken, when we endorsed Harnad's treatment of the formation of categorical representations (Section 4.5). And, as pointed out there, there is good evidence that artificial neural networks are able to learn and use such representations, if they are provided with a series of possible category exemplars together with feedback as to which are 'correct' or 'incorrect'. There would seem to be no difference in principle between this way of using feedback to train neural networks and the way in which human beings learn to categorise elements in the world with which they interact.

The argument from meaning, used above to defeat the possibility of a 'conscious computer', does not therefore apply to the possibility of a conscious robot. But this represents only a limited step forward. As we have seen, there is good evidence that the computation of meaning is conducted by the *unconscious* brain and that consciousness is not required for that computation to influence behaviour (consider, for example, Groeger's experiment, described in Section 4.4). Thus our discussion so far rules out the syntax-only computer, but not the behaving robot, as a model for the unconscious brain; but it has nothing to say about whether a behaving robot would be conscious or not.

One line of argument which suggests that a behaving robot would not be conscious is the following.

The appropriate set of behavioural responses, to which behaviourists appeal as the true 'meaning of meaning', itself depends upon the way in which the 'stimulus' is perceived. How I respond to the drawing in Fig. 10.1 will differ dramatically depending on whether I see it as a vase or as two facing profiles. This difference does not depend upon changes in the 'stimulus' on the retina, since perceptual shifts of this kind occur even if the pattern of retinal stimulation is kept constant. Nor is this just a classroom trick performed by clever psychologists. Few of us have not at some time or other taken fright at the sight of something that is in fact totally innocuous: a menacing figure lurking behind a tree that suddenly transforms itself into a bush. Interpretation in this way of the 'stimulus' as *this* or *that* is an integral part of virtually all perception. Yet, the allocation of at least some behavioural responses becomes possible only *after* perceptual interpretation is complete (and it changes when interpretation changes). I cannot, for example, talk about the picture in Fig.10.1 as a vase until I have seen it as one. It is these perceptual qualities that lie at the heart of the Hard Problem. If, on at least some occasions, behavioural dispositions have to wait upon the formation of a percept, then the intentional qualities of the percept cannot be explained in terms of these dispositions.

So, while we may grant robots the power to form meaningful categorical representations at a level reached by the unconscious brain and by the behaviour controlled by the unconscious brain, we should remain doubtful whether they are likely to experience conscious percepts. This conclusion should not, however, be over-interpreted. It does not necessarily imply that human beings will *never* be able to build artefacts with conscious experiences. That will depend on how the trick of consciousness is done. If and when we know the trick, it may be possible to duplicate it. But the mere provision of behavioural dispositions is unlikely to be up to the mark.

## 10.4  Functionalism

The most common contemporary approach to the problem of consciousness is generally known as 'functionalism'. Essentially, this is what I have described in the previous section as the 'conscious robot' position: the hypothesis that, if one duplicates in a robot all those functions which, in a human being, are associated with conscious experience, then the robot would also have conscious experiences—no matter what the robot is made of. So dominant is this position in cognitive science, artificial intelligence and philosophy that it is hard to make a contrary voice heard at all. But I have come to the view that functionalism is false. (Notice, by the way, that this is not a comfortable view for me to come to. For my own hypothesis concerning the survival functions of conscious experience, set out in Chapters 7 and 8, is functionalist. I leave till later the search for a way out of the dilemma thus posed.)

My reasons for the conclusion that functionalism is false turn on the results of a particular set of experiments on the phenomenon of 'synaesthesia'. This is a condition in which stimuli presented in one sensory modality give rise to sensations in another. Although synaesthesia may involve many different combinations of senses, one of the most common is 'word–colour synaesthesia' or 'coloured hearing'. In this condition, when the synaesthete hears or sees a word, she sees in addition, in her mind's eye, a colour or multicoloured pattern. I say 'she', by the way, not for reasons of political correctness, but because the great majority of synaesthetes are women. Synaesthetes are in other respects normal. The details of their synaesthetic experience are varied and idiosyncratic. The condition tends strongly to run in families. But, even within a family of, say, coloured hearing synaesthetes, different family members have different specific experiences. So one may respond to the word 'train' with a bluish-green experience and another to the same word with an orange experience, and so on. Synaesthetes almost universally report that they have had their synaesthesia for as long as they can remember. Once they discover that few other people have this kind of experience, they tend not to talk about it to anyone. They fear, with justice, that they will be regarded as queer or crazy. And, indeed, the scientific community has only recently begun to take seriously the reports they give of their experiences.

Before I describe the results of our experiments, let me state the doctrine of functionalism in a form in which it is particularly imperilled by them. As we know, the crux of the 'Hard Problem' of consciousness lies in the phenomena of perception—qualia. Consider, as a specific version of the Hard Problem, this question: how should one explain the difference between two subjective experiences of colour, say of red and green? Functionalism approaches a question of this kind in the following way.

It starts by eliminating from the question the qualia—of red and green—as such. For these, it substitutes as the explicandum the repertoire of responses by which the experiencing individual demonstrates, *behaviourally*, the capacity to discriminate between red and green. This repertoire would include, e.g. pointing to a red (green) colour when requested to do so, using the word 'red' ('green') appropriately in relation to the colours red and green, stopping (going) at red (green) traffic lights, stating that a lime is green and a tomato, red, and so on. Next, functionalism seeks an understanding of the mechanisms by which these behavioural 'functions' are discharged. This understanding may be sought at a 'black-box' level, as in the box-and-arrow diagrams familiar in cognitive psychology, neural networks, computer simulations and so on; or it may be sought in the circuitry of the actual brain systems which connect the inputs to the outputs of each of the discriminating behavioural functions. A full 'function' for a given difference between qualia then consists in a detailed account of the corresponding differences in inputs, in outputs, and in the mechanisms that mediate between input and output. As a shorthand, I shall describe such a full function as taking the form 'input-mechanism-output'. (The argument is essentially unchanged if one interprets full functions in a more sophisticated manner, as including, for example, feedback from output to input or other additional cybernetic machinery.) If a full functional account is given, then, according to functionalism, there is no further answer that can be given to the original question: what is the difference between the subjective experiences (the qualia) of red and green? To continue asking this question in the face of a complete functionalist account would, so the doctrine holds, be a meaningless activity. For, according to functionalism, qualia just *are* the functions (input-mechanism-output) by which they are supported.

Note that, even though functionalism is willing (at least in some of its forms) to take into account the detailed circuitry of the brain that mediates between input and output as part of the full description of a function, it does so only *as circuitry*. The tissue out of which brain circuits are made (neurons, membranes, synapses and so on) and the means by which the circuits operate (passage of impulses along axons, release of neurotransmitter into the synapse, etc.) are regarded within functionalism as irrelevant. In principle, the functionalist holds, one could mimic the circuitry with any materials to hand, and the result, in terms of either conscious or unconscious processing, would be the same. Same functions, same processes: if the relevant brain process attains consciousness, so would the same function no matter what material was used to carry it out.

From this formulation of functionalism one can draw the following, 'primary', inference: (1) *For any discriminable difference between qualia, there must be an equivalent discriminable difference in function.* There is also a 'complementary' inference: (2) *For any discriminable functional difference, there must be a discriminable differenced between qualia.* Clearly, there are ways in which this second, complementary inference may be false. There are many forms of behaviour which are not accompanied by qualia at all. So, for example, the pupils of one's eyes constrict if illumination increases and dilate if it decreases; but one is not normally aware of either of these changes in pupil size. However, in the case of a behavioural domain which *is* normally accompanied by qualia, whenever functionalism draws the primary inference, it should also draw the complementary one.

Let us apply these inferences again to the example of red and green. The primary inference is that (within the domain of colour vision), if someone claims to have different red and green experiences, then there must be different functions (input–mechanism–output) to support this claim. The complementary inference would be that (within the domain of colour vision), if someone manifests different functions, then there must be different qualia accompanying them. The two inferences together constitute a claim for identity between qualia and functions within the domain of colour vision. Functionalism at its strongest generalises this identity claim across all qualia within each domain and all domains of conscious experience.

There is a related but nonetheless separate strand of functionalist thought. This treats the functions that give rise to qualia as providing benefit to the behaving organism. This strand is particularly evident in discussions of the evolution of qualia. The claim here is that evolution works by selection of behavioural functions that contribute (in the usual way) to Darwinian survival, and thus by selection of the neural mechanisms which mediate those functions. The evolution of qualia themselves, on this view, occurs only parasitically by linkage to such functions. From this view one can draw a further inference. (3) *One would not expect to find qualia which adversely compete with the functions to which they are linked.*

A final word about functionalism is this: functionalism is proposed in two different flavours (I say 'flavours' rather than 'forms', since the nuances are often quite subtle). In one flavour, qualia are reduced to so little beyond the functions with which they are linked as to be virtually eliminated. This is more or less Dan Dennett's position in his book *Consciousness Explained*. In the other, the separate existence of qualia is explicitly acknowledged, but all empirical data are treated as requiring explanation in terms only of the functions with which they are linked. So, as we have seen, Stevan Harnad argues that qualia are epiphenomena: they are caused by functions and their underlying mechanisms, but have no causal effects of their own. In either flavour, qualia are left with no substantive properties of their own.

## 10.5   Experiments on synaesthesia

At the Institute of Psychiatry in London, we have been using neuroimaging techniques to study word–colour synaesthetes. Our data appear to contradict what I called above 'the complementary inference', and also to demonstrate qualia with behavioural effects that are adverse to the functions with which they are linked (contrary to inferences 2 and 3, above). This evidence constitutes a serious challenge to functionalism in both its flavours. I shall therefore describe the experiments here in some detail.

The starting point for any study of synaesthesia lies in the synaesthete's own report of her experience. However, if the arguments advanced here are to hold, it must be the case that the report is veridical, in two senses. First, the report must be more than mere confabulation—there must be *something* that is separate from the report and is reliably reported. Second, the reported experience must be *perceptual*. Otherwise, we could not base arguments about qualia upon it.

Over the last decade evidence has accumulated to support these assumptions.

First, Simon Baron-Cohen, Laura Goldstein and their colleagues in London demonstrated the reliability of reports of word–colour synaesthesia. Their subjects gave essentially identical reports of their colour experiences in response to a list of words at a year's interval, with no prior warning that they would be retested at that time. In a group of non-synaesthetes retested over a period of just a month, the similarity of reported word–colour associations was strikingly inferior.

Second, the perceptual nature of the synaesthetic experience has been well-documented in experiments by 'Rama' Ramachandran and Ed Hubbard in San Diego. I give here just one example of their findings. This depends on the phenomenon known as 'visual pop-out'. It is characteristic of visual perception that items in a display with a feature that differs from other 'background' items 'pop out' from the background—that is to say, they are seen automatically and involuntarily as being different, and they are grouped together as being separate, from the background. Exploiting this feature of perception, Ramachandran and Hubbard presented subjects with a black-against-white display of 2s and 5s, computer-generated so that the latter were mirror images of the former. The 2s were disposed among the background 5s so as to form a triangle (Plate 10.1). Non-synaesthetes found it hard to detect the triangle. In contrast, number-colour synaesthetes, for whom 2s and 5s gave rise to different colour sensations (e.g. red and green), at once saw the triangle, which stood out in one colour against a background of a different colour. It is virtually impossible to account for this and similar phenomena except by giving credit to the synaesthetes' own reports: that they have a perceptual experience of colours when they see black and white number displays just as they do when they inspect coloured surfaces.

This evidence from Ramachandran's perception experiments is supported by our neuroimaging data. For this work we (Julia Nunn and other colleagues) used the technique of functional magnetic resonance imaging (fMRI). When a particular brain region is active, it uses up oxygen. This is then replenished by an increase in the supply of oxygen delivered to the region via the blood supply. Using fMRI it is possible to distinguish between signals from oxygenated and deoxygenated haemoglobin (the carrier of oxygen in the blood), and so to detect brain regions that are particularly active at a particular time. Functional MRI is usually done by subtraction. That is, you measure activation in your experimental condition of interest, e.g. listening to words, and in a control condition, and you subtract the latter from the former. The results of this subtraction give you the pattern of activation that is specific to the experimental condition of interest.

We used this method to detect brain regions activated by simply hearing spoken words. In our study, the control condition consisted of a series of tones. So, the subjects listened to alternating blocks of words and tones, each block lasting 30 seconds. In non-synaesthete controls, as you would expect, the activation caused by spoken words occurred in the auditory cortex and language areas, as it did also in a group of coloured-hearing synaesthetes. However, the synaesthetes (but not the non-synaesthetes) showed an additional area of activation in the visual system. The location of this activation coincided perfectly with the area that is selectively activated by colour (Plate 2.1). This area—known as V4 or sometimes V8—is determined in fMRI by subtraction of the activation patterns produced by monochrome patterns from those produced by coloured versions of the same patterns. The patterns most often used are called 'Mondrians', since they resemble the abstract paintings of the artist, Piet Mondrian (Plate 7.2). Coloured, but not black-and-white, Mondrians activate V4. So, just as one would expect from the synaesthetes' own reports, the same region is activated in their brain by heard words, as is activated by seen colours (Plate 10.2). These findings, like those in Ramachandran and Hubbard's experiments, support the hypothesis that synaes-thetic colour experiences are truly perceptual in nature. The synaesthetic experi-ence, then, at least in the cases of word- or number-colour synaesthesia, is reliable, veridically reported and perceptual.

The colour experiences of synaesthetes, in addition, provide a particularly uncluttered example of the general truth (Chapter 2) that perceptual experiences are constructed by the brain, and are only (at best) indirectly related to the states of affairs in the 'real world' that cause them to be constructed. The perceptual experiences of colour, in word–colour synaesthetes, are reliably, automatically and involuntarily triggered by *spoken words*. Thus they bear *no* relationship to the wave-length properties of light reflected from surfaces which normally provide the exter-nal basis for experienced colour. This leaves no room for doubt that synaesthetic colours are constructs of the brain, nor any room for interpretation within a 'naïve' or 'direct' perceptual realist framework. For such an interpretation even to get off the ground, there has to be at least a resemblance between the state of affairs in the external world that gives rise to the percept and the percept itself (though this begs the question of what could possibly be meant by 'resemblance' in this context). Clearly, no such resemblance exists when a synaesthete reacts, say, to the heard word 'train' with a greenish-blue experience. When qualia of this kind are experienced, therefore, they cannot be construed as direct perception of *any* state of affairs in the real world.

These experiments demonstrate yet again, by the way, that the 'privacy' of conscious experience offers no barrier to good science. Synaesthetes claim a form of experience that is, from the point of view of most people, idiosyncratic in the extreme. Yet it can be successfully brought into the laboratory.

## 10.6    Function vs tissue

Section 10.4 presented a formulation of functionalism without contrasting it to any alternative approach to qualia. In the context of our experiments on synaesthesia, the most relevant contrast is with what I shall call, for want of a better word, the 'tissue' approach. (The term 'physicalism' is also used in this sense.) The 'want of a better word' reflects the fact that this alternative to functionalism has been articulated far less clearly than functionalism itself. Indeed, it is not clear that it has ever been fully articulated at all.

As we have seen, functionalism more or less inevitably leads to the conclusion that, if a system displays behaviour of a kind that, in us, is associated with conscious experience, then the components out of which the system is made are irrelevant (as one among many examples, see Igor Aleksander's book, *How to Build a Mind*). The contrary, tissue, view, however, holds that there is something special about the physical components from which brains are made that provides a necessary condition for consciousness to arise. This view (which we consider in its own right later) may stress the physics of these components, as in Hameroff and Penrose's quantum gravitational theory of consciousness (see Chapter 16), or their biology, as in Koch and Crick's search for genes underlying the evolution of the neural correlates of behaviour. Views of this kind are sometimes explicitly proposed as superior to functionalism, as by Hameroff and Penrose, but more often it is left unclear whether or not they are compatible with functionalism. Similarly, on the functionalist side, some thinkers (e.g. Harnad) concede the possibility that, for a complete account of consciousness, the actual mechanisms that the brain utilises may be a crucial addition to its functions, whereas others scorn the whole idea as relying upon 'wonder tissue', in Dennett's caustic phrase.

Despite its relative lack of conceptual articulation, I shall here use as the contrast to functionalism, the tissue approach. This choice is dictated by a useful parallel that the contrast offers to the two most plausible accounts of synaesthesia. These hold that synaesthesia is based upon either (1) early and strong associative learning, or (2) an unusual form of 'hard wiring' in the synaesthete brain. The parallel recognises equivalences between, on the one hand, associative learning and functionalism and, on the other, hard wiring and the tissue approach.

Recall that synaesthetes generally report that they have had their synaesthesia for as far back as they can remember. They do not normally report any specific learning experience that might have led to their associating a particular word with a particular colour. However, such learning may have taken place at a sufficiently early age to fall into the period of infantile amnesia. Thus, one possible explanation for synaesthesia is that the individuals concerned formed exceptionally strong and enduring associations between words and colours at an early age. This is the associative learning account of synaesthesia. Since the general process of associative learning offers no problems for functionalism, neither does a specific associative learning account of synaesthesia.

The alternative, hard-wiring, account is that the synaesthete brain has abnormal projections that link one part of the brain (the sensory system in which the inducing stimulus is processed) to another (the sensory system in which the synaesthetic percept is experienced). So, in the instance of word–colour synaesthesia, there would be a projection, not existing in the non-synaesthete brain (nor even in the brains of individuals with other types of synaesthesia), from the parts of the brain which process heard and/or seen words to the colour-selective regions of the visual system. This abnormal projection might arise because the synaesthete has a genetic mutation which promotes its growth. Alternatively, a genetic mutation might prevent the extra projection from being 'pruned' during early development, a time at which the brain normally shows an abundance of connections that are no longer present in the adult brain. The likelihood of a genetic basis for synaesthesia is strengthened by the fact that there is a strong tendency for the condition to run in families, and especially in the female line.

There is at present no way directly to test the hard-wiring hypothesis (though recent developments in MRI are bringing this prospect closer), since this would require anatomical investigation of the brain. What we have tried to do, therefore, is to test the associative learning hypothesis. To do this, we performed two experiments.

In the first experiment, we trained non-synaesthetes on a series of word–colour associations and then tested them with fMRI to see whether their pattern of activity in response to spoken words had come to resemble the pattern spontaneously displayed by synaesthetes (as shown in Plate 10.2). We made strenuous efforts to ensure that the subjects had formed strong associations between the words and the colours. First, we gave them extensive over-training outside the MRI scanner. We were concerned that, nonetheless, the contextual shift from the training environment to the scanner would weaken these associations. We therefore retrained the subjects once they were in the scanner. Finally, since the synaesthete experience is perceptual, we asked our subjects to 'imagine' the colour associated with each word, and also included as a comparison a condition in which they were asked only to 'predict' the colour. We anticipated that, if the associative learning hypothesis of synaesthesia is correct, then these non-synaesthete subjects should show, particularly in the 'imagine' condition, at least some activation in the V4 region where the synaesthetes showed activation in response to spoken words

In all, four sets of activation patterns to words were gathered from these non-synesthete subjects. Two were gathered prior to retraining: 'pre-predict' (with instructions to predict the associated colors) and 'pre-imagine' (with instructions to imagine them). Two further sets were gathered after retraining in the scanner: 'post-predict' and 'post-imagine'. No activation was seen in any of these conditions in the V4 region activated by words in the coloured hearing synaesthetes. These negative results did not represent any general failure of activation, as might happen for example if the subjects simply did not attend to the stimuli, since there was clear activation in the auditory cortex and regions of the brain concerned with language, such as Broca's area, presumably reflecting the active processing of heard words.

This experiment on word–colour associations in non-synaesthetes weakens the possibility that synaesthetic colour experiences result from normal associative learning. If that were so, the non-synaesthetes given over-training on word–colour associations and listening to the words in the scanner should have shown at least some activation in the V4 region.

Conceivably, however, synaesthetes differ from non-synaesthetes in the *nature* of their associative learning process. Perhaps, in them, this is unusually strong. If so, one might more easily train synaesthetes than non-synaesthetes on an association which is not spontaneously present in the synaesthetes.

To test this possibility, in our second experiment we used training methods similar to those used in the first, but for word–colour associations we substituted melody–colour associations. Neither our synaesthete nor our control subjects had any pre-existing colour associations to the melodies. These were chosen from classical works, by Chopin or Mozart for example. We trained both word–colour synaesthetes and non-synaesthetes before testing them as before in the MRI scanner; and we again retrained them in the scanner. If synaesthetes have generally strong associative learning processes, then they (but not the controls) would be expected to show, after training, responses to melodies in the same V4 region activated by words in these subjects. However, the results showed no significant differences in activation patterns between the synaesthetes and controls; and in neither case was there significant activation in the V4 region. There was again clear activation in the auditory system, so the lack of activation in the visual system could not be attributed to a failure to attend to the stimuli. Thus these results lend no support to the hypothesis that synaesthetes might show particularly effective associative learning. In addition, they clearly distinguish between the brain activation patterns elicited by the kind of sensory association that the synaesthetes spontaneously report (word–colour) and the kind they deny (music–colour).

## 10.7   Implications of synaesthesia for functionalism

It is always difficult to reject a hypothesis on the basis of negative findings alone. Clearly, we cannot rule out the possibility that, despite the considerable effort we put into over-training non-synaesthetes on word–colour associations in the first experiment, or both synaesthetes and non-synaesthetes on melody–colour associations in the second, we were unable to achieve the strength of the early learning which hypothetically underlies word–colour associations in synaesthesia. Perhaps there is something special about the period of early learning which cannot be duplicated in adult subjects. Nonetheless, the complete absence in these experiments of any activation in the colour-selective regions of the visual system, except in the case of spontaneous synaesthete word–colour associations, casts considerable doubt on the hypothesis that the latter are the fruit of normal associative learning.

Given this (albeit weak) conclusion, we are left by default with the hard-wiring hypothesis. This supposes that synaesthetic perceptual experience arises because of 'sparking over' of neural excitation from one pathway (the inducing pathway) to another (the induced pathway) to which the inducing pathway is abnormally connected. In word–colour synaesthesia colours are usually triggered by both auditory and visual presentation of words. The most important feature of the trigger usually lies in the first syllable of the word, whether spoken (when it is called a 'phoneme') or seen on the page (a 'grapheme'). This evidence suggests that the inducing pathway most likely consists in regions in which the auditory and visual representations of phonemes and graphemes are jointly represented. Our fMRI data do not directly throw further light upon the inducing pathway. Nor would they be expected to do so. Recall that the fMRI method depends on the possibility of comparison or subtraction between experimental and control conditions or groups. But the inducing pathway is presumably activated to a similar degree whether words are presented to synaesthetes or non-synaesthetes. So comparison between the activation patterns observed in these two groups of subjects is uninformative.

Our fMRI results do, however, sharpen up hypotheses concerning the likely route from the inducing to the induced pathway. The word–colour synaesthetes in our experiments responded to spoken words by activating the colour-selective region of the visual system *without* activation at any earlier point in the visual pathways, such as V1 or V2 (see Plate 4.1), although these regions *are* activated when subjects are presented with coloured visual stimuli. This pattern of results—similar activation in more central parts of the visual pathway, but V1/V2 more clearly activated by the more 'normal' route of stimulation—has been reported also in studies of colour after-images, motion after-effects and illusory motion (see Plate 13.1 for an example of such an illusion). In contrast, *imagining* colours is *insufficient* to activate either of these regions, V1/V2 or V4. These contrasting patterns of activation are consistent with the common introspection that after-images and after-effects are true visual percepts, whereas merely imagined visual features are not. (You should try this contrast out for yourself. As with many other assertions in this book, careful observation is all you need do your own experimental detective work.)

Overall, then, these results suggest that activation of modules in the visual system specialised for the analysis of particular visual features, such as colour or motion, is both necessary and sufficient (not requiring supplementation by activity in regions earlier in the visual pathway) for the conscious experience of that visual feature. Data tending to the same conclusion have been reported by Dominic ffytche and his colleagues for hallucinatory experiences of colour in certain patients with eye disease, in whom V4 activation again accompanied the illusory experience. From this point of view, then, word–colour synaesthesia can be regarded as an example of illusory experience in which the triggering stimulus (words) occurs with very high frequency, as compared to triggers for other illusions, e.g. colour after-images or motion after-effects, which occur with much lower frequency. In all these cases, however, once the relevant visual module (V4 for colour, V5 for motion) is activated, the illusory experience occurs automatically. These results, then, have strong implications for determining (in Francis Crick's phrase) the 'neural correlate of consciousness'. We deal with this issue in Chapter 13.

A further important aspect of our findings is that we saw activation in the word–colour synaesthetes presented with spoken words in V4 only in the *left* hemisphere. Given the lateralisation of cortical language systems also to the left hemisphere, this left-lateralised activation in synaesthesia may relate to the fact that it is speech sounds rather than sounds in general which elicit the synesthete's colour experiences. Thus the abnormal projection which hypothetically underlies word–colour synaesthesia appears to travel from left-lateralised cortical language systems directly (without involvement of regions lower in the visual system; see above) to left V4.

A final result from our fMRI study of word–colour synaesthetes deserves mention. The data from the Mondrian experiment showed good agreement in the area activated by colour as between synaesthetes and non-synaesthete controls— but only in the *right* hemisphere. In this hemisphere, both groups showed activation of V4. However, left V4 was activated by coloured Mondrians only in non-synaesthetes. Thus, in the synaesthetes, left (but not right) V4 was activated by spoken words and right (but not left) V4 was activated by coloured Mondrians. These data raise the interesting possibility that, in word–colour synaesthesia, the putative abnormal projection from left cortical language systems to left V4 prevents the normal dedication of the latter region (alongside its right-sided homologue) to colour vision.

Taken together, these results and our inferences from them paint the following picture. Word–colour synaesthetes are endowed with an abnormal extra projection from left-lateralised cortical language systems to the colour-selective region (V4) of the visual system, also on the left. Whenever the synaesthete hears or sees a word, this extra projection leads automatically to activation of the colour-selective region. Activation of this region is sufficient to cause a conscious colour experience. The exact nature of that experience presumably depends upon the particular set of V4 neurons activated. Importantly, there is *no* evidence that the experienced colour plays any functional role in the synaesthete's auditory or visual processing of words. (In the next section, indeed, we consider evidence that the experienced colour may actively interfere with such processing.) *Thus, there is no relationship between the occurrence of the synaesthete's colour experiences and the linguistic function that triggers them.* This conclusion is incompatible with the functionalist analysis of conscious experience.

## 10.8 The alien colour effect

The data reviewed in the previous section tend strongly to the conclusion that word–colour synaesthesia is based upon an abnormal, probably genetically determined, projection hard-wired into the brain. Conversely, these data lend no support to the hypothesis that this condition results from any special form of associative learning. This section describes additional experimental data which further weaken the associative learning hypothesis. These data come from a study of a sub-group of word–colour synaesthetes who experience what I have termed the 'alien colour effect', or ACE for short. In this phenomenon, the names of colours induce a colour experience that is different from the colour named. So, for example, the word 'red' might give rise to the experience of green, 'blue' to the experience of pink, and so on. For a given synaesthete, the ACE may affect all, some or just a few colour names.

As is the case for synaesthesia in general, the ACE appears to have been present for as long as the synaesthete can remember, that is, back to early childhood. Now, consider the opportunities for associative learning that this situation provides. A young child with the ACE would frequently encounter circumstances in which someone makes a statement of the kind: 'see the red bus coming round the corner'. From statements such as these, the child has normal opportunities to learn the visual colour to which the word 'red' applies. Synaesthetes do indeed learn colour names normally: as adults they show normal colour perception and normal colour naming. Yet, in the example given above, as well as seeing a red bus come round the corner just after being told about the bus, the child with ACE would also experience a different colour, e.g. green, upon hearing the word 'red'. Thus she must frequently encounter opportunities for associative learning provided by chains of events such as: the word 'red' followed by an experience of green and then the sight of a red bus. If the first part of this chain, the word 'red' followed by a green experience, were due to associative learning in the first place, one would expect it to be unlearnt by these further associative learning opportunities. This, certainly, is what happens in countless experiments on so-called reversal learning with both animal and human subjects. Thus, the existence of the ACE is incompatible with the associative learning account of word–colour synaesthesia.

Given the scope of the conclusions we seek to draw from these phenomena for functionalism, it is important to validate the ACE experimentally. To do so, we modelled our approach on the 'Stroop interference effect', encountered in the previous chapter (Section 9.3). This is demonstrated most easily in experiments in which the subject merely has to name, as quickly as possible, the colour of the 'ink' in which a series of letters is displayed. (It used to be real ink, but the experiment is now normally done using a computer; nonetheless, everyone continues to call it the ink colour.) In a control condition, the letters are a simple row of Xs. The critical experimental condition is one in which the names of colours (e.g. the word 'red') are displayed in ink of an incongruent colour (e.g. green). The subject has to disregard the colour name 'red' and answer 'green', since this is the colour of the ink. The speed of naming the ink colour in which incongruent colour names are written is reliably slower than the speed of naming the ink colour for a row of Xs.

This is the 'Stroop effect'. It is thought to arise because of the difficulty the subject has in ignoring the colour name when attempting to retrieve the name of the ink colour.

We reasoned that something similar should happen in subjects with the ACE even when they are asked to name just the row of Xs. Suppose this row is printed in red ink. The subject retrieves the name 'red' preparatory to uttering it. But, in a subject with the ACE, the name 'red' gives rise to an experience of green (or pink, or stripy orange and blue—it doesn't matter). The green experience gives rise to a tendency to utter, instead of 'red', the word 'green'. This should interfere with the utterance 'red' and so slow down colour naming. We anticipated, however, that this might be a small effect, so we also tested our subjects in a full Stroop paradigm.

We first assessed a group of colour-word synaesthetes for the degree to which they displayed the ACE (as the percentage of colour names which caused 'alien' colour experiences). On the basis of these scores subjects were assigned to one of three groups: with 0–35%, 35–70% and 70–100% ACE. We also tested a group of non-synaesthete controls. We measured speed of colour naming in a conventional Stroop test, using Xs as the control condition and incongruent colour words (ink colour different from colour name) as the Stroop condition. The results (Fig. 10.2)

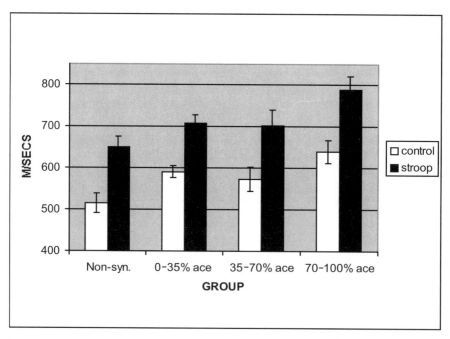

**Fig. 10.2** Mean reaction times and standard errors for naming the 'ink' colour of rows of Xs (control condition) or of incongruent colour names (Stroop condition) in groups of coloured hearing synaesthetes with varying percentage of the alien colour effect (ACE). Non-syn: non-synaesthete group. From Gray *et al.* (2002).

were very clear. As the degree to which the ACE occurs increased, so colour naming was slowed.

These results confirm the reality of the self-reported ACE, showing once again that such reports are a reliable source of information in synaesthesia. The greater the percentage ACE reported, the slower was colour naming. This effect, furthermore, was observed as clearly in the control condition, in which the subject had only to name the ink colour in which four Xs were presented, as in the Stroop condition. The additional conflict between ink colour and colour name inherent in the latter condition was not required to bring out the effect of the ACE upon the speed of colour naming. Indeed, the Stroop effect, as such, was unaffected by the ACE. This pattern of results presumably indicates that, in subjects with the ACE, the basic process of retrieving the name of the ink colour is sufficient (because the name leads automatically to the experience of a different colour) to slow down colour naming. Quantitatively, the degree of this ACE-induced slowing (if one compares full ACE colour naming speed to that of the non-synaesthetes; Fig. 10.2) was about the same as the size of the Stroop effect itself. Note that the interference caused in colour naming by the ACE must precede the subject's overt utterance of the colour name. We may therefore infer from this pattern of results that the degree of interference in colour naming caused by the percept of an incongruent colour is as great when this is induced by subvocal retrieval of the colour name as when it is perceived by the normal visual route.

The reality of the ACE, demonstrated in this experiment, casts further doubt on the possibility that word–colour synaesthesia could be the result of any associative learning process. Every time a colour name occurs in association with the perception of the colour named, and also in conjunction with the alien colour experience triggered by the name, as presumably occurred in the experiment reported here, there is an opportunity for normal associative learning processes to reverse the aberrant association that putatively underlies the ACE. Yet the ACE persists unchanged from childhood to adulthood. It is extremely unlikely therefore that the ACE is established as the result of an initial stage of normal associative learning. By extension, it is also unlikely that word–colour synaesthesia in general rests upon such an associative basis.

## Conclusions

Overall, the results of these experiments, together with their various strands of supporting data and argument, give rise to the following conclusions.

1. Word–colour synaesthesia does not result from aberrant associative learning.
2. Word–colour synaesthesia is most likely due to an extra, abnormal, left-lateralised projection from cortical language systems to the colour-selective region (V4) of the visual system.

3. On this analysis, excitation in synaesthetes by heard or seen words of cortical language systems 'sparks over' to activation of the colour-selective region of the visual system.

4. Activation of the colour-selective region of the visual system is sufficient to lead, automatically and involuntarily, to the conscious experience of colour, with the specifics of the colour experience depending upon the particular pattern of neuronal firing caused in V4 by the sparking over.

5. The occurrence of the synaesthetic colour experience in word–colour synaesthesia plays no functional role in relation either to speech or language perception or to colour vision. An intriguing gloss on this conclusion is provided by Ramachandran and Hubbard's description of a grapheme-colour synaesthete with a form of colour blindness, who "claimed to see numbers in colours that he could never see in the real world ('Martian colours')". Such 'Martian' colours imply that, if a pattern of V4 neuronal firing induced in synaesthesia differs from any caused via the normal visual pathway, it can nonetheless give rise to a colour experience specific to the pattern *per se* and not to any visually linked functional relationships.

6. The occurrence of the synaesthetic colour experience in the alien colour effect has behaviourally *dys*functional effects (as shown by the slowed naming of colours).

These conclusions are incompatible with a functionalist account of word–colour synaesthesia. This condition provides a clear counter-example to what I called above the 'complementary inference' from functionalism: namely, that, for any discriminable functional difference, there must be a corresponding discriminable difference between qualia. Within the behaviour of any given word–colour synaesthete there is a clear functional separation between the seeing of a colour presented via the normal visual channel, on the one hand, and the perception of that same colour triggered by a word. Yet, apparently, neither the qualia nor their neural bases (as tested in our fMRI experiments) produced by these two functional routes differ. It is, of course, difficult to affirm a lack of difference in qualia with any certainty. However, to examine this issue, we have worked with a small number of word–colour synaesthetes with sufficient artistic talent to depict their colour experiences in response to specific words (see cover illustration). We are currently applying fMRI to these subjects to determine just how closely the activation patterns elicited in V4 by a given word and its corresponding picture resemble one another. This is a difficult experiment that may lie beyond the technical limitations of current neuroimaging techniques. But we hope that it will provide a route by which to test objectively this key assumption in the argument: that, in word– colour synaesthesia, similarity or even perhaps identity of qualia can occur despite disparate functional routes underlying them.

There is an apparent escape hatch for functionalism in our finding that, in coloured hearing synaesthetes, left V4 is devoted to synaesthetic colours and right

V4 to visually detected colours. The sensitivity of fMRI does not allow us to assert that this observation represents complete lateralised separation between the two functions. But, given that the different lateralisations were observed in the same subjects within a single scanning session, they cannot be dismissed as artefact. Thus one might try to salvage the functionalist account of coloured hearing synaesthesia by asserting that the two functions (elicited by spoken words or seen colours) do not in fact share qualia, since one is associated with qualia generated in left V4 and the other, with qualia generated in right V4. However, this line of defence takes as axiomatic what ought to be an empirical hypothesis: namely, that different neural processing produces different qualia. Yet subjectively, to the synaesthete, both are experienced as colour. Indeed, one may also interpret the different lateralisation of colour produced visually and synaesthetically as providing an even stronger counter-example to functionalism. For there is considerable evidence that activity in V4 in either hemisphere is sufficient for the experience of colour. Thus an opponent of functionalism might argue that, in coloured hearing synaesthetes, colour experiences are produced by two routes which differ in *all* critical respects: input, output and the site (left or right hemisphere) of the strongest neural correlate of the consciousness of colour.

It may appear that, in adopting this joint line of attack upon functionalism, I am trying to have my cake and eat it too. The argument needs, therefore, to be spelt out carefully. There are three terms that have to be put together in any understanding of the relations between qualia (Q), functions (F) and brain processes (B). The complementary inference drawn from functionalism states that, if F1 differs from F2, then (provided that F1 and F2 belong to a domain of processing associated with qualia) F1 must be associated with Q1 and F2 with Q2, such that Q1 differs from Q2. As noted earlier, in most version of functionalism functions are specified in terms of abstract processes alone (the box-and-arrow diagrams of cognitive psychology being a familiar example); however, in others they are specified in terms of actual neural processes in the brain. In the latter case, F1 is mediated by B1 and F2 by B2. Assuming a case (like that of word–colour synaesthesia) in which Q1 and Q2 are the same even though F1 and F2 differ, we can therefore envisage two possibilities: (1) that B1 and B2 do not differ, or (2) that they do. Both of these patterns of results run counter to the complementary inference and therefore to functionalism. However, they differ in that the first alternative places the fault line in functionalism between functions, on the one hand, and qualia-plus-brain processes on the other; whereas the second places the fault line between functions-plus-brain processes, on the one hand, and qualia on the other. We anticipated the former outcome to our experiments. The latter, which is the result observed, is equally inimical to functionalism but perhaps inimical to physicalism (the tissue approach) too, in that qualia appear to be stripped by it of any necessary connection to *either* specific functions *or* specific brain processes.

Our findings also run counter to functionalist expectation in a second respect. Harnad (in his paper on 'Turing indistinguishability') has argued that qualia can be selected in biological evolution only in virtue of the fact that they are epiphenomenally linked to functions that have survival value. It is difficult to see, on this basis, how the ACE could ever arise. The understanding of language, in audition and vision, clearly has survival value, as does colour vision. One can also see that a neural linkage between language systems and colour vision could provide survival value, for example, by facilitating the naming of colours. But no natural account emerges along these lines of why this neural linkage should give rise to the perception of colours triggered by words in word–colour synaesthesia. Such an arrangement is at best functionally neutral. Still less does this functionalist account offer any explanation of how the alien colour effect, which is (as we have seen) actively dysfunctional, could have arisen during evolution. Functionalism supposes that qualia are fully dependent upon the functions with which they are associated. If that is so, it should be impossible for qualia *to compete negatively with those very same functions*. Yet, in the case of the alien colour effect, that is just what they appear to do.

There will perhaps be a temptation to dismiss these findings on the basis that they depend upon 'illusory' perception. I have myself, above, drawn a parallel between word–colour synaesthesia and other illusory experiences of colour and motion. In particular, these all appear to rest upon the same neural foundation (discussed more fully in Chapter 13), namely, activation of that part of the visual system which is responsible for the analysis of the specific visual feature concerned (colour, motion), without activation in earlier parts of the visual pathways. However, to dismiss our findings on this basis would be to misunderstand how normal vision works. In a very real sense, this too is illusory. Thus, for example, in the particular case of concern to us here, that of colour vision, it is universally agreed that colours, as such, are not properties of the objects that we perceive as being coloured (see Chapter 7). The basis that such objects provide for the brain's construction of colours lies in the light reflectances of their surfaces as a function of the wavelengths of light that fall upon them. There is no known relationship (other than correlational) between these reflectances, whether measured on the surfaces themselves or as computed by the brain, and the qualia by which they emerge into conscious perception. The phenomenon of word–colour synaesthesia therefore provides an empirical basis upon which to ask an ancient philosophical question: why should not colour qualia have been used normally, as they are used unusually by word–colour synaesthetes, to model in consciousness auditory inputs (words) rather than visual inputs (reflectances)?

This question, of course, takes us to the heart of the Hard Problem of conscious experience. Until we can go beyond correlation to mechanism in understanding how qualia come to be allocated to function, that problem will remain. The considerations advanced in this chapter render it less likely that the allocation of qualia in word–colour synaesthesia is determined solely or even at all by function as such. And, given that functionalism purports to provide a completely general account of how conscious experiences relate to brain activity, even one such counter-instance, if it can be firmly established, should be sufficient to overthrow it. The consequences that would flow from such an overthrow might be dramatic. Pretty well every contemporary account of consciousness is functionalist in both concept and detail. That tally includes my own theory, as sketched out in Chapters 7 and 8, so creating a conceptual tension that will hover around the rest of the book (for a resolution, see Section 20.3).

It is, of course, too soon to come to such a dramatic conclusion. The data base is extraordinarily slim. Indeed, to the best of my knowledge, ours are the first studies that have explicitly sought to put functionalism to the test of experiment. Nonetheless, it is not too soon to ask this question: if functionalism were to be overthrown, what might take its place? The answer is far from clear. We next need to look at some possibilities.

# CHAPTER 11

# From Cartesian theatre to global workspace

One swallow doesn't make a summer and one experiment doesn't overthrow a theory, especially one as entrenched as functionalism. But the price of this entrenchment has been high. Leaving aside purely philosophical argument, the fundamental postulates of functionalism have never been put to proper scrutiny. However, the experiments on synaesthesia, described in the previous chapter, brought these postulates at last into the laboratory. At the very least, our results must cast doubt on their viability. So we need to cast around for possible alternatives to functionalism.

Our starting point remains the brain, as the only physical underpinning to consciousness known for certain. But, as pointed out in the previous chapter, the brain can be considered in many ways. To recapitulate, it is (1) a system which (2) interacts with an environment and (3) is made up of physicochemical components; these components are (4) biological cells, more specifically (5) neural cells. The approaches we considered in the previous chapter regarded the brain only under aspects (1) and/or (2). In the next few chapters we look at approaches based upon the remaining aspects.

We leave until Chapter 16 an approach that takes the physics of the brain seriously—so seriously, in fact, that it places governance of the making of qualia among the fundamental laws of physics. Curiously, I am aware of no theory that takes biology equally seriously. There has been no attempt to explain consciousness by properties attaching to biological cells generally, including those *outside* the nervous sytem. Thus, here we consider only nerve cells—the brain as studied by neuroscientists. How do these scientists conceive of the problem of consciousness?

It is actually rather difficult to answer this question. Until the late 1980s it was rare for neuroscientists to discuss the problem of consciousness at all. The two great exceptions to this rule, Charles Sherrington and John Eccles, were both extremely eminent, as though only they dared break a strong taboo. However, their transgressions did little to encourage others, as the dualism they both espoused was, and still is, badly out of scientific and philosophical fashion. This was compounded in Eccles' case by his giving a role in brain function to the Holy Ghost. The dam broke more widely in 1987, with the publication of *Mindwaves*, a volume edited by two Oxford neuroscientists, Colin Blakemore and Susan Greenfield. Even today, however, neuroscientists are normally reluctant to espouse general positions concerning consciousness. Pressed on the topic, they tend to deny that there is any special problem of consciousness, or to align themselves with the functionalism described in the previous chapter. One looks in vain for any statement of a position that would give to brain tissue *per se* the kind of overarching role in conscious experience that functionalism gives to functions. So Dennett's fears of 'wonder tissue' are—at least until the physicists get into the act in Chapter 16—groundless.

The chief preoccupations of the neuroscientists have been, at bottom, correlational. A general pattern has been the following. A neuroscientist first proposes that certain functions are critical for consciousness. But, in doing so, he bases his specific postulates upon data and concepts taken, not from neuroscience itself, but from experimental psychology, cognitive science or just plain 'folk psychology'. He then searches in the brain for those regions and systems that 'mediate' the critical functions. Since no specifically neuroscientific argument is used to justify the initial postulate, this approach adds nothing theoretically to its functionalist starting point. The same essential logic can also proceed in reverse. A neuroscientist first observes experimentally that a particular brain region or system discharges a particular function; he considers the function to be one which, in normal human experience, is associated with consciousness; so, he concludes, this region or system plays an important role in consciousness. But, in whichever direction the logic proceeds, the validity of the conclusion is entirely dependent upon the assumption that a particular *function* is critical for, or critically dependent upon, conscious experience. All the neuroscientist adds is a location in the brain (human or animal) where the putatively critical function is discharged. *Location, location, location* may be the right slogan for selling a shop, but it throws little light on the problem of consciousness.

The neuroscientific trail then, at least as at present trodden, leads at best to a three-way set of correlations: between functions, brain regions or systems that mediate the functions, and conscious experiences. Let's explore this terrain in a little more detail.

## 11.1  Is there a Cartesian theatre?

The first question is whether one can in fact locate consciousness, or any of its features, in one part of the brain at all. There is a vocal claim, especially from Dan Dennett and Marcel Kinsbourne, that consciousness is an attribute of the activity of the whole brain. Indeed, they lampoon the contrary view—that some activities in the brain bear a more privileged relation to conscious experience than others—as the search for a 'Cartesian Theatre'.

As originally formulated by Descartes, there are indeed strong reasons to reject this concept. For Descartes, when the material brain has done its materialist job, it enters into two-way communication with a quite different, non-material stuff, the *res cogitans* (or psyche or soul or spirit—there are many synonyms). He thought the locus for this communication lay in the pineal gland, better known today for its role in controlling the hormone, melatonin. So it made sense to speak of brain activities 'entering' consciousness (*res cogitans*) in a particular place (the Cartesian Theatre) and at a particular time. Eccles retained this dualist notion, merely moving the Theatre from the pineal gland to the cells of the cerebral cortex and replacing Descartes' 'animal spirits' by modern neurophysiology. No-one has ever produced a satisfactory account of how two such very different stuffs—material and psychic—can interact, whether in the pineal or anywhere else. Attempts to do so pose seemingly insurmountable problems for the unified theory of the universe sought by physics. Thus dualism is today almost entirely abandoned. However, the demise of dualism does not entail demise of the hypothesis that some parts of the brain stand in a closer relation to conscious experience than do others. Despite Dennett's lampooning, I shall continue for a while to call this the 'Cartesian Theatre' hypothesis—but stripped of its dualist overtones.

The metaphor of the Cartesian Theatre is intuitively very natural. It permeates the thinking of all of us, including scientists who would be mortally offended to be told they are dualists. Take vision. It is natural to think in terms of non-conscious goings-on in the retina (stimulated, shall we say, by light reflected from a rose) and the optic nerve that carries signals from the retina to the visual cortex; natural, also, to speak of other non-conscious goings-on that carry signals from the motor cortex to the arms and hands with the consequence that the rose is picked. Somewhere in between these inputs and outputs the image of the rose appears to 'enter consciousness'. In our discussions of colour vision and coloured-hearing synaesthesia (Chapters 7 and 10), we saw reasons to locate the conscious perception of the colour of the rose in an area called V4 (Plate 4.1). Given that we perceive the rose, not just as a patch of colour, but also as having shape, a position in three-dimensional space, a scent, etc., there may be better reasons to locate the conscious perception of the rose-as-a-whole somewhere else, further down the line from V4. (This is the 'binding' problem, to which we return later.) But *somewhere*, surely, the non-conscious input must be transformed into this conscious percept, and this must take place at *some time* in the chain of events leading from light-reflected-from-rose-on-retina to the picking of the rose. Visual scientists not only speak like this all the time, but write their papers that way too. The main difference (*res cogitans* apart) from Descartes is that, whereas he had a definite idea as to where (the pineal gland) and therefore when this 'entry into consciousness' takes place, today we know that we don't know.

But, according to Dennett and Kinsbourne, the whole metaphor of the Cartesian Theatre is disastrously wrong. Most mercilessly lampooned are the audience (who's there to watch?) and curtain-up time (the entry into consciousness). The standard charge in regard to the audience is that of infinite regress. If the theatre of consciousness needs to be watched by a homunculus inside the brain, does the homunculus have a still smaller homunculus to help him do his watching? We deal with this issue in a more general manner later. First we need to take on the issue of time: does it make any sense to speak of material 'entering consciousness' at a precise moment in time?

Dennett and Kinsbourne argue persuasively that such talk makes no sense at all. Here are some of the points they make. But note that these take on a somewhat different significance within the perspective we adopted as early as Chapter 2. Two relevant aspects of that perspective are, first, that the brain does not receive direct percepts of the world 'out there', but rather constructs that world; and, second, that 'consciousness comes too late'—all conscious experiences lag behind both the events to which they correspond and the immediate, non-conscious responses to which these give rise. However, let us first look at Dennett's arguments from the common-sense point of view (which he too is keen to reject, but in favour of a different replacement): that events take place just as they seem to do to conscious experience. Within that framework, certain paradoxes arise.

A good example is based on apparent motion or 'phi', described by Max Wertheimer in 1912. In the simplest case, phi refers to the fact that, if two or more small spots separated by a small distance are each briefly lit up in succession, then you perceive just one spot moving between the positions of the two. Phi is now so familiar that it is the basis of countless neon sign advertisements, not to mention motion pictures. Dennett (in his book, *Consciousness Explained*) concentrates upon a variant of phi, demonstrated in 1976 by Kolers and von Grünau, in which the two spots are each of a different colour. A red spot flashes briefly on the left side of the display and shortly afterwards (the distances and intervals, of course, have to be appropriately adjusted) a green spot flashes briefly on the right. What you see is a single spot which travels from left to right, changing colour from red to green half way through its trajectory. (Type 'colourphi' into Google and you will find several illustrations; I liked *http://www.mdx.ac.uk/www/ai/rss/phi/ColourPhi.html*.) How can it be understood within a common-sense framework? This supposes that, first, the red spot on the left of the display enters consciousness and then, a little later (about 200 milliseconds later in Kolers' experiment), it is followed into conscious experience by the green spot on the right.

Here is Dennett (*loc. cit.*, p. 115) on the ensuing paradox:

> Unless there is 'precognition' in the brain (an extravagant hypothesis we will postpone indefinitely), the illusory content, *red-switching-to-green-in-midcourse*, cannot be created until *after* some identification of the second, green spot occurs in the brain. But if the second spot is already 'in conscious experience', wouldn't it be too late to interpose the illusory content between the conscious experience of the red spot and the conscious experience of the green spot? How does the brain accomplish this sleight of hand?

Dennett's answer to this question is that there is no sleight of hand—because there are no conscious experiences, of red spot, green spot, spots moving and changing colour, or anything else. Out must go the Cartesian Theatre, the audience for which the show is staged, and the very show itself. In their place Dennett proposes a model termed 'Multiple Drafts'. The notion is that as inputs arrive in the brain it strives to make the best sense possible of them and changes its 'draft' inter-pretations with each new development, revising or abandoning the old drafts as required in the light of the new information. So the interpretation 'red spot on the left' is eventually replaced by 'red spot on the left moving to the right and changing colour to green'. The final draft leads to behavioural output, e.g. a verbal report to the effect 'I saw a red spot change colour to green in midcourse as it moved from left to right'. But there is no independent event of consciously seeing this multicoloured trajectory. In Dennett's words (p. 128):

> ...retrospectively the brain creates the content (the judgment) that there was intervening motion, and this content is then available to govern activity and leave its mark on memory.

But the brain does not, according to Dennett bother to fill in the qualia:

> ...that would be a waste of time and (shall we say?) *paint*. The judgment is already in, so the brain can get on with other tasks!

To my mind, this is just a way (the functionalist way) of dodging the issue. It is that very conscious experience, to which Dennett denies independent existence, that we seek to understand. (This full-bodied denial is actually quite hard to pin on Dennett. He explicitly refuses (p. 459) to answer the question: *'What, in the end, do you say conscious experiences are?'* But the only reasonable interpretation I can place on what he writes is that he throws the qualic baby out with the bath-water.)

There are two inferences, one temporal and one spatial, that, without prejudice to the reality of qualia, one might draw from these data and arguments.

The first, temporal, inference is that, on a sufficiently fine-grained temporal scale, it is impossible to allocate a precise time to a conscious experience. Consider the difference, in the Kolers and von Grünau experimental set-up, between presenting the subject with just a red spot on the left of the display, and present-ing a red spot on the left followed 200 milliseconds later by a green spot to the right. Does the conscious experience of the red spot on its own in the first case have a time of occurrence that is 200 milliseconds earlier than the experience of the same spot when (a fact that cannot be known by the subject until after the event) it is followed by a green spot on the other side of the display? But how could this occur? If a precise time is allocated to the conscious experience of the red spot on its own (taking account only of the relatively fixed delay between retinal impact and feature extraction higher up the visual system), then it is hard to quarrel with Dennett's conclusion that the brain would need powers of precognition to delay the experience only on those occasions when the green spot follows. So a precise time cannot be allocated to the experience of the red spot. And, since there is nothing unusual about red spots, this conclusion must apply to all visual percepts.

Just in case you thought that this is a problem only for vision, Dennett (p. 143) draws attention to an equally compelling tactile illusion. This is the 'cutaneous rabbit', described by Frank Geldard and Carl Sherrick in 1972:

> The subject's arm rests cushioned on a table, and mechanical tappers are placed at two or three locations along the arm, up to a foot apart. A series of taps in rhythm are delivered by the tappers, e.g. five at the wrist followed by two near the elbow and then three more on the upper arm. The taps are delivered with interstimulus intervals between 50 and 200 msec. So a train of taps might last less than a second, or as much as two or three seconds. The astonishing effect is that the taps seem to the subject to travel in regular sequence over equidistant points up the arm—as if a little animal were hopping along the arm.

On 'catch' trials just the five taps on the wrist are delivered, without the rest. The subject now perceives all the taps as occurring on the wrist—there is no incipient movement up the arm. The implications of this experiment for touch are exactly the same as those of colour-change phi for vision. Without the added but unwelcome ingredient of precognition, there can be no allocation of a precise time to the conscious perception of the taps on the wrist. We may reasonably, therefore, conclude that it is impossible in general, in any sensory modality, to allocate precise times of occurrence to conscious experiences. Later in the chapter I shall try to show that one can accept this inference while nonetheless not obscuring the reality of conscious experience.

The second, spatial, inference is one that Dennett draws from the first. Essentially, the argument is as follows. Since the neural activity related to *the experience of* (Dennett would say, to *the judgement that there is*) a red spot or a tap on the wrist is constantly on the move throughout the brain, then, if there is no precision in the time of occurrence of the conscious experience, there can also be no specific place in the brain where it takes place. I shall question this inference in a moment. But first let us see how Dennett pursues his argument. Here is part of his description (p. 134) of the Multiple Drafts model as applied to vision.

> Visual stimuli evoke trains of events in the cortex that gradually yield discriminations of greater and greater specificity. At different times and different places, various 'decisions' or 'judgments' are made; more literally, parts of the brain are caused to go into states that discriminate different features, e.g. first mere onset of stimulus, then location, then shape, later color (in a different pathway), later still (apparent) motion, and eventually object recognition. These localized discriminative states transmit effects to other places, contributing to further discriminations, and so forth. The natural but naïve question to ask is: Where does it all come together? The answer is: Nowhere. Some of these distributed contentful states soon die out, leaving no further traces. Others do leave traces, on subsequent verbal reports of experience and memory, on 'semantic readiness' and other activities of perceptual set, on emotional state, behavioral proclivities, and so forth. Some of these effects—for instance, influences on subsequent verbal reports—are at least symptomatic of consciousness. But there is no one place in the brain through which all these causal trains must pass in order to

deposit their content 'in consciousness'. As soon as any such discrimination has been accomplished, it becomes available for eliciting some behavior, for instance a button-push (or a smile, or a comment).

## 11.2   An egalitarian brain?

The Multiple Drafts model is splendidly egalitarian. It is egalitarian, first, with regard to location: all brain regions are equal. The only differences allowed are quantitative and evanescent. An intense 'discriminative state' has bigger behavioural effects, a less intense one has smaller effects. Intense states are capable of influencing verbal report, which is 'at least symptomatic' of consciousness. (A useful word, 'symptomatic', for one unsure whether or not there is a real disease of consciousness in the head.) Placed in a context that assumes there are indeed real conscious experiences, this model would relate these to whatever assemblage of neurons placed into temporary alliance are firing together more intensely than any another at a given time. This 'moment of fame' (another of Dennett's captivating phrases) for that assemblage then lasts only so long as it remains the strongest focus of activity around. But what that fame buys for the assemblage, in Dennett's own context, is not qualia, but the capacity to affect behaviour more dramatically, more widely and (via memory) for longer periods. It is difficult to get away from the impression that, at heart, Dennett is as much a Radical Behaviourist as Howard Rachlin. It is Howard, you will recall (Chapter 10), who sees the difference between a hearing and a deaf person sharing a room with a Mozart string quartet as consisting in their later 'verbal behaviour'.

The Multiple Drafts model is equally egalitarian when it comes to behaviour. It completely ignores all the fine distinctions I (and many others before) have drawn between behaviour which is or is not accompanied by conscious experience, or which occurs before or after the accompanying experience, or which is sometimes but sometimes not accompanied by conscious experience. A 'button-push' (which we saw in Chapter 2 is almost certain to occur before any relevant conscious experience), results in Dennett's view from exactly the same set of processes as the subsequent verbal report which is 'at least symptomatic' of consciousness.

It is on this (erroneous) basis that Dennett is able to dismiss a possible explanation of changing-colour phi.

Might this phenomenon arise, he asks (p. 122) 'because there is *always* a delay of at least 200 msec in consciousness?' 'No' he replies…

…suppose we ask subjects to press a button 'as soon as you experience a red spot'. We would find little or no difference in response time to a red spot alone versus a red spot followed 200 msec later by a green spot (in which case the subjects report color-switching apparent motion). There is abundant evidence that responses under conscious control, while slower than such responses as reflex blinks, occur with close to the minimum latencies (delays) that are physically possible. After subtracting the demonstrable travel times for incoming and outgoing pulse trains, and the response preparation time, there is not enough time in 'central processing' in which to hide a 200 msec delay. So the button-pressing response would have to have been initiated before the discrimination of the second stimulus, the green spot.

QED. There is no question that Dennett's concluding sentence in this passage is correct. In fact, the button-pressing response would be initiated before the subject became conscious even of the *first, red spot*. As we saw in Chapter 2, and as Max Velmans has exhaustively reviewed, that is what happens whenever a subject is asked to make a manual response as fast as possible: consciousness of the stimulus comes too late to affect the response. So this thought experiment, which could easily be carried out in practice and would surely produce just the results that Dennett anticipates, just doesn't speak to the issue of the subject's conscious awareness of *either* the red *or* the green spot.

Despite Dennett's critique, then, it remains possible that one might account for colour-changing phi in terms of the general lateness of conscious experience. For this to be possible, however, we would need much more information than is currently available about the actual temporal course of the formation of conscious experience. How variable, and over what limits, is its lateness? What triggers the beginning, duration and end of a given conscious 'moment'? Within such a moment, do the components retain any temporal order at all, or are they all necessarily simultaneous? Answering these questions will not be easy. But they do not seem to be in principle immune to empirical study. Depending on the answers they receive, one can envisage an account of colour-changing phi in which the different conscious experiences depend upon, e.g. the time at which an integrated conscious 'moment' is triggered, and the duration over which it extends. At the moment this is no more than an exercise in hand-waving. But it is preferable to the solution counselled by Dennett: that of giving up altogether on the notion that conscious experience has a reality independent of behaviour.

There is in any case an alternative possible account of colour phi, but one which will perhaps appear incoherent until Chapter 13. There we consider evidence that the necessary and sufficient neural conditions (the 'neural correlate of conscious-ness') for the conscious perception of a visual feature (motion, colour, form, etc.) lie in activity in just and only that region of the brain which is specialised for the feature: V4 for colour, V5 for motion and so on. This inference is consistent with the results of our studies of coloured hearing synaesethetes, which you will recall (Chapter 10) showed that experiences of colour evoked by spoken words were associated with activity in the visual system restricted to the colour-selective region, V4. This evidence from neuroimaging studies is complemented by purely behavioural (or 'psychophysical') experiments from Zeki's laboratory (reviewed in his article in 2003 in *Trends in Cognitive Sciences*). These have demonstrated a strik-ing asynchrony in the time it takes for different visual features to achieve conscious perception. In particular, colour is perceived some 80 milliseconds before motion.

Armed with this knowledge, I have just re-inspected the demonstration of colour phi at *http://www.mdx.ac.uk/www/ai/rss/phi/ColourPhi.html*. What I see is not (as the customary description of the phenomenon would have it) a single spot that *changes colour as it moves*, but rather a spot that changes its colour and a *separate sensation of movement*: I never see a colour change in mid-trajectory. This percept is consistent with the neuroimaging and psychophysical evidence briefly sketched above. But, of course, that very consistency may well have biased my introspection. It is precisely for that reason that the great introspectionist schools that dominated psychology at the end of the nineteenth century collapsed in spectacular disarray. Nonetheless, taken together with the experimental evidence upon which the arguments in this book are largely based (but which the introspectionist schools of psychology scorned), a tenable account of colour phi begins to emerge. The brain first creates the conscious perception of colour and colour change in the spot; some 80 milliseconds later it creates the conscious perception of motion of the spot. These two percepts sit (at least in my experience—try it for yourself!) side-by-side.

Let us continue our scrutiny of the Multiple Drafts model. Mary Phillips, Andy Young and I have extended this scrutiny to the laboratory. We used the technique of functional magnetic resonance imaging (fMRI; see Chapter 10) to ask the question: how does brain activity differ between consciously and unconsciously made discriminations? The Multiple Drafts model, as well as rather similar ideas proposed by Susan Greenfield in her book *The Private Life of the Brain*, leads to the following prediction: the brain activity that accompanies the conscious discrimination should be the *same in kind* as the activity that accompanies a corresponding unconscious discrimination, only *more so*. This prediction captures two features of the Multiple Drafts model. First, there should be no Cartesian Theatre, so no new region should 'light up' in fMRI just because the subject becomes conscious of something. Let's call this the 'no Cartesian Theatre' hypothesis. This is the *same in kind* part of the prediction. Second, the Multiple Drafts model attributes behaviour 'symptomatic of consciousness' to more intense patterns of brain activity. Greenfield uses the analogy of a pebble thrown into a pool of water. Small pebbles produce small ripples, big pebbles big ripples. Entry into consciousness is the privilege of the currently biggest pattern of ripples in the pool. I shall call this the 'biggest kid on the block' hypothesis. It leads to the *more so* part of the prediction.

To test these predictions we took advantage of two previous findings.

First, the brain discriminates clearly between facial expressions depicting the emotions of fear and disgust (Fig. 11.1). The experiment is very simple. The subject (inside the MRI scanner) merely observes a series of faces of different identities (over a 30-second block of time) all expressing the same emotion. In one condition, blocks of faces bearing a fearful expression alternate with blocks with neutral expressions. Subtraction of the 'neutral' pattern of brain activity from the 'fearful' one gives you the pattern that is specific to fear. Similarly, from blocks of disgusted expressions that alternate with neutral ones you can extract the pattern

(a) 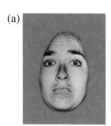 (b)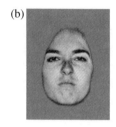

**Fig. 11.1** Facial expressions of fear (a) and disgust (b), after Ekman and Friesen (1976), shown by Phillips *et al.* (1997) to activate different brain regions (see Fig. 11.2).

of activity specific to disgust. When this experiment is done, it turns out that two quite different regions are activated by fearful and disgusted facial expression, respectively. Fearful expressions activate a region called the amygdala; disgusted expressions, a region called the insula (Figs 11.2 and 18.6). There is, conversely, no activation in the amygdala in response to disgust, nor any in the insula in response to fear. There is other evidence of a variety of kinds which strongly suggests that these two regions do not merely participate in the detection of particular kinds of facial expression, but take a much more general role in the emotions with which each is associated. It has been repeatedly demonstrated, for example, that the

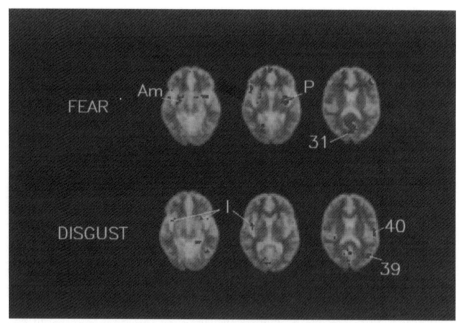

**Fig. 11.2** Different areas activated in fMRI by facial expressions of fear (*upper row*) and disgust (*lower row*) of the kind illustrated in Fig. 11.1. The right side of the image corresponds to the left hemisphere of the brain. Am: amygdala. P: putamen. I: insula (see Fig. 18.5). 31, 39, 40: Brodmann areas so numbered. Unpublished data from our laboratory confirming results initially reported in Phillips *et al.* (1997).

amygdala plays a critical role in mediating the response to a cue (e.g. a light or a tone) that an animal such as a rat has learnt to associate with a painful shock to the feet. There is little reason to doubt that such a cue causes in the rat an emotion of fear just as it would do in a human being. As to the insula, Maike Heining has shown in our laboratory that disgusting smells and sounds activate it in the same way as facial expressions of disgust.

The second previous finding was that one can present facial expressions like those illustrated in Fig. 11.1 in such a manner that the subject has no conscious awareness of the face but nonetheless shows an appropriate emotional reaction. The main trick is that the facial expression (the 'target') is presented for a very short time, typically about 30 milliseconds, and is immediately followed by a visual mask, that is, a display which prevents conscious perception of the target. Ulf Dimberg, in Stockholm, has successfully applied this technique in a number of experiments. In one, for example, he made use of the fact that, when people see a facial expression of emotion, they spontaneously and unconsciously mimic it. By measuring changes in the activity of the facial muscles, he showed that, even though his subjects were at chance in naming the emotional expression on a masked target face, their own faces mimicked the masked expression.

People, therefore, can discriminate between facial expressions of emotion unconsciously as well as consciously. This gave us the opportunity to test the 'Cartesian Theatre' predictions. If the Multiple Drafts model is correct, then presenting subjects with masked expressions of fear and disgust should activate the same regions as presentations of unmasked expressions—the amygdala for fear, the insula for disgust—but to a lesser degree. We therefore used fMRI to compare four conditions. In all of them, a mask (a face bearing a neutral expression) followed the target face; but it only actually served as a mask in two of them. The four conditions differed according to the nature and the duration of the target face: these were either fearful or disgusted, and either presented for a long enough time for easy conscious perception (170 milliseconds) or for so short a time (30 milliseconds) that conscious detection was at chance. The results of this experiment are presented in Fig. 11.3. They show, first, the expected activation by consciously perceived targets of the amygdala for fearful expressions and the insula for disgusted expressions. But, second, there was *no* activation of these regions when the masked targets were presented. Clearly, this on its own might show merely that our masked targets were totally without effect, either on behaviour (we were unable in these experiments to measure behaviour in the scanner) or on brain activity; or, at any rate, that our apparatus was insufficiently sensitive to detect any such activity. However, both masked targets clearly activated *other* brain regions. Furthermore, the activated regions differed between masked fear and masked disgust (see Fig. 11.3). So the brain not only reacted to these masked faces but discriminated between them.

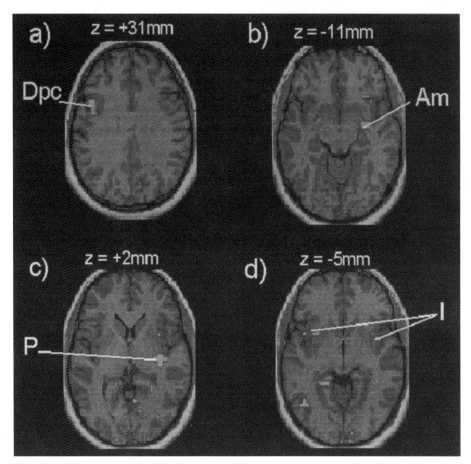

**Fig. 11.3** Different areas activated in fMRI by facial expressions of fear (a, b) or disgust (c, d) when these were presented below (a, c) or above (b, d) the threshold of conscious recognition. The emotional expressions were presented for 30 (a, c) or 170 (b, d) milliseconds, followed immediately in both cases by a 100-millisecond face bearing a neutral expression. The right side of the image corresponds to the left hemisphere of the brain. Am: amygdala. I: insula. Dpc: dorsolateral prefrontal cortex. P: putamen. Reprinted from *NeuroImage*, Phillips *et al.*, copyright (in press), with permission from Elsevier.

This pattern of results is at variance with the predictions from the 'biggest kid on the block' hypothesis. But neither does it offer any support for the Cartesian Theatre model. If that were correct, we should have seen an additional area of activation, common to both the fearful and the disgusted expressions, light up in the condition in which these expressions were consciously perceived, but not in the masked condition. We saw no such area. However, these results call for qualification. We have not yet demonstrated, for example, that the discrimination by the brain of the masked target faces is truly a discrimination between emotions (as distinct, say, from one between the patterns of lines that make up the different emotional expressions). For this inference, we have relied upon other work, such as Dimberg's on facial mimicry. There are also contrary reports in the literature, in which it is claimed that the amygdala *is* activated by unconsciously detected fear stimuli. We have fully replicated our findings and we believe that our experiments were better conducted—but we would say that, wouldn't we? And, even if our findings are correct, they may not apply outside the domain of emotional expression that we have investigated. An elegant experiment conducted by Moutoussis and Zeki, for example, used fMRI to compare brain activity when subjects discriminated behaviourally between faces and houses that they could see consciously or which had been masked. They found activity in the same regions in both cases, but more so during the conscious discrimination—just as the 'biggest kid on the block' predicts.

Nonetheless, if we put together these results with arguments deployed earlier in the book, I believe we can rule out at least the strong egalitarian form of the Multiple Drafts model or Susan Greenfield's equivalent hypothesis. It is not the case that, when it comes to consciousness, all brain tissue and brain systems are equal. It would be remarkable indeed if the difference between action (not normally accompanied by consciousness) and fully-fledged perception (invariably so accompanied) were not paralleled by differences in how the brain systems that mediate action and perception, respectively, relate to conscious experience. And it is unlikely to be the case that the difference between brain activity that (in some sense yet to be determined) achieves consciousness and that which does not is quantitative only. Suppose one could measure activity in the brains of Venus and Serena Williams as they battle it out at Wimbledon. It would be surprising if the most intense activity in their brains were not in the action systems controlling the limbs that put them in the right place on the court and drive their rackets. But it is just this type of brain activity of which one is not normally (perhaps ever) conscious. However, to reject the 'biggest kid on the block' postulate of the Multiple Draft model does not require us to revert to Cartesian dualism, or even to the Cartesian Theatre. Indeed, as noted above, our results were incompatible with either model.

## 11.3    Executive functions

Having exorcised both Cartesian dualism (too much psyche) and Multiple Drafts (too little), let's move on to consider attempts to localise at least some aspects of conscious experience to particular regions of the brain. These attempts fall broadly into two categories, which however are not necessarily mutually exclusive and, indeed, sometimes blend into one another. One starts from the belief that so-called 'executive' functions play a critical role in conscious experience; the other, from perception, and especially vision (because vision has been the most intensively studied part of perception). The approach from executive functions is considered in this and the next chapter; we come to 'visual awareness' in Chapter 13.

We first consider, in this and the next chapter, the hypothesis that conscious experience bears a particularly close relationship to those brain systems which mediate executive functions. This term refers, broadly, to systems which manipulate information as distinct from representing that information directly. Systems of this kind were inferred initially from the results of behavioural experiments. Powerful new neuroimaging techniques are now gradually localising them to specific regions of the human brain, but for the most part they still retain a largely hypothetical status. 'Working memory', for example, is a system which selects a particular piece of information that, unaided, would rapidly decay from short-term memory and maintains it in an active state by recursive rehearsal. A common situation requiring working memory is when you are told a novel telephone number that you will need to dial in a few minutes time. One way of maintaining the number in memory is to repeat it aloud to yourself over and over again. Another, more common way is to carry out this same rehearsal routine, but subvocally—'in your head'. Working memory refers to the system that manages this rehearsal process. It enters into a huge array of normal human activities. Mental arithmetic, as another example, often requires you to carry in your memory an intermediate step in a multi-staged operation, such as long division. Another postulated executive process, Tim Shallice's 'supervisory attentional system', is somewhat similar in concept, but concerned with selecting one among a set of potentially conflicting *action* programmes and maintaining it in an active state. 'Action' in this context includes the production of speech or the pursuit of an internal train of thought. Thus this system, too, would be expected to play a role in many forms of human activity.

We need not go into further detail regarding these executive functions or the systems that mediate them, since hypotheses allocating to them a critical role in consciousness share critical common features, as do the arguments against them.

Throughout this book I have stressed perception as the locus of the Hard Problem of consciousness. If there were no qualia, there would be no such problem. For that reason, most of our discussion has centred on cases in which qualia are especially salient: in the perception of the public 'real' world 'out there'. In contrast, the executive function approach to consciousness generally takes its examples from those more private regions of consciousness in which we think, imagine, do mental arithmetic, solve problems, and so on. (See Chapter 1, where this distinction between the public and private spaces of consciousness is first made.) Activities such as these do not require direct, ongoing interaction with the public world.

Now, the more private regions of consciousness also involve qualia—that is what it means to call them conscious. Take the example, paradigmatic for working memory, of remembering for a period of time a novel telephone number. One way of remembering the number is simply to do so. You tell me the number, I go away and do something else without further awareness of the number, later on you ask me for it, and *lo!* I tell you. The other way is for the number to keep coming back

to my mind every few seconds over the intervening period of time, either spontaneously or because I adopt the strategy of deliberately repeating it to myself subvocally. The difference which makes the second way 'conscious' is that I hear the
telephone number 'in my head' in much the same (but not identical) way as if I
spoke it aloud. The number comes, so to speak, clothed in phonetic qualia. So the
problem of qualia is posed in these private regions of consciousness just as it is in
the more public places. All the same questions arise: how does the brain create
qualia, why does it need to do so, what differences to information processing do
qualia make, and so on?

Just as qualia are present in both the public and the private spaces of conscious
experience, so are executive functions present in both. But, reversing the case for
qualia, these appear more salient in the private spaces. Suppose, for example, that
you are lying on the grass gazing at the sunset. That simple act of perception of the
public world starkly poses the Hard Problem: whence the conscious visual appearance of the sunset? But there seems to be little if anything in the way of executive
function, no mental operations to be managed. You just sit there and look. Such
simple, qualia-dominated moments are harder to find when one is not in direct
interaction with the world out there. Purely internal qualia are evanescent or
require just that special rehearsal of working memory to prevent them from
becoming so. The exceptions to this rule (marching pink elephants, say, after years
of excessive alcohol abuse or a dose of LSD) have the smack of the pathological
about them.

It is perhaps for reasons like these that emphases upon the private spaces of
consciousness, and upon executive functions as their dominant characteristic, tend
to go hand in hand. The resulting models of consciousness may be taken in two
ways, weak and strong. The weak version accepts simply that executive functions
are applicable to the management of the contents of consciousness. One may
indeed rehearse a telephone number clothed in conscious qualia. Therefore, however the brain creates the contents of conscious experience, it must do so in a way
that allows them to be manipulated by executive functions. The strong version is
to treat one or other executive function as critical to the very process that brings
the contents of consciousness into being.

The strong version of the executive function approach to consciousness can, I
think, be weakened, perhaps even discounted, by way of a double dissociation. The
first side of the dissociation is that executive function can occur without its being
applied to conscious experience. Thus, as noted above, one may hold a telephone
number in one's memory without conscious rehearsal. Indeed, if we could not
unconsciously select one among other possible unconscious items to hold in short-
term memory, or one among other possible actions to unconsciously perform, it is
doubtful that we could survive in a fast-moving world. The flip side of the dissociation is that one may have conscious experiences in which executive functions
play little or no apparent role—witness gazing at sunsets. Still more telling is the

automatic nature of much conscious experience. Not only does it not appear to arise from manipulation by executive function, it is strongly resistant to such manipulation. Take, for example, 'coloured hearing' synaesthesia, explored in detail in Chapter 10. The colours experienced by the synaesthete when she hears words come unbidden and unstoppable.

The weak version of the executive function approach looks much more promising. It seems constitutive of conscious experiences that they are *available* to be manipulated by executive functions. At the very least, we can speak about them; indeed, in our human species, such reportability is the best empirical test we have of the very occurrence of conscious experience. We can therefore also think about them, by talking to ourselves. We can deliberately strive to bring conscious experiences to memory, imagine them, rehearse them etc. We can also choose to respond to them in a wide range of different ways. Having sipped a mouthful of vintage wine I can drink some more, put the wine away because I don't drink in the middle of the day, hand the bottle to a guest, declare the wine to be French, or just enjoy the taste. So we may conclude—along with pretty well everyone who has ever written on the subject—that conscious experiences are not only available to executive functions, but supremely available, and probably to any and all such functions.

## 11.4   The global workspace

This general view has led to the concept that consciousness provides a 'global workspace' (Bernard Baars' term), underpinned by a 'global neuronal workspace' (Jean-Pierre Changeux and Stanislas Dehaene). This very influential idea has a number of important aspects. But take care, as you read on, lest the words 'global workspace' (borrowed as they are from the language of digital computing) lull you into the false sense that we have moved beyond the mysteries of consciousness into something easier to comprehend. For the most part, the term 'global workspace' acts as a simple place-holder for 'consciousness'. Sadly, a mere change of vocabulary doesn't make problems go away.

With this caution in mind, the chief characteristics of the global workspace are as follows.

*First*, the *global availability* to executive function of conscious experience contrasts with the 'encapsulation' of unconscious processes. The latter are specialists at doing just one thing well. My eyes may automatically swivel towards a moving stimulus detected unconsciously in peripheral vision; but, if the swivelling fails to bring the stimulus into conscious vision, that system's repertoire of responses is exhausted. A masked fearful face, as in the experiments described earlier in this chapter, may cause in me an incipient feeling of fear and an incipient facial grimace; but it does nothing to help me track the cause of my disquiet. Non-conscious systems of this kind are often called 'modules' that are 'domain-specific' (limited to handling only one kind of information), 'encapsulated' (they don't communicate well with each other or with the general global workspace) and 'automatic' (give them the right trigger and they just do what they are specialised to do). Modules of this kind can turn up in surprising places.

Before I describe one such surprising place, try out the following experiment for yourself. Count the number of 'F's in the following sentence: 'finished files are the result of years of scientific study combined with the experience of years'. How many did you get? You'll find the right answer, and the reason that most people get it wrong, in the footnote[1]. This little experiment is part of the evidence that so-called 'function' words are to some degree isolated from other aspects of language. Words of this kind ('and', 'or', 'but' and so on) serve only a syntactic function but have no additional semantic content. And, as you have perhaps just demonstrated for yourself, it can be remarkably difficult to select function words for conscious processing.

I once had a striking personal demonstration of the encapsulation of function words. I am fluent in French and a skilled touch typist. I was spending a year in Paris lecturing in French. I used to type up my lecture notes in French—except that, when I came to read what I had typed, many of the function words came out in English. So, in a perfectly normal French sentence, the word 'et' would be substituted by its English equivalent 'and'. In my head, I had heard 'et', but my fingers ran off the function routine they were most used to: a, n, d. And I was unaware of what my fingers were doing till I read what I had typed. Worse, even when I realised what was going on, the same thing happened regularly every week.

*Second*, global availability is purchased at the price of a sharp restriction—a *bottleneck*—on the range of processing to which consciousness can simultaneously be deployed. This phenomenon was first emphasised by Donald Broadbent, whose book *Attention and Perception* (1958) started the so-called 'cognitive revolution' (replacing the earlier Behaviourist régime) in psychology. Since then there has been a huge range of experimental demonstrations of the bottleneck. Again, there is a sharp contrast between conscious and unconscious processing.

Suppose you are walking down a crowded city street. The brain does an excellent job of unconsciously and simultaneously controlling your walking, your balance on a slippery pavement, your zig-zag path through the maze of other pedestrians, your noticing from the corner of your eye the movement of passing traffic, your body temperature—and so on and on. All of these processes go on perfectly well at the same time. But try to read a book and at the same time solve a problem in mental arithmetic! So strong is this contrast that a common

---

[1]   There are 6 'F's. If you counted fewer, that is probably because you ignored—didn't perhaps even see—the Fs in the three repetitions of 'of'.

way of experimentally demonstrating that a particular task requires conscious, or 'controlled', processing is to show that it is subject to interference from a simultaneously performed task.

The limits on simultaneous conscious processing are not absolute. The method of 'dual task interference' can be used to pinpoint the type of conscious processing employed in a particular task. Two tasks that both make use of visual mental imagery, for example, show a greater degree of mutual interference than when one uses visual mental imagery and the other, auditory rehearsal. Data of this kind have led Alan Baddeley, who first developed the concept of working memory, to distinguish the auditory rehearsal loop, as used in remembering a telephone number, from a 'visual scratch pad', as used say in imagining a rotating triangle. But, even given this kind of fractionation of the 'global workspace', the limits upon simultaneous conscious processing are sharp compared with the omni-present multiplicity of simultaneous unconscious processes. This distinction is often made, in a further borrowing from computer-speak, by saying that unconscious processing is parallel and conscious processing, serial.

*Third*, the particular form of executive process that is *attention* seems to play an especially critical role in determining the contents of consciousness. Philip Merikle goes so far as to conclude that 'perception with and without awareness, and perception with and without attention, are equivalent ways of describing the same process distinction' (Merikle and Joordens, 1997, p. 219). A nice illustration of what he means is an experiment by Mack and Rock on what they call 'inattentional blindness'. The design of their experiment is illustrated in Fig. 11.4 and described in the legend to the figure. Subjects were required to judge which were longer, the horizontal or vertical arm of the crosses in these visual displays. This is a sufficiently difficult task that they needed to concentrate their attention very hard upon the crosses. In consequence most subjects became effectively blind to words (like 'flake' in Fig. 11.4) also presented clearly and prominently on the displays— they claimed not to have seen them at all. However, as in other cases in which awareness of a visual stimulus is blocked, e.g. by backward masking or after damage to the brain producing 'blindsight' (Chapter 2), other tests showed that the subjects' brains had in fact analysed the words to a relatively high level. So, for example, when asked to complete three initial letters, '*fla*...', with the first word that came to their heads (a 'stem completion' task), subjects came up with the very word, *flake*, that they had just denied seeing.

*Fourth*, for an item to enter into global workspace a *critical duration* appears to be necessary. This is the basis of the backward masking procedure we have now seen at work in several experiments. If a visual target, such as a word, picture or face, is presented for, say, 30 milliseconds and then followed by a mask, it is not consciously perceived; if it is presented for 150 milliseconds and followed by the mask, it is consciously perceived. The function of the mask is not merely to curtail the duration for which the target is displayed. If one presents the target for

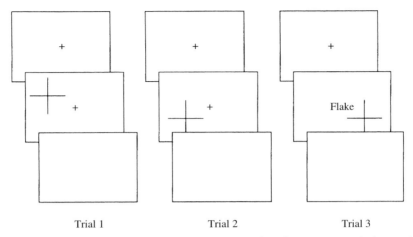

Trial 1                    Trial 2                    Trial 3

**Fig. 11.4** Example of the methodology used by Mack and Rock (1998) to study inattentional blindness (for explanation, see text). On trials 1 and 2, the observers initially viewed a fixation display for 1500 milliseconds (ms). The fixation display was followed by a 200 ms presentation of a display with a large cross in one quadrant, which in turn was followed by a 500 ms presentation of a blank display. Each cross was constructed so that either the vertical arm was longer than the horizontal arm or *vice versa*; and on each trial the observers were required to report whether the horizontal or vertical arm of the cross was longer. Trial 3 was the critical trial in these experiments. On this trial, the sequence of events was the same as had occurred on trials 1 and 2, except that the display with the cross in one quadrant also contained a word located at the centre of the display. Following presentation of this display, the observers first reported whether the horizontal or vertical arm of the cross was longer, and they were then asked whether they saw anything on the screen other than the cross. The surprising finding is that approximately 60% of the participants in these studies were 'blind' to the presentation of the word. When asked whether they had seen anything other than the cross, they indicated that they had noticed nothing other than the cross and that the sequence of events seemed similar to the sequence of events on the two preceding trials. Thus, based on these reports of their conscious experiences, it appears that many of the observers were unaware of the word presented at the centre of the display. From Merikle *et al.* (2001).

30 milliseconds but without the following mask, it *is* consciously perceived. Rather, the mask must also curtail the continued analysis of the target that the brain is otherwise poised to make even after it has disappeared from view. To achieve this, masks are carefully designed to overwrite that analysis with other stimuli that call upon the same type of processing. So, for example, to mask a fearful facial expression in our fMRI experiments we used a different facial expression.

Edmund Rolls and his colleagues at Oxford University have shown this process at work in face-selective neurons in the temporal lobe of the monkey brain (homologous to the region—the fusiform gyrus—in the human brain activated by faces in fMRI experiments). When a face was presented for 50 milliseconds and followed by a mask, the neurons fired for about the same short period of time. But when the same brief stimulus was not followed by a mask, the burst of firing lasted for as long as a third of a second. One may anticipate, therefore, that the brain processes responsible for causing conscious perception must display this capacity for long-lasting, self-sustaining activity after the triggering stimulus has disappeared. An interesting question is whether this is the same capacity that underlies the general role of perception in constructing a model of the relatively enduring features of the world (see Section 8.3).

*Fifth*, conscious processing confers additional potential *flexibility* on behaviour. This is to some extent a restatement of the first point above. The central intuition of the global workspace model is that items in consciousness may affect behaviour in a great variety of ways. In contrast, items susceptible only of unconscious processing remain encapsulated—they are connected to only a limited set of functions especially appropriate to the type of information processed. This general difference has been made concrete in a number of specific experimental tasks in which conscious processing enables greater flexibility of performance.

An example is one of Merikle's experiments on the Stroop effect introduced in Section 9.3. In this version of the task the subject has to name the ink colour (red or green) of a target that is not itself a word. The target is always preceded by a 'prime', which is the word 'red' or 'green'. As we have seen, the basic Stroop effect is that, if the prime is incongruent with the target (the word 'red' followed by a target in green ink), naming the colour is slowed down relative to congruent pairings of prime and target. However, when the probability of an incongruent pairing is made much greater than that of a congruent pairing (e.g. 75% incongruent), then subjects presented with these stimuli in a fully visible manner are able to take advantage of this regularity: they are now faster to name the ink colour when it is preceded by the 'wrong' word. That is, they learn a new strategy for dealing with the task. If the prime is presented masked so that no conscious perception of the word is possible, the basic Stroop effect is still obtained, showing that unconscious analysis is able to detect the difference between the words 'red' and 'green'. However, in this masked condition, subjects are unable to learn and use the rule that on 75% of trials the correct response is the one opposite to the prime word. They continue to respond slower on incongruent trials. Thus conscious awareness of the words confers extra flexibility on performance.

Another example is the 'Jacoby exclusion task'. This again makes use of the backward masking procedure. The duration of the word before it is masked is either 50 milliseconds, too short for conscious perception, or 150 milliseconds allowing conscious perception. The subject is then given the same stem-completion task used in Mack and Rock's experiment (Fig. 11.4), but with a twist. The stem must be completed by any word *other* than the one just presented. So, suppose the presented word was *frigid* and the stem for completion therefore *fri*. It is OK to complete the stem with *fright*, *fringe* or *Friday*, but not with *frigid*. Presented with *frigid* above the threshold of awareness, subjects follow this instruction well. But presented with it below threshold, they not only fail to follow instructions, they complete the stem with *frigid* more often than under control conditions in which there is no word presented at all. So, as in Merikle's Stroop experiment, the brain processes the word unconsciously well enough to know what it is, but (in the absence of conscious awareness) is unable to alter its basic pattern of responding to it. Note that both these examples imply that the extra flexibility that conscious processing confers is that of *inhibiting* a prepotent response to a stimulus in favour of a different one. This is an important aspect of what is normally meant by the voluntary control of behaviour or, in more dramatic language, 'free will'.

*Sixth*, only items in the global workspace are available for report. As in the case of executive functions generally (Section 11.3), one may take this relationship between reportability and the contents of consciousness in a weak or a strong version. The weak version states simply that, for an item to be reportable, it must be consciously perceived. The strong version has been stated by Larry Weiskrantz as follows: 'it is the very achieving of the ability to make a commentary of any particular event that is what gives rise to awareness'. Adoption of this thesis does not necessarily limit consciousness to the only species that has language. To be sure, in the human case, reports are almost always couched in language. However, as we have seen in a number of experiments, it is possible to obtain 'reports' also from animals. Thus Logothetis trained monkeys to press a button to report which of two visual stimuli in binocular rivalry they saw at any given time (see Plate 6.2). So one could adopt the strong version and still look for consciousness in animals. But I know of no reason why the strong version should apply any better to the executive function of commentary than to other executive functions.

*Seventh*, a special relationship is claimed between global availability and *voluntary or intentional behaviour*. Essentially the same relationship is claimed in the archetypal narrative of consciousness, which however we saw in Chapter 2 to be in many situations hopelessly wrong. Nonetheless, the claim contains certain elements of truth. To begin with, once an item is consciously perceived, it potentially becomes the target of a great variety of forms of action; we have considered a number of examples of this kind above. This variety of potential forms of action is one of the hall-marks of voluntary behaviour. The difference between the cases where the claim for a special relationship between consciousness and voluntary behaviour is false and where it is true probably lies in the time scale. Rapid, immediate action is carried out by unconscious processes. But it would be odd indeed to call all such action 'involuntary'. As we saw in Chapter 2, that would mean, for example, that the return of a serve at Wimbledon is an involuntary act. However, for strategic planning of complex and enduring programmes of action, the manipulation in consciousness of its elements seems to be an essential component. By now, however, we should have learned to distrust introspection unless it is backed up by other evidence. And, even in this case, much of the problem solving that goes into complex planning is performed unconsciously. What appears to happen is that the elements that go into the planning, or pose the problem, are contemplated in consciousness; and subsequently the results of the planning or the solution to the problem are re-entered into consciousness. Everything in between takes place unconsciously. Nonetheless, it is likely that the availability of the elements of the plan or problem to the global workspace is in some way critical to the success of the overall planning operation.

A further interesting relationship between conscious awareness and intentional behaviour has been pointed out by Weiskrantz in his discussions of blindsight. This, you will recall, is the condition in which, after damage to the primary visual cortex, the patient is unable consciously to see shapes or objects in the blind part of his visual field, but nonetheless achieves high levels of performance if required to point to the stimulus or 'guess' at some of its attributes. Thus the patient has many residual visual functions. But he never engages *spontaneously* in behaviour that is visually guided towards objects in his blind field. Nick Humphrey, then a student of Weiskrantz's, observed the same lack of spontaneous visually guided behaviour in a monkey with blindsight after damage to primary visual cortex like that which causes this condition in human beings.

## Conclusions

The concept of the global workspace has gained wide currency. But I fear it derives much of its charm by the license it affords to talk, in an apparently acceptable scientific and technical language, about matters that are in fact known largely from common or garden introspection. Perhaps it might have more substance if we could uncover its neural underpinnings (if any). We turn to this task in the next chapter.

# CHAPTER 12

# The global neuronal workspace

In the previous chapter I set out a number of characteristics of a dominant contemporary metaphor for consciousness, the 'global workspace'. To account for these characteristics in neuronal terms, a central hypothesis has been proposed by Bernard Baars at Berkeley, California, in his 1989 book, *A Cognitive Theory of Consciousness*, and by Jean-Pierre Changeux, Stanislas Dehaene and Lionel Naccache in Paris. Here is how the Paris group expresses the hypothesis (Dehaene and Naccache, 2001, p. 13; their italics):

> Besides specialized processors, the architecture of the human brain also comprises *a distributed neural system or 'workspace' with long-distance connectivity that can potentially interconnect multiple specialized brain areas in a coordinated, though variable manner.* Through the workspace, modular systems that do not directly exchange information in an automatic mode can nevertheless gain access to each other's content. The global workspace thus provides a common 'communication protocol' through which a particularly large potential for the combination of multiple input, output, and internal systems becomes available.

We'll come in a moment to consider the specific long-distance connections that the Paris group has in mind. First, however, we need to give some thought to the notion of a 'common communication protocol'.

## 12.1   The common communication protocol

This is a seductive idea. All these specialised modules are talking to themselves in obscure local dialects that no other module understands. But the clever multi-lingual global workspace translates them into English and so can juxtapose and compare what each is saying. Having carved out a more general truth from the hubbub, the workspace then performs a reverse translation and communicates that truth to whichever modules need to know it. The idea is all the more seductive because part of the underlying analogy is again drawn from the familiar digital computer. The modules tick away, each in its own low-level machine code, while the global workspace uses a high-level computer language (like *Java*) that can be translated into all possible machine codes. Or, going straight to the brain, you can think of the modules as using local and highly specific neuronal circuitry to compute body temperature for the thermostat located in the hypothalamus, or time of day so that the clock in the suprachiasmatic nucleus can control diurnal rhythms, and so on. The global workspace, in contrast, is equipped with its postulated long-distance connections, and these make use of much more flexible circuitry able (as we shall see) to go into rapidly changing, dynamic patterns.

So seductive, indeed, are these ideas that they now probably constitute the dominant view in both cognitive and neuroscience of how consciousness works. So I hate to throw a spanner in the works—but I shall.

The aim of the game is to explain consciousness. Indeed, the characteristics of the global workspace are all derived from what consciousness feels like. If this derivation is not direct, then it comes (in an important advance beyond unaided introspection) from experimental demonstrations which themselves depend upon assessment (usually by verbal report) of whether or not the subject of the experiment was aware or not of this or that experimental manoeuvre. This appeal, explicit or implicit, to introspection contributes further to the seductiveness of the notion of a common communication protocol. For that is what normal conscious experience is like. It doesn't matter whether an item of information has come into awareness through vision, audition or any of the other senses, it doesn't matter whether I sense my bodily state via a tenseness in the muscles of my stomach or the dryness of my palms or the feeling of hunger in my palate, it doesn't matter whether my inner thoughts are dominated by words, images or a snatch of music—all of these can co-exist, be juxtaposed, compared and so on momentarily in the medium of my conscious awareness. So the seductiveness of the 'common communication protocol' is well founded: it is a good model for consciousness, because that's just what consciousness feels like. But, at the same time, the concept has been domesticated into plausible, everyday science by the analogy with high-level computer languages; and one can see in principle how the ordinary doings of neurons might provide such a common communication medium.

Here, now, is the spanner. We are hunting for something for consciousness *to do*. Provision of a common communication protocol indeed looks like something that consciousness can do, and do well. But if this job is already being done by a neuronal language, then why do we need consciousness to do it *as well*? This brings us back, of course, to the Hard Problem. But part of my task in this book is, like Ulysses, to tie you to the mast so that you are not too readily tempted by the siren calls of easy ways out of the Problem. So, just as we did for functionalism in general (Chapter 10), we need now to ask of neuroscientific functionalism: does it treat conscious experience as having a reality in its own right? Does it explain how neuronal firings (whether they provide a common communication protocol or anything else) can *create* qualia, or does it merely redescribe qualia in neuroscientific terms? Just to put neuronal firings and conscious experience in correlation with one another, in no matter how sophisticated a manner (and that includes, of course, my own version of functionalist global workspace theory, outlined in Chapters 7 and 8), does not on its own provide a solution to the Hard Problem.

## 12.2   Some neuronal specifics

Now that you are tight bound to the mast, we can sail on. Let's look in more detail at proposals for a *neuronal* global workspace: that is, for the way the brain acts as the global workspace defined functionally in the previous chapter.

We have in fact already considered one of these in Chapter 11, namely, the Multiple Drafts model of Dennett and Kinsbourne and Susan Greenfield's very similar proposal. We rejected that model as being too egalitarian: it failed to take account of the fact that not all brain functions have an equal chance of entering consciousness. Some functions never enter consciousness, some do whenever they occur, and many do only some but not all of the time. The Multiple Drafts model, in effect, deals only with this last case: now you see it, now you don't. Other models, however, chart a mid-course between the egalitarianism of Multiple Drafts and the unique, privileged locus that is the Cartesian Theatre. Unlike the Multiple Drafts model, they accept that only some forms and loci of brain activity achieve consciousness. However, within this set of *potentially* conscious brain activities, they agree with Multiple Drafts in treating conscious awareness as belonging to just that particular activity which, at any given moment, is strong enough to dominate all others. There is in fact a consensus emerging around models of this kind. These models also incorporate a solution to the binding problem forcefully advocated by the German neuroscientist, Wolf Singer. This finds the neural basis of binding in temporal synchrony between the firing of neurons located even in widely separated regions of the brain.

Two particularly influential models are those proposed by Dehaene and his colleagues in Paris, and by Gerald Edelman (Nobel Prize winner for his work in immunology) and Giulio Tononi in their book, *A Universe of Consciousness*. Rather than discuss these or other models separately, I here present a synthesis to illustrate the consensus. ('Consensus', of course, does not mean 'truth', nor does good scientific practice take it even as evidence of truth.) Key features of the consensus are as follows.

The neural underpinning of the global workspace itself is said to lie in long-distance connections between different regions of the cerebral cortex. These cortico-cortical connections are called 'tangential' or 'horizontal'[1] to distinguish them from the ascending and descending connections that each region of the cortex has with subcortical brain regions such as the thalamus; and also from connections internal to each region that provide the local basis for the particular computations carried out there. Almost all the tangential connections are reciprocal, that is, if region X receives from region Y it also sends to that region. The

---

[1]   The terms 'tangential' or 'horizontal' are also often used to refer to connections *within* an area (e.g. connections between orientation columns in visual area V1), not fibres connecting different areas. However, I shall conform here to the usage of Dehaene and Naccache.

neocortex has a distinctive six-layered architecture (Fig. 12.1). The tangential projections mostly originate from the pyramidal cells of layers 2 and 3; and these layers are particularly prominent in regions of the prefrontal and parietal cortex (Figs 12.2 and 15.1). The regions linked by tangential projections manage between

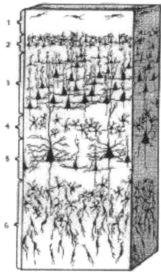

**Fig. 12.1** The neurons of the cerebral cortex are arranged in distinctive layers. From Kandel *et al.* (2000).

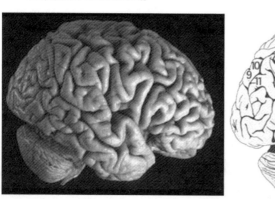
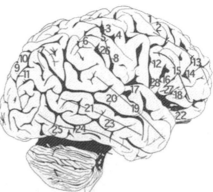

**Fig. 12.2** Superolateral surface of right cerebral hemisphere, showing sulci and gyri. 1: Superior frontal gyrus. 2: Superior frontal sulcus. 3: Central sulcus. 4: Precentral gyrus. 5: Postcentral gyrus. 6: Supramarginal gyrus. 7: Angular gyrus. 8: Postcentral sulcus. 9: Parieto-occipital sulcus. 10: Superior parietal lobule. 11: Intraparietal sulcus. 12: Precentral sulcus. 13: Middle frontal gyrus. 14: Inferior frontal sulcus. 15: Inferior frontal gyrus. 16: Anterior ascending ramus of lateral sulcus. 17: Transverse temporal gyrus. 18: Anterior horizontal ramus of lateral sulcus. 19: Superior temporal gyrus. 20: Superior temporal sulcus. 21: Middle temporal gyrus. 22: Stem of lateral sulcus. 23. Inferior temporal sulcus. 24: Inferior temporal gyrus. 25: Preoccipital notch. 26: Posterior branch of lateral sulcus. 27: Triangular part of inferior frontal gyrus. 28: Opercular part of inferior frontal gyrus. From Williams *et al.* ***http://www.vh.org/adult/provider/anatomy/BrainAnatomy/Ch5Text/Section02.html***

them all the functional domains thought to bear a critical relationship to conscious awareness: perception, action, memory, emotion and attention. In this way, the global workspace is able to deal with material in all these domains. But that is not to say that material in these domains is always conscious, only that it may become conscious if other conditions are satisfied.

The most important of these other conditions is this. Given that the neurons hosting a pattern of neural activity have the appropriate anatomical connections to permit entry into the global neuronal workspace (now defined as the network of tangential cortico-cortical connections), this pattern must attain a sufficient degree and duration of self-sustained activity to do so. The details of how this level of activity is achieved differ somewhat from model to model. But essentially they all call upon some form of reverberatory circuit involving feedback, harking back in this respect to a concept (the 'cell assembly') proposed half a century ago by the great Canadian psychologist, Donald Hebb. Dehaene and Naccache (2001, p. 19) illustrate this general idea with the diagram shown here as Fig. 12.3.

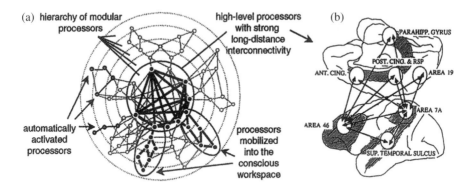

**Fig. 12.3** Neural substrates of the conscious workspace proposed by Dehaene and Naccache (2001). (a) Symbolic representation of the hierarchy of connections between brain processes (each symbolized by a circle). Higher levels of this hierarchy are assumed to be widely interconnected by long-distance interconnections, thus forming a global neuronal workspace. An amplified state of workspace activity, bringing together several peripheral processors in a coherent brain-scale activation pattern (*black circles*), can coexist with the automatic activation of multiple local chains of processors outside the workspace (*white circles*). (b) Possible anatomical substrate of the proposed workspace: long-distance network identified in the monkey and linking dorsolateral prefrontal, parietal, temporal, and anterior cingulate areas with other subcortical targets.

Some reverberatory circuit or other will almost certainly have to form part of the finished story, if only to account for the temporal course of the contents of consciousness. You will recall both that there is a delay before a stimulus at one of the sense organs is able to gain entry into consciousness, and that such a stimulus has to be presented for a minimum duration if entry is to be gained at all. These intervals are of the order of tens or hundreds of milliseconds, much longer than the duration of any immediate neural response to stimulation. Thus, some way has to be found for neural activity to keep circulating for long enough to bridge between these immediate responses and the temporal durations required for conscious experience. The major difference between the different models then lies in the circuits to which they give most emphasis in this role.

Those theorists, including Dehaene and his colleagues, who focus upon executive functions, such as working memory, look especially to the frontal lobes. In support of this view, they point to a large number of neuroimaging studies that show activity in the prefrontal cortex and anterior cingulate area (see Fig. 18.7) in tasks that demand the application of executive functions. Further support comes from experiments demonstrating 'delay' neurons in monkey frontal cortex. In these experiments neurons have been shown to keep firing during a delay between the presentation of a stimulus and the time at which the animal is allowed to make an appropriate response. Firing patterns of this kind are just what you would expect of a system mediating short-term or working memory. (Though notice that these durations of firing, corresponding to the intervals involved in this kind of 'delayed response' task, go up to many seconds, well beyond the durations required to account for simple conscious perception.)

A major role is also allotted to the parietal cortex (Figs 12.2 and 15.1), because of the role this region seems to play in attention. Damage to the parietal cortex, most often caused by stroke, can cause the syndrome of contralateral neglect. In this, the patient can lose awareness of everything on the side of the world, including his own body, opposite to the lesion. (In most brain functions, the right hemisphere of the brain controls activity in relation to the left side of the world, and *vice versa*.) That this is probably due to a disturbance in attentional function is indicated by a phenomenon known as 'extinction'. If the lesion (as is most common) affects the parietal cortex in the right hemisphere, then the patient may be aware of a stimulus to, say, the left hand provided that this is the only stimulus presented. But, if the left and right hands are stimulated simultaneously, the patient loses conscious awareness of the stimulus on the left. The simultaneous right-sided stimulus thus appears to block the left-sided one from attention. This blockage affects only conscious processing, since a variety of tests demonstrate considerable unconscious processing of the unfelt stimulus. A plausible interpretation of this pattern of results is that, for a stimulus to enter consciousness, it requires a kind of attentional 'amplification' provided by the parietal cortex. Such amplification could be provided by way of a reverberatory circuit between the somatosensory system and the parietal cortex, in line with Dehaene's model of the neuronal global workspace.

Dehaene and Naccache (2001, p. 19) characterise this general type of process as one in which 'active workspace neurons send top-down amplification signals that boost the currently active processor neurons, whose bottom-up signals in turn help maintain workspace activity'. In this formulation, 'top-down' refers to the brain regions that mediate executive functions and 'bottom-up', to those that contain active perceptual representations or motor programs. Another vocabulary often used to describe essentially the same notions is that of 'feed-forward' and 'feed-back' circuits. This vocabulary fits the anatomical architecture of the perceptual systems particularly well. Plate 12.1, for example, illustrates the way in which visual information, after first being received in the retina, passes along the successive modules of the visual system. Each module both sends information further up the line ('feed-forward') and receives information back ('feed-back') from these later modules. Note that 'feed-back' in this sense does not have the same meaning as it does when an engineer talks of 'feedback' in a simple servomechanism of the kind we considered in Chapter 3. 'Feedback' in that original sense requires that the signal fed back be compared to a desired set-point so as to control the output of the system. To distinguish between the two uses, I shall preserve a hyphen in 'feed-back' when it means, as here, simply the existence of an anatomical connection heading back in the direction of a sensory input. It is, of course, possible that a given 'feed-back' connection carries out a 'feedback' function; but that remains to be seen.

Edelman and Tononi emphasise a different form of interconnectivity as critical for the selection of one rather than other trains of neural activity for entry into the global workspace (*scilicet* consciousness). They call this 're-entry'. Essentially the notion is one of dynamically shifting temporary alliances. Imagine a number of trains of activity going on simultaneously in different assemblies of cells, each distributed across a range of brain regions and modules. They are each able to access the long-distance interconnections of the global workspace. They are, therefore, all in a position to interact with one another. The interactions between any two pairs of cell assemblies can be mutually inhibitory or excitatory. As a result of these interactions, some of the cell assemblies are weakened, but others enter into a mutually self-sustaining larger assembly of cells. Eventually, the overall pattern shakes down into one super-assembly which, for the moment, dominates the entire workspace. That moment is the moment during which the contents instantiated in the temporarily dominant cell assemble enter consciousness.

Edelman and Tononi have gone on from this core concept (which bears many similarities to the more general, but less well specified, Multiple Drafts model) to formulate their ideas mathematically. Using computer simulations of appropriate neural networks, they show that a system of this kind can work in principle. More importantly, their mathematical treatment enables them to investigate the degree to which their proposed system depends upon differences in underlying anatomical 'architecture'. By this I mean features like the nature of the circuitry, the length of the connections, the paths traversed through the network before a signal

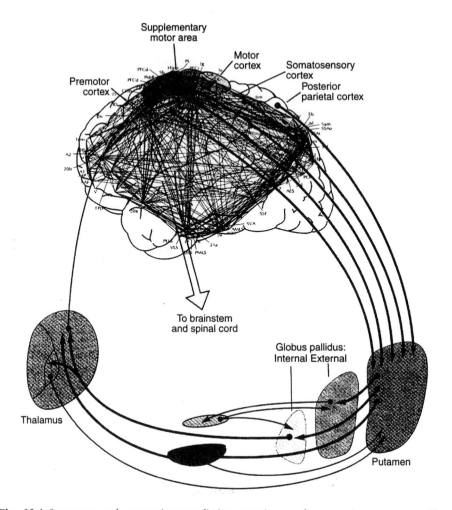

**Fig. 12.4** Structures and connections mediating conscious and unconscious processes. The thalamocortical system, which gives rise to the 'dynamic core', is represented by a fine meshwork of cortical and thalamic areas and re-entrant connections. The functionally insulated routines that are triggered by the core and return to it travel along parallel, polysnaptic, one-directional pathways that leave the cortex, reach the various components of the basal ganglia and certain thalamic nuclei and finally return to the cortex. The large arrows represent connections to the brain stem and spinal cord that mediate motor input. From Edelman and Tononi (2000).

sent out by one set of neurons is returned to its origin, and so on. They model features of this kind both in the abstract and by taking into account what is known about the real architecture to be found in different regions of the brain. Comparing the two leads to a particularly interesting result: the anatomical architecture of the thalamocortical and limbic systems (Fig. 12.4) is better able to sustain dynamic

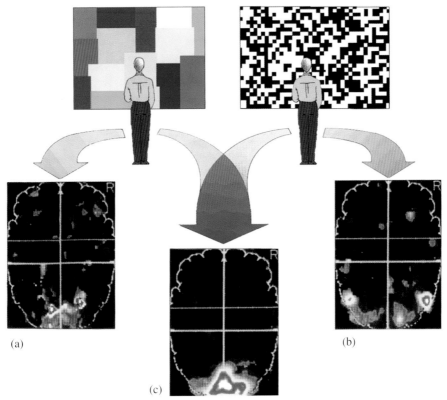

**Plate 2.1** The regions of increased cerebral blood flow in the human brain when subjects view (a) a multi-coloured Mondrian (see Plate 7.2) display and (b) a pattern of moving squares. Highest increases are shown in white, red and yellow. The regions of high cerebral blood flow are indicated in horizontal slices throughout the cerebral cortex. Note the difference in location between the area activated by the colour stimulus (human V4) and the one activated by the motion stimulus (human V5). Note that area V1 and the adjoining area V2 were active with both stimuli, suggesting that both colour and motion signals reach V1 and are distributed from it to the specialized visual areas V4 and V5. From Zeki (1993).

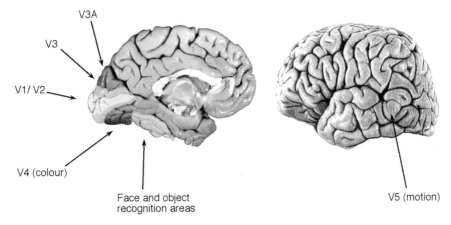

**Plate 4.1** The location of visual areas in the human cortex (cf. Plate 2.1). From Zeki (1999).

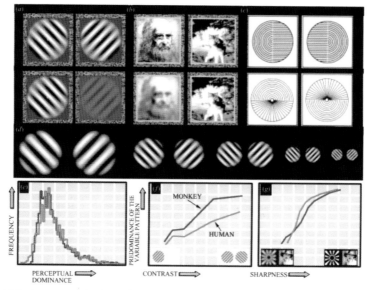

**Plate 6.1** (a) Grating patterns of orthogonal orientation that are usually employed in the study of binocular rivalry. Varying the strength of the patterns (e.g. as shown here, their degree of contrast) changes the predominance of each stimulus. Strong stimuli remain suppressed for shorter periods. (b) Rivalling complex patterns. The strength of such stimuli can be manipulated, as shown, by the degree of blurring. (c) 'Caneja' patterns, used to demonstrate that rivalry does not occur just between the two eyes or the two hemispheres but at a higher level of perceptual integration. When these patterns are presented dichoptically, rivalry occurs between percepts of concentric circles or lines (horizontal in the top display, radial in the bottom). (d) Exclusive dominance of a pattern during rivalry depends on both the size and spatial frequency of the stimulus. Stimuli of low spatial frequency (*left*) that are much larger than patterns of higher spatial frequency (*right*) can still yield frequent phases of exclusive dominance. (e) Distribution of alternation phases for human and monkey subjects. (f, g) Both humans and monkeys (see Plate 6.2) show the same predominance-strength functions for two different stimulus types. From Logothetis, Single units and conscious vision. *Philosophical Transactions of the Royal Society B*, 353, 1801–18 (1998).

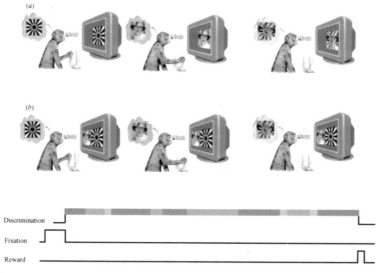

**Plate 6.2** (a) Non-rivalry; (b) rivalry. The monkeys were taught to pull and hold the left lever whenever a sunburst-like pattern ('left object') was displayed, and to pull and hole the right lever upon presentation of other figures ('right objects'). In addition, they were trained not to respond on presentation of a physical blend of different stimuli ('mixed objects'). During the behavioural task, individual observation periods consisted of random transitions between presentations of left, right and mixed objects. A juice reward was delivered only after the successful completion of an entire observation period. During rivalry periods, the monkeys indicated alternating perception of the left and right objects (see Plate 6.1e–g). From Logothetis, Single units and conscious vision. *Philosophical Transactions of the Royal Society B*, 353, 1801–18 (1998).

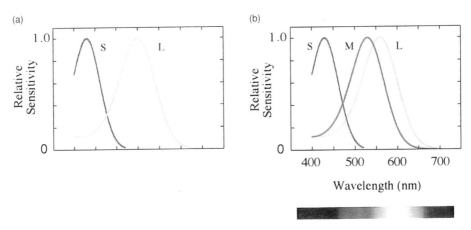

**Plate 7.1** (b) The sensitivities of the long-wave (L), middle-wave (M) and short-wave (S) photopigments found in the retinae of humans and of Old World primates. (a) The sensitivities of the pigments thought to have been present in ancestral mammals. From Mollon (1999).

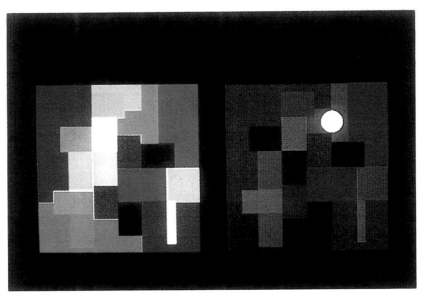

**Plate 7.2** A 'Mondrian' design. *Right*: If the polygon marked by a white circle is viewed in isolation through a small aperture, with the rest of the design obscured, it is seen as white or grey. *Left*: Viewed with the rest of the design visible, the polygon is seen as green. From Zeki (1993).

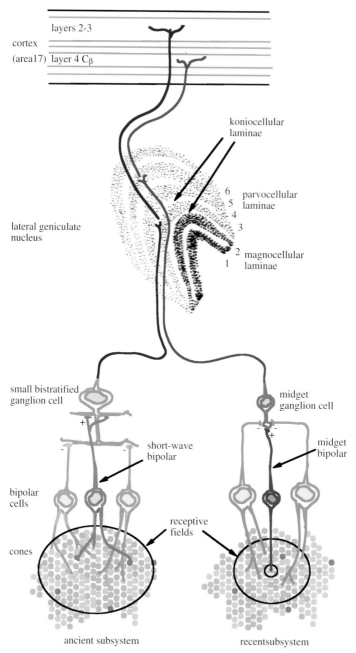

cortex (area17)

layers 2-3

layer 4 C$_\beta$

koniocellular laminae

lateral geniculate nucleus

6
5 parvocellular laminae
4
3
2 magnocellular laminae
1

small bistratified ganglion cell

midget ganglion cell

short-wave bipolar

midget bipolar

bipolar cells

cones

receptive fields

ancient subsystem

recentsubsystem

**Plate 7.3** The two subsystems of primate colour vision. A schematic of the photoreceptor matrix shows the S, M and L cones (see Plate 7.1) in blue, green and orange, respectively. The phylogenetically ancient subsystem (*left*) draws opposed inputs from the S cones, on the one hand, and from the L and M cones on the other. Its signals are carried by the small bistratified ganglion cells and the koniocellular laminae of the lateral geniculate nucleus (LGN). The recent subsystem (*right*) compares the signals of the L and M cones. Its signals are thought to be carried by midget ganglion cells and the parvocellular layers of the LGN. From Regan *et al.*, Fruits, foliage and the evolution of primate colour vision. *Philosophical Transactions of the Royal Society B*, 356, 229–83 (2001).

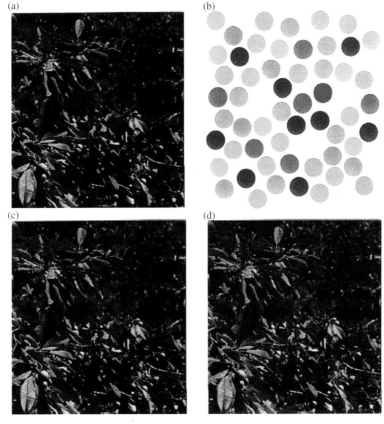

**Plate 7.4** (a) Fruits of *Manilkara bidentata* (Sapotaceae) photographed in the forest canopy at Les Nouragues. The species *Alouatta seniculus, Ateles paniscus* and *Cebus apella* all eat these fruits. (b) Typical stimulus array from a laboratory visual search task: the task might be to press one button if the orange circle is present, and a different button if the orange circle is absent. The chromaticity of the orange target circle is the same as the chromaticity of a fruit in (a), and the chromaticity of the distractors were drawn from the chromaticities of leaves in (a). The same photograph as it would appear (c) to a protanope (a colour-blind individual who lacks the L or red photopigment) and (d) a deuteranope (who lacks the M or green photopigment), illustrating the importance of trichromatic colour vision for locating the fruit. From Regan *et al.*, Fruits, foliage and the evolution of primate colour vision. *Philosophical Transactions of the Royal Society B*, 356, 229–83 (2001).

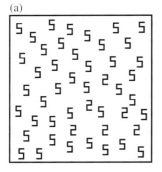
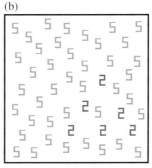

**Plate 10.1** The displays used by Ramachandran and Hubbard (2001) to demonstrate visual 'pop-out' in coloured grapheme synaesthetes. (a) When presented with a matrix of 5s in which a triangle composed of 2s is embedded, control subjects find it difficult to discern the triangle. (b) However, coloured grapheme synaesthetes who see, for example, the 5s in green and the 2s in red detect the embedded triangle much more rapidly.

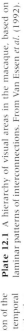

**Plate 12.1** A hierarchy of visual areas in the macaque, based on laminar patterns of interconnections. From Van Essen *et al.* (1992).

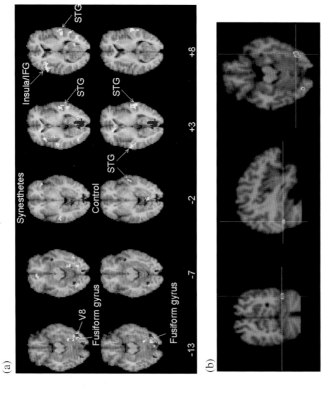

**Plate 10.2** (a) Activation maps of coloured-hearing synaesthetes and controls in response to heard words, combined with the results of a colour activation mapping study (Howard *et al.*, 1998). The data shown are 5.5-mm axial slices, between Talairach z planes −13 and +8 mm, for synaesthetes (*upper row*) and controls (*lower row*). Yellow: heard words *minus* tones. Blue: coloured Mondrian (see Plate 7.2) patterns *minus* monochrome Mondrians. Red: cluster common to both heard words and coloured Mondrians. The coordinates of this cluster correspond very closely with those reported by Hadjikhani *et al.* (1998) for V8, the colour selective region of the visual system. The right side of the image corresponds to the left hemisphere of the brain. STG: superior temporal gyrus. IFG: inferior frontal gyrus. (b) Orthogonal views of the site of overlap (red cluster in A) between activation in coloured hearing synaesthetes by heard words, and in non-synaesthetes by coloured Mondrian patterns. Left to right: coronal, sagittal and axial planes. From Nunn *et al.* (2000).

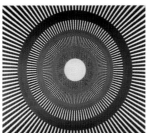

**Plate 13.1** An illusion of motion. *Enigma*, by Isia Levant. Palais de la Découverte, Paris. From Zeki (1999).

Quantum theory describes the bizarre properties of matter and energy at near-atomic scales. These properties include: (1) QUANTUM COHERENCE, in which individual particles yield identity to a collective, unifying wave function (exemplified in Bose–Einstein condensates); (2) non-local QUANTUM ENTANGLEMENT, in which spatially separated particle states are nonetheless connected or related; (3) QUANTUM SUPERPOSITION, in which particles exist in two or more states or locations simultaneously; and (4) QUANTUM STATE REDUCTION or 'collapse of the wave function', in which superpositioned particles reduce or collapse to specific choices. All four quantum properties can be applied to the seemingly inexplicable features of consciousness. First, quantum coherence (e.g. Bose–Einstein condensation) is a possible physical basis for 'binding' or unity of consciousness[a]. Second, non-local entanglements (e.g. 'Einstein–Podolsky–Rosen correlations') serve as a potential basis for associative memory and non-local emotional interpersonal connection. Third, quantum superposition of information provides a basis for preconscious and subconscious processes, dreams and altered states. Lastly, quantum state reduction (quantum computation) serves as a possible physical mechanism for the transition from preconscious processes to consciousness[b,c].

What is quantum computation? In classical computing, binary information is commonly represented as 'bits' of either 1 or 0. In quantum computation, information can exist in quantum superposition, for example, as quantum bits or 'qubits' of both 1 and 0. Qubits interact or compute by entanglement and then reduce or collapse to a solution expressed in classical bits (either 1 or 0). In the Orch OR model, quantum computation occurs in microtubules within the brain's neurons. Microtubules are polymers of the protein tubulin, which in the Orch OR model transiently exist in quantum superposition of two or more conformational states (Fig. I). Following periods of preconscious quantum computation (e.g. on the order of tens to hundreds of milliseconds) tubulin superpositions reduce or 'self-collapse' at an OBJECTIVE THRESHOLD (hence OBJECTIVE REDUCTION) due to a quantum gravity mechanism proposed by Penrose[b,c].

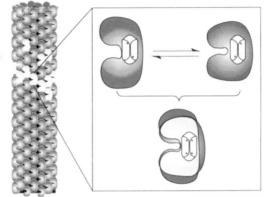

**Fig. I.** Microtubule structure shown at left: a hollow tube of 25 nm diameter, consisting of 13 columns of tubulin dimers arranged in a skewed hexagonal lattice. Each tubulin molecule can switch between two (or more) conformations (top right: blue, red), coupled to London forces in a hydrophobic pocket. Each tubulin can also exist in quantum superposition of both conformational states (bottom right: gray). According to the Orch OR model, dipole interactions among tubulin states in the microtubule lattice process information classically and by quantum computation.

*TRENDS in Cognitive Sciences*

Microtubule-associated protein (MAP-2) connections provide input during classical phases, thus tuning or 'orchestrating' the quantum computations (hence orchestrated objective reduction or 'Orch OR'). Each Orch OR quantum computation determines classical output states of tubulin, which govern neurophysiological events, such as initiating spikes at the axon hillock, regulating synaptic strengths, forming new MAP-2 attachment sites and gap-junction connections, and establishing starting conditions for the next conscious event[d–g].

These events are suggested to have subjective phenomenal experience (what philosophy calls 'QUALIA') because in the Penrose formulation superpositions are separations in fundamental spacetime geometry. In a pan-protopsychist philosophical view, qualia are embedded in fundamental spacetime geometry and Orch OR processes access and select specific sets of qualia for each conscious event[h].

**References**

a Marshall, I.N. (1989) Consciousness and Bose–Einstein condensates. *New Ideas Psychol.* 7, 73–83

b Penrose, R. (1989) *The Emperor's New Mind*, Oxford University Press

c Penrose, R. (1994) *Shadows of the Mind: A Search for the Missing Science of Consciousness*, Oxford University Press

d Penrose R. and Hameroff S.R. (1995) What gaps? Reply to Grush and Churchland. *J. Conscious. Stud.* 2, 98–112; http://www.consciousness.arizona.edu/hameroff/gap2.html

e Hameroff, S.R. and Penrose, R. (1996) Orchestrated reduction of quantum coherence in brain microtubules: a model for consciousness. In *Toward a Science of Consciousness: The First Tucson Discussions and Debates* (Hameroff, S.R. et al., eds), pp. 507–540, MIT Press [Also published in *Math. Comput. Simulation* (1996) 40, 453–480; http://www.consciousness.arizona.edu/hameroff/or.html.]

f Hameroff, S.R. and Penrose, R. (1996) Conscious events as orchestrated spacetime selections. *J. Conscious. Stud.* 3, 36–53; http://www.u.arizona.edu/~hameroff/penrose2

g Hameroff, S. (1998) Quantum computation in brain microtubules? The Penrose–Hameroff 'Orch OR' model of consciousness. *Philos. Trans. R. Soc. London Ser. A* 356, 1869–1896; http://www.consciousness.arizona.edu/hameroff/royal2.html

h Hameroff, S. (1998) 'Funda-mentality': is the conscious mind subtly linked to a basic level of the universe? *Trends Cognit. Sci.* 2, 119–124

**Plate 16.1** Microtubule structure shown at left: a hollow tube of 25 nm diameter, consisting of 13 columns of tubulin dimers arranged in a skewed hexagonal lattice. Each tubulin molecule can switch between two (or more) conformations (top right: blue, red), coupled to London forces in a hydrophobic pocket. Each tubulin can also exist in quantum superposition of both conformational states (bottom right: gray). According to the Orch OR model, dipole interactions among tubulin states in the microtubule lattice process information classically and by quantum computation. From Woolf and Hameroff (2001).

In our approach, quantum computing by the Orch OR mechanism occurs within pyramidal cell dendritic cytoplasm, but is linked to synaptic membrane events by well-established SECOND MESSENGER chemical cascades activated by METABOTROPIC RECEPTORS (Fig. I). Acetylcholine, operating through the metabotropic muscarinic receptor, serves to activate the second messenger, PHOSPHOINOSITIDE-SPECIFIC PHOSPHOLIPASE C (PI-PLC), which in turn activates two protein kinases: PROTEIN KINASE C (PKC) and CaMK II (Ref. a). These protein kinases then add phosphoryl groups to specific sites on the microtubule-associated protein-2 (MAP-2) molecule. Serotonin, norepinephrine, glutamate and histamine also activate PI-PLC (but to lesser degrees than acetylcholine) via subpopulations of their own metabotropic receptors, leading to additional phosphorylation of MAP-2.

MAP-2 phosphorylation at these particular sites acts to decouple MAP-2 from microtubules and from actin[b-d], the net effect being to isolate microtubules from membrane and environmental influences (Fig. Ib). PI-PLC activation also directly isolates actin molecules from the neuronal membrane[e], further isolating microtubules embedded in actin gel. We suggest that these mechanisms of isolation initiate phases of quantum coherent superposition in microtubules, and then the Orch OR mechanism, resulting in phenomenal consciousness.

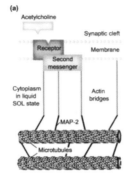

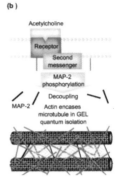

*TRENDS in Cognitive Sciences*

**References**

a Siegel, G.J. *et al.* (1998) *Basic Neurochemistry: Molecular, Cellular and Medical Aspects,* Lippincott–Raven

b Sánchez, C. *et al.* (2000) Phosphorylation of microtubule-associated protein 2 (MAP2) and its relevance for the regulation of the neuronal cytoskeleton function. *Prog. Neurobiol.* 61, 133–168

c Johnson, G.V.W. and Jope, R.S. (1992) The role of microtubule-associated protein 2 (MAP-2) in neuronal growth, plasticity, and degeneration. *J. Neurosci. Res.* 33, 505–512

d Woolf, N.J. (1999) Dendritic encoding: an alternative to temporal synaptic coding of conscious experience. *Conscious. Cognit.* 8, 574–596

**Fig. I.** Neuronal cytoplasmic interior switching between (a) classical 'Sol' state, in which membrane and receptors communicate with microtubule information processing, and (b) quantum 'Gel' state in which quantum computations in microtubules are isolated from membrane interactions. Acetylcholine binding to muscarinic receptors (b) acts through second messengers to phosphorylate MAP-2, thereby decoupling microtubules from outside environment. According to our model, such transitions between Sol/classical and Gel/quantum states occur roughly every 25 ms (i.e. around '40 Hz').

e Tall, E.G. *et al.* (2000) Dynamics of phosphatidylinositol 4,5-bisphosphate in actin-rich structures. *Curr. Biol.* 10, 743–746

**Plate 16.2** Linking isolated microtubule quantum computation to neural membrane mechanisms. From Woolf and Hameroff (2001).

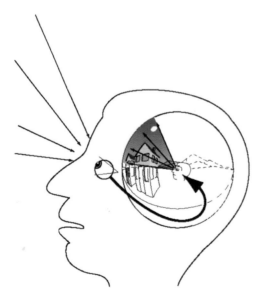

**Plate 17.1** The image from the retina is projected into the perceptual sphere from the centre outward in the direction of gaze, as an inverse analogue of the cone of light that enters the eye in the external world, taking into account eye, head, and body orientation in order to update the appropriate portion of perceptual space. From Lehar (in press).

patterns based upon re-entry than is the architecture of the basal ganglia. This difference maps neatly onto the fact that the former systems are concerned with perception and the latter, with action. Given the much closer relations between consciousness and perception than between consciousness and action, this is an encouraging observation.

These mathematical studies look as though they may lead to a rigorous method for classifying different kinds of feed-back systems. For the moment, it seems probable that, despite their different terminology, the interactions between top-down and bottom-up processes described by Dehaene and the re-entrant circuits analysed by Edelman and Tononi are much the same thing. Theoretical simulations have shown that both can give rise to temporal synchrony between individual 'spikes' (the basic unit of neuronal information processing) in neurons at a distance from one another. Synchronised firing can arise either because both neurons are the recipients of feed-forward influences from the same neurons earlier in the processing stream, or because of their own reciprocal connections, or both.

There are now many experimental demonstrations of such temporal synchrony, operating on a millisecond scale and between widely separated regions of the neocortex, for example, between sensory and motor cortices, as well as between neurons within the same informational domain (e.g. the visual cortex) when they both belong to the same perceptually integrated object. We saw an example of the latter kind in Singer's experiment with cats viewing a stimulus that could be perceived either as two transparent gratings sliding diagonally across one another or as a single plaid moving vertically (Fig. 4.3). But, you will recall, the cats in this experiment were anaesthetised. So, while temporal synchrony may, as Singer proposes, play a key role in solving the binding problem, it is not clear that it plays a similar role in the entry into consciousness of the bound percept. The ability of neurons to fire in synchrony at a distance from one another also bids fair to eliminate some of the mystery attaching to Gestalt stimuli, in which the whole determines how the parts are perceived (see Section 16.1). Another potential role for synchronised firing is in aiding the formation of the currently dominant dynamic pattern in the workspace. This is because, if neurons fire synchronously and both project to the same target down stream, this enhances their chances of causing the down-stream neurons to fire in turn.

## Conclusions

The theorists contributing to the emerging consensus are all agreed that the global neuronal workspace differs radically from the Cartesian Theatre.

First, of course, they eschew dualism: the dynamic pattern that wins out in the competition for access to the global workspace is not in consequence miraculously transmuted into an entirely different psychic stuff. I have no desire to quarrel with this eminently sensible assumption. But rejection of dualism does not eliminate the gap dualism was trying to fill. Essentially, the concept of the global workspace represents an increasingly well worked-out exercise in what the Gestalt psychologists called 'psychophysical isomorphism' (equipping the system that produces consciousness with properties equivalent to those found in conscious experience itself; see Section 16.6), now complemented by 'psychoneural' isomorphism as the detailed neuronal machinery of the workplace becomes better defined. But it won't do merely to say that, because the isomorphism is good or even very good, the dominant dynamic pattern just *is* conscious. That on its own explains nothing.

Second, the theorists say, the global workspace differs from the Cartesian Theatre in that there is no uniquely privileged, fixed spot (as was the pineal gland) where the transmutation into consciousness takes place. Instead, there are patterns of neural activity battling it out over networks widely distributed across the brain. The one that wins can be represented in any way across the entire distribution. Furthermore, it is said, the activity that is destined for conscious awareness does not have to be forwarded on to any privileged consciousness spot. It is 'boosted' into consciousness just as it is, where it is, and representing what it represents.

All this may be so; but theatres come in many forms. The diagram used by Dehaene (Fig. 12.3) looks suspiciously like a theatre in the round—a Cartesian Arena, perhaps, defined by the collectivity of tangential neurons. I once saw a production of *Orlando Furioso* in a converted covered market in which the show went on in several different places at once, and the audience moved around. This is not such a bad way to think of Edelman and Tononi's re-entrant circuits busily communicating with one another.

The serious point I am making is this. The global workspace aspires to be a good isomorph of what conscious experience feels like. But one of the things that conscious experience feels like is a display that one is able to inspect. The most dramatic of these displays does not lie in the 'private spaces' of consciousness—the words, numbers, images etc that we are able to call to mind and which executive functions manipulate in relative isolation from the world outside. It lies, rather, in that very world outside. To me, it seems clear that I inspect that world. In that very concrete sense there is an audience looking at, listening to, smelling, tasting and touching the effects, in consciousness, of the dynamic patterns that have won out in the competition for the global workspace. But the concept of the workspace gives no clue as to how this is done, and consideration of its neuronal underpinnings has done nothing to advance matters in this respect. Nor for that matter, once its dualism is stripped away, does the Cartesian Theatre have any kind of explanatory force. But it provides no worse a metaphor for the problem.

# CHAPTER 13

# The neural correlate of consciousness

The central intuition underlying the approaches considered in the last two chapters is that the neural basis of consciousness is directly related to executive functions: that is, to systems which *manipulate* information. The contrasting intuition behind the approaches we now consider is that the neural basis of consciousness lies in systems which directly *'code'* this information—that is, in perceptual systems. This intuition is much more in keeping with the general tenor of this book, given its emphasis that *the* Hard Problem is posed by the brain's ability to create qualia.

The two types of approach are not incompatible. Once the brain has created, by whatever means, qualia, it is clear that they are available to be manipulated by executive functions. This is so, whether a percept lies in the public or private space of consciousness. Thus I may use the processes of attention and deliberate commitment to memory so as to recall the exact shape and colour of a flower seen in a garden; or I may later call these attributes of the flower to mind and describe them to someone else. Indeed, one of the questions we ask in this chapter is whether the same brain regions are activated when such a percept is formed by way of visual stimulation (public space) or is imagined (private space). However, even given this availability of percepts to manipulation by executive functions, there remains a major difference if the two starting intuitions are stated in their extreme forms. For one of them states that the neural activity *proximal* to conscious experience is to be found in executive regions of the brain and the other, in perceptual regions. (For 'proximal', a more contentious vocabulary would say 'the activity which directly enters consciousness'.)

A major proponent of the perceptual approach is Francis Crick. Having solved (together with James Watson) the structure of DNA (by way of the famous double helix), he has since devoted his career to cracking the problem of consciousness (many readers will know his book, *The Astonishing Hypothesis*). He coined the phrase 'the neural correlate of consciousness' (NCC) to describe the neural activity that is proximal to any particular form of conscious experience. The phrase has caught on, and we shall use it here.

Crick's particular interest (and that of the majority of investigators following the same approach) lies in the NCC of specifically visual awareness. He asks the question: what is the proximal activity underlying the visual qualia of colour, motion, shape, etc.? This emphasis on vision is driven, not theoretically, but practically, since so much more is known about this sense, both psychologically and physio-logically, than any of the others. However, there is no reason to think that a solution found for the NCC of vision would be inapplicable in principle to the other senses, though the details, of course, might differ considerably.

Note that this concept of the NCC specifically for vision is incompatible with the notion of a single Cartesian Theatre for *all* conscious experience considered in Chapter 11. Crick's approach implies, in contrast, that there will be multiple foci of neural activity, each proximal to a different type of qualia. However, it further implies (unlike Dennett's Multiple Drafts model, also considered in Chapter 11) that only some forms of neural activity can serve as NCCs. In particular, NCCs should be found in perceptual systems (since one is consciously aware of percepts) but not in systems whose operation does not figure in conscious awareness (ones, for example, that control pupillary dilation or walking).

## 13.1   Activity in V1 and visual awareness

In the last decade or so the concept of the NCC for vision has stimulated a remark-able surge of experimental research. It is too soon to judge properly how the new data will pan out. But some general principles are beginning to emerge, as summarised in this section. Since the data are so new, I shall in this chapter increase the scholastic burden on the text with appropriate references (author's name and date of publication); these can be found at the end of the book in the general list of references. (For a more detailed review, see Rees, Kreiman and Koch, 2002.)

Crick and his colleague, Christof Koch, propose that 'any neurons expressing an aspect of the NCC must project directly... to at least some of the parts of the brain that plan voluntary action—that is what we have argued seeing is for' (Koch and Crick, 2000, p. 1289). From its beginning, then, this approach from perception holds out a welcoming hand to executive functions. However, Koch and Crick's assumptions are not self-evident. For, as we saw in Chapter 2, much voluntary action takes place prior to any conscious awareness of the environment to which the action is directed. Still, for the moment let us accept these assumptions and see where they lead. Guided by a large volume of empirical data, discussed in the previous chapter, Crick and Koch identify the regions of the brain concerned with the planning of voluntary action as lying in the frontal lobes—the prefrontal and anterior cingulate cortex. They therefore propose that the NCC for vision should be located in parts of the visual system which have direct projections to these frontal regions. One implication of this proposal is that primary visual cortex (V1, also known as the striate cortex or Brodmann area 17; see Plates 4.1 and 12.1), should *not* play host to the NCC, since it does not project directly to frontal cortex.

This implication can be restated as a prediction: neural activity in V1 should not be *sufficient* for conscious visual experience. A complementary prediction is that neural activity in V1 may not even be *necessary* for conscious visual experience. It is difficult to test these predictions by the normal route of retinal visual stimuli giving rise to veridical perceptual experience, since V1 is the main gate by which all visual stimuli enter the cerebral cortex. For the same reason, the mere fact that activity is observed in V1 when the retina is visually stimulated is not enough to disconfirm the Crick and Koch predictions. However, a number of experiments using visual stimuli that give rise to *illusory* experiences have provided strong support for the second prediction, of conscious visual experience in the absence of corresponding activity in V1.

Consider first illusory contours, of the kind shown in Fig. 13.1. In the well-known 'Kanizsa' triangle illusion, named after the psychologist who devised it, nearly everyone sees a triangle even though no triangular contours are in fact present in the design. The interior of the illusory triangle, moreover, appears brighter than the surround, though there is in fact no brightness difference. Monkeys, too, respond to such illusory contours—or, at least, neurons in their visual system fire differentially depending on their presence or absence, as seen by a human observer. To show this, Von der Heydt, Peterhans and Baumgartner

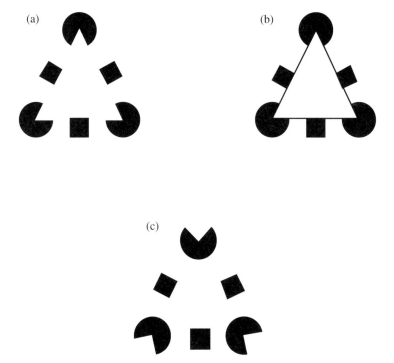

**Fig. 13.1** The Kanizsa triangle and its control stimuli. Reprinted from *NeuroImage*, 3, ffytche and Zeki, Brain activity related to the perception of illusory contours, 104–8, copyright (1996), with permission from Elsevier.

(1984) recorded from neurons in a monkey's brain while it looked at the designs shown in Fig. 13.2. As you can see, designs A, B and D contain illusory lines, and these can be eliminated by quite small changes in the pattern (C). Von der Heydt's group was able to identify neurons in the monkey's brain that fired only when the illusory lines were present. (This result, of course, and the increasing number like it, add weight to our earlier conclusion that animals have conscious experiences that closely resemble the human variety.) The neurons that showed this pattern of response were located in an area known as V2 (or area 18), which lies adjacent to V1 (Plate 4.1). But no such neurons were observed in V1 itself.

More than a decade later these findings in the monkey brain were confirmed with human subjects by ffytche and Zeki (1996). They used positron emission tomography (PET) to compare patterns of brain activity in response to a Kanizsa triangle and to a control figure (shown on the right of Fig. 13.1) in which the illusory triangle was destroyed by scrambling the orientation of the elements (or 'pacmen') composing it. A further control (middle of Fig. 13.1) presented a real triangle, by drawing a black outline round the contours of the illusory one. As in the monkey experiment, ffytche and Zeki observed activity in response to the illusory triangle (after subtraction of the pattern of activity induced by the scrambled control design) in V2 but not V1. The veridical triangle also activated V2 but, surprisingly, to a smaller degree than the Kanizsa triangle itself.

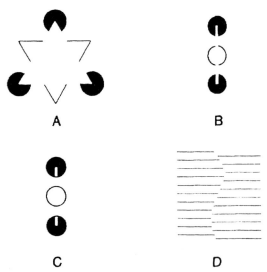

**Fig. 13.2** Illusions of edges used by Van der Heydt *et al.* (1984) to study higher level information processing in V2 cells of monkey cortex. A: A white triangle is seen, although it is not defined in the picture by a continuous border. B: A vertical bar is seen, although again there is no continuous border. C: Slight alterations obliterate the perception of the bar seen in B. D: The curved contour is not represented by any edges or lines. From Von der Heydt *et al.* (1984).

This type of result calls for an important *caveat* concerning the methodological limitations of neuroimaging experiments. These largely rely upon the method of subtraction. In the example just given, activity caused by the scrambled control design (right-hand side of Fig. 13.1) is subtracted from that caused by the Kanizsa triangle to obtain the pattern of activity associated specifically with the conscious percept of the triangle. Thus the statement that no activity was observed in V1 in the subtracted pattern does not entail that this region was silent when the Kanizsa triangle was presented—indeed, it was almost certainly highly active. It means, rather, that there was no activity that *differentiated* between the two conditions: consciously perceived triangle present and triangle absent. Thus, from this type of experiment, one can conclude that the specific percept does not depend upon V1 activity. Nonetheless, it could still be the case that V1 activity is essential for visual perception of *one kind or another*. I shall continue, however, to speak of 'no V1 activity' as shorthand for 'absence of differential V1 activity' in describing results of this kind.

Studies of the perception of motion lead to the same pattern of results as do the experiments on illusory contours. The region of the visual system that responds most selectively to movement is V5 (Plate 4.1). Zeki, Watson and Frackowiak (1993) used PET and an impressive picture named 'Enigma' (Plate 13.1). This causes in most observers a powerful illusion of swirling motion. This illusion was accompanied by strong activation in V5. Somewhat stronger activation of V5 was also obtained when subjects viewed veridical motion. But the two stimuli differed in that real motion also activated V1, but illusory motion did not. Nor did Enigma activate V2. Putting this result together with the experiments on illusory contours, it seems that these activate V2 but not V5, illusory motion activates V5 but not V2, and neither activates V1.

Thus illusory percepts seem to depend upon activity in just the one visual area that is selective for the feature (contour or motion) concerned. On the basis of results like these, Zeki (1993; and see Zeki and ffytche, 1998) proposed that activity in such a feature-selective region is sufficient on its own for that feature to enter consciousness, so downgrading the role played in the Crick and Koch hypothesis by the frontal cortex. The phrase 'sufficient on its own' in the Zeki-ffytche hypothesis needs, however, to be interpreted with care. It implies that no activity is required in regions *other than the feature-selective region* for consciousness of the feature to be achieved. It does not, however, exclude the possibility that a relatively low level of activity in the feature-selective region is 'sufficient' only for *unconscious* processing of the feature. And, as we shall see, this appears to be the case. Both the Zeki and ffytche and the Crick and Koch hypotheses agree, however, that activity in V1 is not necessary for conscious visual experience, as indeed the data indicate. When Zeki's subjects observed veridical motion, however, V1 was activated. Activity in V1, then, may provide a basis for the brain to distinguish between illusory and veridical conscious experiences. This distinction is subjectively trans-

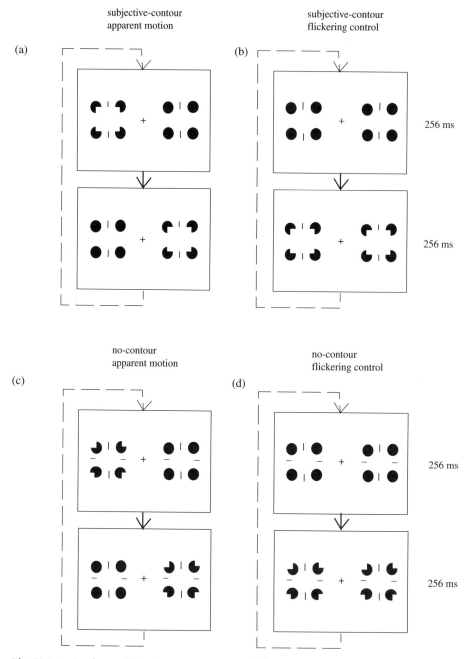

**Fig. 13.3** A stimulus combining illusory contours and illusory motion used by Goebel *et al.* (1998). Four 'pacmen' or four filled circles appeared on the left and right of the fixation cross. Two stimuli were shown repeatedly in sequence, as indicated by the arrows within each panel. (a) Subjects saw one 'Kanizsa' illusory square moving back and forth across the screen. In a first control, subjects saw two Kanizsa squares as stationary and flickering (b). In two others the pacmen were turned around, eliminating the apparent square with (c) or without (d) apparent motion remaining.

parent when viewing Enigma: one perceives swirling motion but one is also aware that nothing is really moving. It is difficult to determine, however, whether this distinction is directly perceptual or results from the more abstract knowledge that pages in books just don't move in this way.

Wolf Singer's group (Goebel *et al.*, 1998) took this line of research one step further by combining illusory contours and illusory motion in a study using fMRI. Their stimulus was a Kanizsa square (Fig. 13.3). When this was flashed first on one side of the display and then on the other, subjects saw a square moving back and forth (although there was no movement and no square—just four stationary pacmen). Viewing this display led to activity in V5 *and* V2 (relative to a control condition in which the illusion was destroyed by turning the pacmen around), but again not in V1. As in Zeki's experiment, however, V1 was activated by veridical motion stimuli.

Another way of producing a sense of motion is the well-known 'waterfall illusion'. Gaze for a while at a waterfall and then shift your gaze to a smooth surface—a nearby rock will do nicely. You are likely to see what looks like a waterfall moving *up* the rock. This illusion belongs to a general class of after-effects which occur in many sensory modalities. Whenever prolonged stimulation gives rise to a particular type or direction of experience and then comes to an abrupt end, there is a strong tendency for you to have exactly the opposite experience even in the absence of appropriate stimuli. Tootell *et al.* (1995) used fMRI to study a motion after-effect similar to the waterfall illusion. After gazing for a while at a pattern of expanding (or contracting) rings, the subject was shown a blank stationary stimulus, which appeared to contract (or expand), taking the direction opposed to what had been inspected. This illusory motion was accompanied by strong activity in V5, none in V1, and some in regions lying between the two on the ascending visual pathway.

After-effects of this kind arise because of 'adaptation'—a kind of fatigue—in the firing rate of the population of cells that undergo the initial prolonged stimulation (by the waterfall, for example). One can observe the adaptation itself as a reduction in the sensory impact of the initial, prolonged stimulus. A familiar example is the ticking of a clock that is always there and which you cease noticing at all (until it stops). Huk and Heeger (2002) used fMRI to measure adaptation to the motion of a 'plaid' (see Fig. 4.3 for an illustration of this stimulus) which appeared either to move steadily in one direction or (as a control) repeatedly to change direction. Adaptation would be expected to show up as a pattern of decreasing activation with prolonged movement of the plaid in one direction. This is exactly what happened in V5. As discussed in Chapter 4, plaid stimuli are in fact composed of two separate gratings. These slide over one another in orthogonal directions which sum algebraically to give the resultant direction of the apparent plaid. Huk and Heeger further showed that adaptation in V5 was specific to the apparent motion of the plaid, not to that of the gratings. As in the other experiments discussed above, these effects were strongest in V5, absent in V1 and intermediate in regions between the two. We may conclude, therefore, that V1 is not involved in the perception of apparent motion or motion after-effects; that V5 *is* involved in these percepts; and that the involvement of V5 corresponds to the subjective report (e.g. movement of a plaid, not two gratings) of what is consciously seen.

The same general story applies also to colour vision. In Chapter 10 I discussed at length our experiments (Nunn *et al.*, 2002) applying fMRI to the study of 'coloured hearing', in which synaesthetes see colours when they hear words. These subjects show activation of the colour-selective region of the visual system, variously known as V4 or V8, when they listen to words, with no accompanying activation in V1 or other areas lower down the visual pathway (see Plate 10.2). Notice that, in this experiment, since the words were presented by way of the auditory not the visual pathway, truly *no* V1 activity accompanied the synaesthetic experience of colour. Colours perceived in the normal way, in contrast, activate V4 *and* V1. Colour after-images (e.g. seeing a red after-image after gazing at a green patch) also activate V4, but V1 less so (Hadjikhani *et al.*, 1998). Thus the findings for veridical and illusory colour closely parallel those for veridical and illusory motion.

A further extension to this consistent pattern of results comes from an experiment by ffytche *et al.* (1998), who used fMRI to study a group of patients suffering from the 'Charles Bonnet syndrome'. This is a condition, occurring after sudden deterioration in normal vision (due to a detached retina or glaucoma, for example), in which the patient experiences vivid involuntary visual hallucinations. The content of the hallucinations differs from patient to patient. In this experiment, each patient described the hallucinatory experience and indicated its start and finish while lying in the MRI scanner. There was an excellent correlation between the content of the hallucinations and the region of the visual system activated. So, hallucinations of colour were accompanied by activity in area V4, in the fusiform gyrus; hallucinations of faces, by activity in a closely adjacent part of the fusiform gyrus known to be specialised for the perception of faces; and hallucinations of objects, by activity in a further region of the fusiform gyrus known to have *this* specialisation. In no case was there activity in V1. There was also no activity in the frontal cortex, supporting Zeki's hypothesis that activity in these specialised regions of the visual system is sufficient on its own to give rise to the appropriate conscious experience.

Experiments on visual imagery are not so consistent as the data on illusory percepts and visual after-effects. However, they give rise to the same general pattern of results. Imagined visual percepts are generally accompanied by activity in the visual area specialised for the visual feature imagined. So, imagined motion is accompanied by activity in V5 (Cohen *et al.*, 1996; Goebel *et al.*, 1998), as are veridical and illusory motion. Imagined faces and places are similarly each accompanied by activity in just those regions (in the fusiform gyrus and parahippocampal area, respectively) that are activated by direct perception of faces and places (O'Craven and Kanwisher, 2000). Imagined colours, however, seem to provide an exception to this rule. Nunn *et al.* (2002) saw no activity in the colour-selective part of the fusiform gyrus (V4) when their subjects imagined colours. Howard *et al.* (1998) did observe activity in the fusiform gyrus under these conditions, but it was located adjacent to, rather than actually in, the area activated by directly perceived colours. Activity was not detected in V1 in these studies, whether the imagery was of colour (Howard *et al.*, 1998; Nunn *et al.*, 2002) or motion (Cohen *et al.*, 1996; Goebel *et al.*, 1998). This neuroimaging difference between direct perception (V1 activated) and imagery (V1 inactive) finds parallels in a number of studies of patients with brain lesions in whom either direct perception is impaired while imagery is intact, or *vice versa*. However, there are a number of other neuroimaging studies in which V1 was clearly activated when subjects formed visual images of one kind or another (e.g. Chen *et al.*, 1998; Klein *et al.*, 2000). The critical conditions that determine whether visual imagery is or is not accompanied by V! activity await clarification. One possibility, suggested by Kosslyn *et al.*, 1995), is that VI activation occurs if what is imagined requires the high degree of spatial resolution of which only this region of the visual system is capable. However, whatever the ultimate resolution of this issue, it seems reasonable to conclude, as do Mellet *et al.* (1998, p. 137), that V1 activity is 'not mandatory for the visualization of an object or a scene'. And, even when such activity is observed during visual imagery, it is usually more intense during direct perception when this is measured in the same experiment.

The final brick in the wall that separates V1 from conscious experience has been laid in a study of a 'blindsight' patient, 'D. B.', by Larry Weiskrantz and his colleagues from Oxford. D. B. is now 61 years old. At the age of 33 he had surgery to remove a tumour from his brain, resulting in the loss of a large portion of primary visual cortex in the right hemisphere. As a result, he is blind to stimuli in the corresponding portion of his left visual field. Like a number of other such patients, however, he is able to perform significantly above chance when asked to guess at, or point to, stimuli in the affected part of the field (see Chapter 2), but he denies consciously experiencing them. This 'blindsight' is thought to be mediated by other pathways from the retina, not traversing V1 but travelling beneath the cerebral cortex.

Despite the lack of conscious experience of stimuli presented to the blind field, D.B does report conscious experience of after-images when the unseen stimulus in is turned off. Weiskrantz, who is known for his love of puns (it was he who first coined the term 'blindsight'), has named this effect 'prime-sight'. Weiskrantz, Cowey and Hodinott-Hill (2002) carried out a number of experiments to confirm D. B.'s reports of consciously perceived after-images. For example, they presented him with gratings in the blind field that could be either horizontally or vertically oriented. Sure enough, D. B. described his after-images as preserving the orientation in which the gratings had been presented, but usually with reversed contrast (dark for light and light for dark), as would be expected for 'negative' after-images. In other experiments, he reported appropriate colour after-images, even integrating them between the blind and seeing hemifields. So, for example, after looking at a white patch through a green filter covering the good hemifield and a red filter covering the blind one, he reported a dark blue after-image. Such an after-image would be expected if the red and green had been fused into yellow; but, at the time when the red and green stimuli were actually presented to D. B., he was consciously aware only of the green presented to the good hemifield (to which, on its own, the after-image should have been red).

Sometimes a single case studied with care is worth a dozen large experiments. This is an instance in point. D. B. has no V1 to receive stimuli in the blind field, yet these stimuli clearly contribute to his consciously perceived after-images. Similar results were reported by Kleiser *et al.* (2001) in an fMRI study of two other patients with partial V1 damage. Strong visual stimulation (with a high-contrast periodically reversing checkerboard) in the blind field gave rise to conscious visual experience (although weaker in quality than stimulation in the intact field), but without activation of any of the residual V1 tissue.

These results provide excellent support for the Crick and Koch hypothesis that activity in V1 is not necessary for visual awareness. Other strong support comes from fMRI studies of dreaming in normal subjects. Dreams are known to occur in a particular phase of sleep accompanied by rapid eye movements. Despite the strong visual experience likely to be occurring during this phase of sleep, activity in V1 is strongly suppressed, while other visual areas such as the fusiform gyrus are strongly activated. All in all, then, it is reasonable to take the Crick and Koch hypothesis as having been confirmed.

Yet this conclusion has the flavour of paradox. D. B. is, after all, *blind* to all conscious perception in the visual field corresponding to the damaged region of V1. So how can that region *not* be necessary for visual awareness? One response to this objection is to point out that damage to the eye or retina also causes blindness. Yet one does not therefore conclude that *retinal* activity is proximal to conscious experience. Just as the retina is the gateway by which visual stimuli reach the whole brain, so V1 acts as the general gateway by which these stimuli reach the remainder of the neocortex. There is no paradox, therefore, in supposing that only after passage through both these gates can visual stimulation enter, at some still higher point, into consciousness.

Activity in V1, then, is not necessary for visual awareness. Is it sufficient? Again the answer appears to be 'no'. Neuronal responses in V1 to visual stimuli are sensitive to a range of features that are absent from conscious visual perception; and, conversely, they are insensitive to other features of which one is normally conscious. Examples of both kinds of dissociation can be found in colour vision.

The human ability consciously to perceive flicker is much poorer for colour than it is for brightness. So, if two colours of equal brightness alternate with one another faster than about ten times a second, one sees, not two colours, but a single fused one. Monkeys, similarly, fail to discriminate between a steady yellow and alternating red and green (which fuse to give yellow), if the alternation takes place at a rate greater than about fifteen times a second. Gur and Snodderly (1997) recorded from 'colour-opponent' neurons in monkey V1; these are cells whose firing is increased by one wavelength of light (e.g. in the yellow region of the spectrum) but decreased by a complementary wavelength (e.g. in the blue region). These cells were able to follow colours flickering up to 60 times a second, firing in response to one but not the other colour. Thus V1 'knows' something about flickering colour of which conscious perception is ignorant.

Conversely, the colour one consciously perceives in a particular region of visual space is strongly modified by the wavelengths of light detected in neighbouring regions. It is this interaction between adjacent regions of visual space that permits computation of the enduring nature of surface reflectance (see Chapter 7). Neuronal firing in V4 (the colour-selective area) in the monkey brain shows this same interactive effect, but firing in V1 does not. In this case, then, conscious perception (and V4) has knowledge of colour that V1 lacks. Similar dissociations between the information available to V1 and to consciousness have been described for depth perception (Cumming and Parker, 1997) and the orientation of the bars of a grating (He, Cavanagh and Intriligator, 1996).

## 13.2   The frontal connection

Crick and Koch suggested that activity in V1 does not directly participate in the NCC for vision. This hypothesis is strongly supported by the data reviewed in the previous section. But the more general hypothesis from which it derives—that structures contribute to the NCC in virtue of their connections to the frontal cortex—is less clearly supported. In several of the relevant experiments, conscious perception was accompanied by activity in a specialised visual module (for colour, motion, etc.), but *not* by activity in the frontal cortex. These results fit better with Zeki's hypothesis that activity in the specialised module is sufficient for conscious experience of the visual feature coded there, without further need for activity in the frontal cortex (or anywhere else).

Recall, however, that Zeki's hypothesis does not require that, whenever a feature-specialised module is activated, conscious experience of the feature *must* ensue. In accordance with this *caveat*, a study of two patients with blindsight after damage to V1 demonstrated that visual motion (a rotating spiral) and coloured pictures of objects caused activity in V5 and V4, respectively, but with no reported awareness of these stimuli (Goebel *et al.*, 2001). Similar findings have been reported in patients who suffer from left-sided unilateral neglect after damage to right inferior parietal cortex. In such patients conscious perception of a stimulus in the left visual field is extinguished by another stimulus simultaneously presented in the right (see Chapter 15). Despite this loss of conscious perception, fMRI experiments (Rees, Wojciulik *et al.*, 2000; Vuilleumier *et al.*, 2001) have demonstrated activity in both primary visual cortex (V1) and higher visual modules appropriate to the extinguished stimuli (e.g. faces, houses) being presented. Activity in these modules appears, then, not to be sufficient for visual experience but, nonetheless, not to require additional activity in other regions.

A natural inference from this pattern of results is that activation of the specialised visual modules must reach a sufficient degree of intensity for conscious experience to occur. This possibility is supported by the findings of Moutoussis and Zeki (2002). They presented to each eye stimuli (faces or houses) that were of opposite colour contrast (e.g. red against a green background vs green against a red background), but otherwise identical. When viewed binocularly, these contrasting stimuli fuse and become invisible to conscious perception. Nonetheless, they continued to activate (in fMRI) just those areas of the fusiform gyrus which previous work (e.g. ffytche's study of patents with the Charles Bonnet syndrome, described above) had suggested to underlie the conscious perception of faces and houses respectively. Conscious perception of these stimuli (achieved by presenting to both eyes identical stimuli of the same colour contrast) was associated with activation in the same regions, but of greater intensity. Just such a role for the relationship between the degree of neural activity and conscious perception is predicted by Dennett's 'biggest kid on the block' hypothesis (see Chapter 11).

Strictly speaking, the Crick and Koch hypothesis is structural only. It specifies that an area responsible for the NCC should possess an anatomical projection to the frontal cortex. In agreement with this postulate, the various regions identified in the previous section as participating in the NCC for vision (V4, V5, etc.) do all project to the frontal cortex. But the existence of this anatomical connectivity does not entail that every conscious perception be accompanied *while it is in progress* by activity in the frontal cortex. In an equivalent distinction, one may propose (as indeed I did in Section 11.3) that consciousness permits manipulation by executive processes of its current contents, without thereby endorsing the hypothesis that these processes form a necessary part of the chain of events that actually create the contents of consciousness.

Indeed, it is not clear that current neuroimaging methods allow the latter hypothesis even to be tested. Suppose there is indeed a particular set, $S$, of neural executive processes responsible for the entry into consciousness of *any and all* of its contents. So, as well as activity in V4 determining the conscious experience of colour, activity in V5 determining the experience of motion, etc., there must invariably also be activity in system $S$. This is a modified form of the Cartesian Theatre hypothesis considered in Chapter 11. But how could we detect activity in

*S*? A neuroimaging experiment that detects, say, activity in V4 in response to coloured designs does so by comparing this activity with that elicited by black and white versions of the same designs. Thus, the contents of consciousness change as chromatic and achromatic designs alternate, and so does the area activated in the visual system (now V4, now elsewhere). But the subject of the experiment is always conscious of *something*, so *S* itself must always be active—and therefore undetectable by this method of comparison.

What, then, are we to make of the fact that, in many neuroimaging experiments, frontal lobe activity has nonetheless been detected in association with conscious experience? It seems likely that this activity reflects the particular kind of manipulation by executive processes (rehearsal in working memory, selective attention, preparation for delayed action, etc.) to which, in a given experimental paradigm, the contents of consciousness are subjected. Consistent with this view, the specific frontal region in which such activity has been detected varies considerably from experiment to experiment. No specific region has been found to be always active when and only when there is conscious visual perception, as required by the hypothesis that it serves the function of system *S*.

We are left, then, in a scientifically uncomfortable position. The hypothesis that there is a 'System *S*' in the frontal lobes (or indeed anywhere else) lacks empirical support from neuroimaging studies; but it also cannot be rejected, as activity in *S* might simply be undetectable. Now, the fact that a hypothesis is currently untestable does not mean that it is wrong. Of course, if there is no way even in principle to test it, then it falls outside science altogether. But it is too soon to come to this pessimistic conclusion. Instead, let us have recourse to other arguments, drawn from the phenomenology of conscious experience. Some of these arguments have been deployed already, in Section 11.3.

In particular, the automatic and involuntary nature of at least some conscious experiences argues strongly against a necessary role for executive functions of the kind mediated by the frontal lobes. A good example lies in the automatic (unbidden and unstoppable) experience of colour in response to words in coloured hearing synaesthesia (Chapter 10); another is the experience of illusory motion when one views the Enigma picture (Plate 13.1). I leave it to readers to supplement these examples, as I believe will be readily possible, with others of their own. Now, automaticity is exactly contrary to what takes place when one deliberately uses executive processes to manipulate the contents of consciousness, e.g. when doing mental arithmetic or rehearsing a telephone number, both operations that are accompanied by activity in the frontal lobes.

Executive functions are unlikely, then, to be a necessary or 'constitutive' component of conscious experience. But rejection of this hypothesis risks endorsement of its apparent polar opposite: that one perceives 'raw' sensory stimuli before they have undergone cognitive processing. The constructivist view of conscious perception adopted in this book (see Chapter 2)—that the brain simultaneously constructs and endows with meaning the world we perceive—is decidedly inhospitable to such a 'raw' alternative (though we shall find a more hospitable environment for it when we consider the bodily senses in Chapter 18). We need, therefore, to explore a middle ground, one that combines 'bottom-up' processing (from the sense organs inward) with 'top-down' processing (from cognitive construction outward) into a seamless whole. We look for that middle ground in the next chapter.

# CHAPTER 14

# Bottom-up vs top-down processing

The approaches to the neural basis of conscious experience considered in the three previous chapters sway between two seductive sirens: one calling down from the top, the other calling up from the bottom. Top-down processing emphasises executive functions located in the frontal lobes, as in the global neuronal workspace of Chapter 12; while bottom-up processing emphasises the posterior cortex modules which mediate the basic ingredients of perception, as in Zeki's hypothesis (Chapter 13). In this chapter we look at the possibility that both approaches are correct, but need to be combined in ways we have not yet considered.

## 14.1 Bottom-up and top-down combined

Some such combination of bottom-up and top-down processing is, in fact, central to the constructivist approach to perception and knowledge adopted at the outset of this book. An early proponent of this approach, Ulrich Neisser, described its application to vision (in his 1976 book, *Cognition and Reality*) as follows (p. 20):

> The cognitive structures crucial for vision are the anticipatory schemata that prepare
> the perceiver to accept certain kinds of information rather than others and thus
> control the activity of looking. Because we can see only what we know how to look
> for, it is these schemata (together with the information actually available) that
> determine what will be perceived.

Neisser's 'anticipatory schemata' represent top-down processing and his 'information actually available', the bottom-up kind.

Ray Jackendoff, in his important 1987 book, *Consciousness and the Computational Mind*, extended this analysis to all the senses to ask the question: what is the level at which informational structures enter consciousness? In his closely-argued answer to this question he arrives at an 'intermediate-level' theory of consciousness. This holds that the contents of consciousness reflect informational structures that are derived from a combination (within each sensory modality) of bottom-up and top-down processing. As he shows, one is not normally aware of sensation unaffected by conceptual interpretation, nor of pure conceptual structure, but only of an admixture of the two that optimises the fit between them. To test this proposition for yourself, try to experience a spoken word (any one will do) as either sound without meaning or meaning without sound. It is just possible with effort to achieve the former, by repeating the word over and over again (making of it a Buddhist-style mantra). But the ensuing loss of meaning ('semantic satiation') is incomplete and short-lived.

There are some apparent exceptions to Jackendoff's rule. Conceptual structure without much in the way of sensation occurs when you have a word 'on the tip of your tongue'. However, this may be one of those exceptions that prove the rule. Tip of the tongue feels as though the brain is busy searching for the missing qualia required to fill a conceptual frame. So it may offer a glimpse of the machinery that works to make Jackendoff's rule operative. Conversely, some sensations are devoid of much in the way of conceptual structure. The inner bodily senses, in particular, offer a number of such examples, as we shall see in Chapter 18.

Earlier in the book (Chapters 7 and 8) I outlined a 'comparator' hypothesis of the selection of the contents of consciousness. This hypothesis incorporates just such an optimised fit between bottom-up and top-down processing as is implied by Jackendoff's analysis. In line with Neisser's treatment of vision, it supposes that conscious percepts (in all sensory modalities) consist in the outputs of a process that compares (1) the 'information available' against (2) 'anticipatory schemata': i.e. (1) information proceeding upwards from the sense organs against (2) predictions as to what form, at this moment and under these circumstances, this information should take (see Fig. 7.1). Those items selected for entry into consciousness are either 'mismatches' from prediction (unpredicted events, or predicted but missing events) or they are 'matches' to predictions that are of particular importance for monitoring the progress of current motor programs. The medium in which these selected items are displayed—that of consciousness—is one that simulates in the constructed perceived world the enduring characteristics of the real (but not directly perceived) external world. For example, in colour vision, consciousness models surface reflectances (of inferred distal objects) rather than wavelengths of incident light (which is what impacts on the sense organ). This medium is multimodal, spatially extended in three dimensions and temporally sequential. (For a detailed account of the hypothesis, see Chapters 7 and 8.)

Note that the proposed comparator function is a hybrid between perceptual and executive processes. At the outset of Chapter 13, I described these processes as directly coding or manipulating information, respectively. So, in working memory, a telephone number (already coded into a form suitable for internal auditory rehearsal) is circulated around Baddeley's 'phonological loop'. But the proposed comparator *both* manipulates *and* directly codes. It manipulates information (sensory information from bottom up, and predictions from top down) in the comparison process, but it also codes that information into its final, consciously perceived form. Note also that the temporal sequence differs between these two types of executive function. In the working memory example, the formation of the conscious percept (the telephone number) precedes its manipulation by working memory (rehearsal of the number 'in the head'). In the comparator system, in contrast, the comparison process is completed prior to entry into consciousness of the final percept. As a further, and most important, distinction, in the working memory example the executive function is *separable* from the role played by conscious perception; thus, working memory can be applied either to conscious or to unconscious items of information. In contrast, the action of the comparator system is *constitutive* of the formation of a conscious percept: *ex hypothesi*, it is only by way of the comparator process that the percept becomes conscious (which is not to deny that other comparator processes play roles in the running of a host of other non-conscious processes).

## 14.2   The hippocampus

Where in the brain might these processes occur? Inherent in the comparator hypothesis is the notion of a negative feedback system. That is to say, the compara-tor seeks to minimise the discrepancies between a series of set-points (the predicted values of the sensory world) and a corresponding series of inputs (the actual values of the sensory world). Not surprisingly, then, the circuitry suggested by the com-parator hypothesis bears a family resemblance to the feed-back and re-entrant connections we met in Chapter 12, when we considered the notion of a 'global neuronal workspace'. But, whereas the various theorists contributing to that notion have emphasised the frontal cortex as the source of feedback, I emphasise the possible role played by a different region of the brain: the hippocampal system (Fig. 14.1). This system has a number of properties which fit it well for a role in the selection of the contents of consciousness, as envisaged in the comparator model.

### Hippocampal cell fields

Anatomically, the hippocampus is well-equipped to interact with the sensory systems of the neocortex. It receives projections from every one of these, via the entorhinal cortex in the temporal lobe (Fig. 14.2). These projections permit convergence between the different sensory modalities. Thus, many hippocampal neurons have multimodal 'fields'—that is, they fire in response to stimuli in more than one modality, or to multimodally presented combinations of such stimuli. But there is an important difference between these hippocampal fields and those encountered in the primary sensory pathways—for example, in the modules of the visual system. These have fixed fields. That is to say, for a given neuron the feature to which it is most respon-sive will always be the same. In V1, for example, the field for a given neuron might consist of an edge oriented in a particular direction in a particular region of visual space; in V4, it might similarly consist of a particular colour in a particular region of visual space. Hippocampal neurons, by contrast, show enormous flexibility.

These neurons fire in a huge diversity of experimental protocols, from running in a complex maze to sniffing odours or sitting motionless awaiting an air-puff to

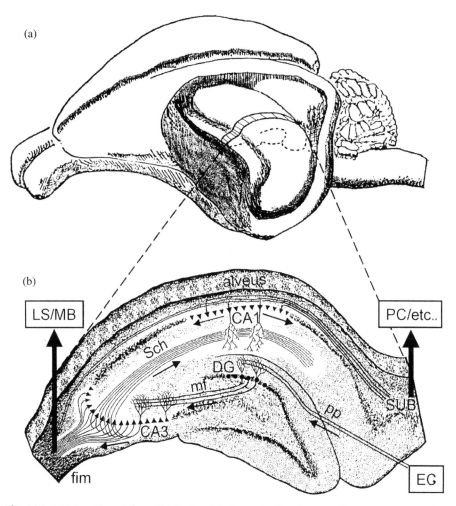

**Fig. 14.1** (a) Dissection of the rabbit brain with the parietal and temporal neocortex removed to expose the hippocampal formation. This shows a nominal lamellar slice through the middle of the hippocampus. (b) Such a slice contains essentially the same circuitry and cell types as the human hippocampus. Input from the medial and lateral entorhinal cortex (EC) enters in the medial and lateral perforant paths (pp), which synapse in middle and outer portions, respectively, of the dendrites of the dentate gyrus (DG) granule cells. These send mossy fibres (mf), which synapse on CA3 pyamidal cells. These, in turn, send output to the lateral septum (LS) and, via the Schaffer collaterals (Sch), to the CA1 pyramidal cells. Area CA1 sends a weak projection out via the alveus and fimbria (fim); and a stronger one to the subiculum (SUB), which in turn sends projections to areas such as the posterior cingulate cortex (PC) and, via the alveus and fimbria, to the mammillary bodies (MB). From Gray and McNaughton (2000).

the eye. This flexibility can be observed, moreover, in a single hippocampal cell. It is possible to impale on an electrode a neuron in the hippocampus of a conscious, behaving animal (most often, a laboratory rat), measure its field in one environment, and then rapidly move the animal to a novel environment. A number of scientists have performed this experiment. They observe that the neuron adopts a quite different field in the new surroundings. So, a cell that fires in response to a specific position in the spatially complex environment of an eight-arm maze may

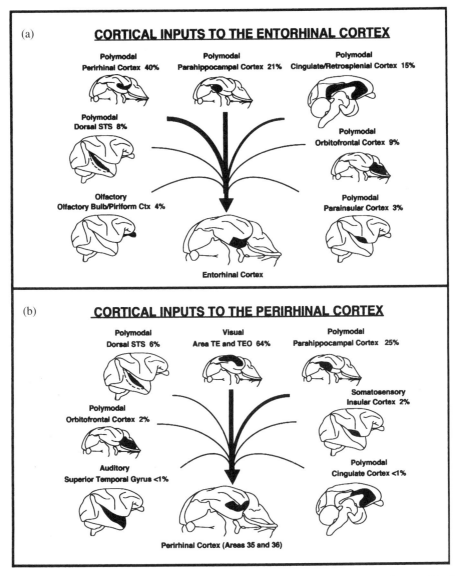

**Fig. 14.2** Cortical inputs to the entorhinal cortex (a) are largely relayed by the perirhinal (b) and parahippocampal (c) cortices. Density of connections is indicated by width of arrows. STS: superior temporal sulcus. TE, TEO, V4: eponymous areas of visual cortex. From Gray and McNaughton (2000).

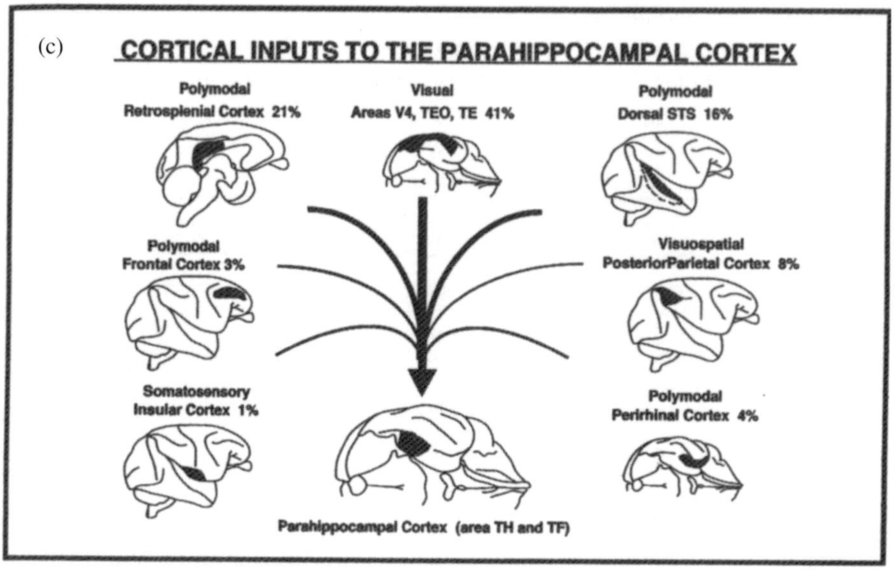

**Fig. 14.2** (*continued*)

also respond to a stimulus associated with the delivery of food in an enclosed box. Furthermore, the second response often occurs immediately the animal is placed into the second environment, so that little if any new learning can be involved. Nonetheless, if the experimenter builds in a particular, arbitrary regularity into the stimuli with which the animal is presented (e.g. in one context, a visually presented square indicates food on the left and a circle, water on the right; but, in a second context, the reverse associations hold), the fields he observes reflect that regularity, no manner what it happens to be. Cells will be found that respond to circles, to food on the left, to circles only in the first context, and so on. It is as though hippocampal neurons are always available for new representational duties. What these turn out to be depends upon the particular environment and the particular events that the animal finds to be of the greatest importance there. This is exactly the kind of flexibility and generality that one would expect of a structure that lies at the heart of a general-purpose comparator system. It is also exactly what conscious awareness feels like: the multimodal contents of consciousness change from moment to moment as either the environment or the attention and concerns of the perceiving subject change.

### Spatial mapping

Very often (so long as the experiment is conducted in a spatially extended environment), the observed hippocampal fields are best defined in spatial terms: as a particular region in the apparatus, or movement in a particular direction across that region. This kind of observation, together with the type of behavioural impairment seen after damage to the hippocampus, led to a theory, proposed in 1978 by John O'Keefe and Lynn Nadel, that the primary function of the hippocampus is to construct a spatial map of the environment. Experiments indicate that this map is generally independent of the momentary relationship of the animal to the places it maps—that is to say, it is a map of 'allocentric' (world-centred) rather than 'egocentric' (body-centred) space. (Use of the term 'map' should not mislead you into thinking that the brain contains a spatially arranged topographical analogue of the space one perceives, in the way, say, that a map of France provides an analogue of that country. The term implies only that there is a consistent 'mapping' between points in space and the firings of particular neurons, or distributed sets of neurons, somewhere or other in the brain. This *caveat* applies also to the later discussion of egocentric spaces.)

There is much controversy about the exact way in which allocentric and egocentric spaces differ, but these details do not affect the argument followed here. A simple example will, I hope, make the fundamentals of the distinction clear. Suppose you have just walked in London from Oxford Circus via Oxford Street, Bond Street and Piccadilly to Piccadilly Circus, and you need to make your way back to Oxford Circus. You might do so by recalling the landmarks you passed on the way and retracing your steps from landmark to landmark. That method relies upon your having learnt a series of steps in egocentric space. It requires that you recall how each landmark looked when you first saw it from one direction, and that you work out how it will look when you return to it from the reverse direction. If this is how you find your way about, you might take the additional precaution of turning round from time to time on the outward journey to see what the landmarks will look like on the return. Alternatively, you might build in your memory a map of the overall spatial relations between the places where you walked. In that case, you would realise that you can take the direct route from Piccadilly Circus to Oxford Circus along Regent Street, even though you did not traverse Regent Street at all on the outward path. In this case, you are using a map of allocentric space (as I did when I wrote these sentences in California, a long way from London). The construction and utilisation of allocentric maps depends critically upon the integrity of hippocampal function. In a recent, but already famous experiment, Eleanor Maguire and her colleagues showed that London taxi drivers, who of course have to do this sort of thing all the time and all over the city, even develop a larger hippocampus for the purpose! Conversely, damage to the hippocampus, in human beings as in the rat, dramatically impairs the ability to find your way around a spatially complex environment.

## Episodic memory

Spatial navigation is not the only important cognitive function in which the hippocampus plays a vital role. It does so also for so-called 'episodic' memory.

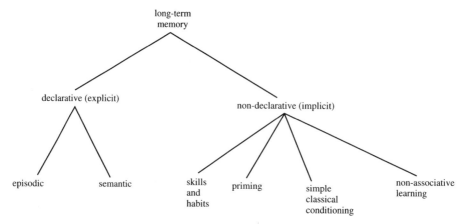

**Fig. 14.3** Classification of long-term memory. Declarative (explicit) memory refers to conscious recollection of events (episodic) and facts (semantic). Non-declarative (implicit) memory refers to a heterogeneous collection of abilities whereby experience alters behaviour non-consciously without providing access to any memory content. From Baddeley (2002).

Just as there are visual processes of which one is aware and others which fail to reach consciousness (Chapter 2), so there are conscious and unconscious processes of learning and memory. A first distinction between types of memory is that between 'short-term' and 'long-term' memory, spanning minutes or years respectively (these temporal indicators are not precise and, in any case, there are intermediate times at which both forms of memory operate in tandem). Working memory, briefly considered in Chapter 11, is a species of short-term memory. The hippocampus comes into play in long-term memory. A classification of suggested sub-species of this form of memory is presented in Fig. 14.3.

The unconscious learning of skills and habits (part of the 'implicit' right half of the tree in Fig. 14.3) is often termed 'procedural learning'. As an example, consider the task illustrated in Fig. 14.4. An asterisk moves erratically from one quadrant to another of a computer screen, and the subject has to follow it by sequentially touching, as fast as possible, the appropriate quadrants with a wand. The movements of the asterisk are sometimes completely random but sometimes follow a set of complex rules. These rules allow prediction of the quadrant to which the asterisk will move next. After a few trials the speed with which the subject touches successive quadrants comes faithfully to reflect the rules: touching the next predictable quadrant is faster than when movement of the asterisk is completely random. Clearly, then, the brain has learned the rules and stored them in memory. But, when questioned, the subject reveals no conscious awareness either of the rules or of the manner in which his behaviour follows them. So procedural memories are not available to conscious recall. In an example more familiar than this laboratory study, you can ride a bicycle because your brain has stored the behav-

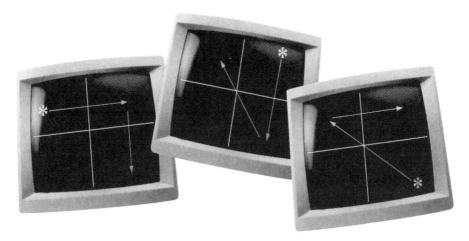

**Fig. 14.4** Method used to study procedural learning. Subjects were presented with a white target stimulus (an asterisk) on a black screen. This target moved between four locations on the screen, which was divided into four equal quadrants by two intersecting white lines. On random trials, movements of the target were completely unpredictable. On pattern trials, target movements were predictable for 75% of cases, i.e. determined following three specific rules: (1) a horizontal target movement was followed by a vertical target movement; (2) a vertical target movement was followed by a diagonal target movement; (3) a diagonal target movement was followed by a horizontal movement. The fourth movement of the target during the pattern trials was unpredictable. From Kumari *et al.* (2002).

ioural rules that keep you upright despite its wobblings. But try retrieving these rules into conscious memory! Another form of implicit learning is priming, in which a stimulus can alter the subsequent response to other stimuli in the complete absence of awareness of its occurrence. We saw an example of this in Marcel's experiments on masked semantic priming (Section 9.3).

The memories termed 'explicit' or 'declarative' (the left half of the tree in Fig. 14.3) are, by contrast, available for conscious recall. Declarative memory is itself broken down into 'semantic' and 'episodic' memory. Semantic memory is memory for facts without explicit recall of a time, place or other autobiographical associations with the occasion on which you acquired the facts. So, to correctly answer the question, 'What is the colour of a ripe banana?', you clearly need to remember something about bananas, and you are clearly conscious of the question and how you reply to it. But you need not (and probably won't) recall a specific occasion on which you bit into a ripe banana, with details of the time, place and circumstances all coming back in an act of conscious recollection. Suppose, however, that I ask you instead, 'What did you have for breakfast today (or last week, or on the day of the murder)?', and you happen to have had a banana. Now you will probably recall that specific episode, with the banana situated pretty firmly into a framework of time, space and general context. This is episodic memory. It is episodic memory that allows you to call to mind last year's summer holiday. It allows me to recall Oxford, magical one winter decades ago with snow so deep that no traffic could move, or Chekhov's *Cherry Orchard* immaculately performed by the Moscow Arts Theatre when I was in my early twenties.

This distinction between the two different kinds of conscious (explicit) memory, has been strongly emphasised by the Canadian psychologist, Endel Tulving since the 1970s (see his retrospective account, published in 2002), but it has only recently attained clear empirical support. This support has come from a variety of experimental paradigms. In one of these, subjects are first asked whether they recognise a series of items, of which they have encountered some but not others before. They are then asked to make a further judgement as to whether they 'remember' a recognised item, in that they have a clear recollection of the circumstances under which it was previously encountered, or merely 'know' that they have encountered it before. It turns out that subjects can make this distinction readily, and in a manner that varies predictably with experimental conditions. I doubt that you will have any difficulty in verifying the distinction from your own experience.

Our lives are enormously enriched by episodic memories—so much so, that it is difficult to imagine life without them. Yet this is just what befalls someone unfortunate enough to sustain bilateral damage to the hippocampus. Such patients become densely amnesic. They no longer form new episodic memories, and also lose access to many (but not all) of their previously stored episodic memories.

It is now generally agreed that the hippocampus does not itself store these memories. The site of storage most likely lies in the temporal lobes of the neocortex, and the storage itself probably takes the form of a changed pattern of connectivity between widely distributed sets of neurons. The hippocampus appears to interact with these neocortical storage sites both when the memory is first laid down ('encoded') and when it is 'retrieved' into consciousness. In agreement with this view, a number of recent neuroimaging studies have demonstrated hippocampal activation when materials, including for example words, pictures, objects or faces, are presented for commitment to memory, or when they are subsequently retrieved from memory. A key factor determining this hippocampal activation is the novelty of what has to be remembered: the greater the novelty, the greater is the degree of hippocampal activation. This pattern of findings is consistent with the comparator hypothesis of hippocampal function. This postulates that the hippocampus is activated proportionately to the degree of mismatch between events and the comparator's prediction (based on past regularities of experience in similar contexts) as to what those events should be. Novel events are therefore expected to activate the hippocampus more strongly than familiar ones.

A clear demonstration of the role played in the retrieval of memories by the hippocampus comes from an experiment with marmosets (a New World primate species), conducted by David Virley and Helen Hodges in my laboratory. The animals were first trained on a series of conditional discriminations. In these, for one pair of identical objects, reward is obtained for choosing the one on the left but, for another, the correct choice is the one on the right. After training was complete, a lesion was placed in the hippocampus, after which the animal was no longer able to perform the discriminations, nor learn new ones. Human amnesics with hippocampal damage show a similar inability to solve this kind of discrimination task. In the final stage of the experiment we transplanted into the damaged hippocampus a line of neural stem cells, developed by our group, which have the remarkable capacity to repopulate and effectively reconstitute the damaged region. A couple of months later the marmosets were tested again, and at once showed good recall of the discriminations that they had learned at the start of the experiment, before the damage to the hippocampus was made. From these results one can conclude that, even during the period of amnesia, the forgotten memories were intact, but inaccessible; and that restitution of the hippocampus provided anew the means to access them.

Most amnesic patients with hippocampal damage have sustained damage also to wider regions of the temporal lobes, in which the hippocampus is situated. Most such patients also display profound impairment in semantic memory as well as episodic memory. Indeed, there is a nearly ubiquitous overlap between impairments in the one and in the other, to the extent that the general view has been that there is but one declarative memory system (Fig. 14.3), but that this manifests itself in two ways, as episodic and semantic memory.

Recently, however, this view has been radically challenged by a report from Faraneh Vargha-Khadem and her colleagues, based upon three unfortunate individuals who suffered damage confined almost totally to the hippocampus and at a very early age (at birth, 4 and 9 years old). These patients are all poorly oriented in place or time, they cannot provide a reliable account of what they have done during the day, they cannot reliably remember messages, visitors and so on. So disabling are these impairments that none of the three can be left alone for any extended period, let alone hold down a job or lead an independent life. Yet, despite the crippling effects of this loss of *episodic* memory, all three of these patients were able to complete school (at the time of testing they were in their 'teens or early twenties) and had scores in the normal range on a variety of tests of information and comprehension. These tests covered facts that they must have learnt after they had sustained the damage to the hippocampus and while their episodic memory for the events of the day (as recounted by their families) was essentially absent. Thus, these patients offer very strong evidence (1) that episodic memory is separate from semantic memory and (2) that it is mediated specifically by the hippocampus.

A further study of one of these patients, Jon, by Eleanor Maguire clearly brings out the contrast between conscious recollection and knowledge of the past, but without such specific conscious recollection. Although Jon had sustained considerable damage to the hippocampus, his residual hippocampal tissue was nonetheless capable of activation as detected by fMRI. In previous work with normal subjects Maguire's group had demonstrated hippocampal activation, particularly in the left hemisphere, during the recall of autobiographical events (that is, events described by the subject as having happened to them personally at some time in the past), as compared to the recall of public events occurring at approximately the same epoch. Despite his generally poor episodic memory, Jon was able to remember a sufficient number of autobiographical events for Maguire to test him in the same experimental paradigm, but with an extra twist. It turned out that Jon spontaneously distinguished between events from his past that he could truly recall and those that he knew about but could not call to mind. This, of course, is the general distinction between remembering and merely knowing which, as noted earlier, is one of the marks of distinction between episodic and semantic memory. The fMRI results showed activation in Jon's hippocampus when he recalled events that he truly remembered, but not when he recalled events that he just knew about. This is good evidence that the hippocampus is involved in the specifically conscious recollection that occurs during the retrieval of episodic memories. This inference is potentially limited by its dependence on data obtained from a patient with a damaged brain. However, the hippocampus was also activated in normal subjects in an fMRI study of remember/know judgements reported by Laura Eldridge and her colleagues. This activation occurred selectively when subjects judged that they had 'remembered' recognised items as compared to just 'knowing' them.

## A common hippocampal computational function?

The hippocampus, then, discharges two major, apparently distinct functions: one in spatial learning and navigation; the other in episodic memory. It would be parsimonious to attribute both to a common underlying computational core. Neil McNaughton and I have proposed that this common core can be found in the comparator function.

Recall (Chapters 7 and 8) that a key output of the comparator system is the detection of error. This may take two forms: something unpredicted may occur; or something predicted may fail to occur. In either case, the system must now move on to correct the predictive circuitry which gave rise to the error. The most general way in which such correction is likely to work is by *contextual disambiguation*. The comparator's predictive circuitry relies upon stored regularities in the subject's previous experience and similarities between relevant past and current conditions. Thus, the faulty prediction is unlikely, in most circumstances, simply to be wrong. Rather, it is likely to be right, but under somewhat different conditions. Nor is it likely to be advantageous simply to delete the circuits that led to the faulty prediction, since the conditions under which that prediction is in fact correct may well recur. In line with this argument, it is generally true that the brain never unlearns anything; it simply stacks up new learning alongside the old—but with each item 'tagged', as it were, as to the right time and/or place and/or circumstances for which it is most appropriate. It is just these kinds of context-rich associations which distinguish the conscious, episodic form of memory from others. Semantic memory, in contrast, is typically memory for what is generally true. To remember that 'Paris was the capital of France on Tuesday last week when the sun was shining' would be idiosyncratic and not particularly helpful.

A further part of the functions of the comparator system, then, is to provide this kind of contextual tagging.

Consider how this might work in the case of retrieval of a conscious memory. Let's take a subject in a paired associate learning experiment. Let's say the subject has been learning three successive lists of pairs of words, in each of which the word 'hook' acted as a cue, first followed by 'money', then by 'ram' and finally by 'Harry'. His task now is to respond to 'hook' by the most recent associate he has learned—'Harry'. It is almost certain that, when he hears 'hook', there will be some degree of activation of all three of the paired associates learned over the three successive lists, not to mention pre-existing associates of 'hook' such as 'nail', 'clasp' or 'cook'. Amid all this confusion, the subject (or rather his brain) has to prefer 'Harry' to all these competitors; and to do so under the contextual description 'third list in this experiment in this laboratory room on this day' (all themselves located within a still more general contextual framework). This is just the kind of task on which patients with damage to the hippocampus fail badly. What McNaughton and I have proposed (see Fig. 14.5 for a more detailed account) is that this process is achieved by way of recursive interactions between the hippocampus and the regions of the temporal lobe in which each of the competing associations are stored. The outcome of these interactions is the utterance of one among the set of possible responses to the cue word, 'hook'. If this is correct, all well and good; if it is incorrect, there is a further round of interaction between the hippocampus and the temporal lobe storage sites, modifying the synaptic connections until the correct response becomes, in this context, dominant. In patients with hippocampal damage, correct recall is often impossible and, in accordance with our theoretical model, the errors made often take the form of intrusions from previous lists or earlier.

A similar analysis can be applied to spatial navigation. Here the problem is to move in a direction which will take you, in a spatially complex environment, from point A, where you are now located, towards point B, where you hope to arrive. But the very nature of space is such that, when you have been at point A before, you are likely to have headed off in many other directions and with many other goals besides B. So, just as in the case of memory, a means is required which will choose between alternative possible actions according to the current contextual demands, and update storage if the choice made proves to be wrong. To this same general problem, then, the same general solution can be provided, only now the

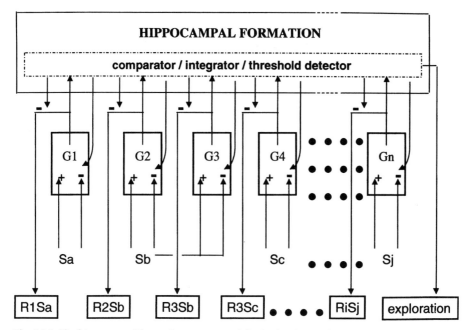

**Fig. 14.5** The hippocampal formation as a general device for the resolution of goal conflict. A goal is defined as a particular combination of environmental stimulus (S) and response tendency (R). Often, two goals will differ in both of these attributes (R1Sa versus R3Sb), e.g. in an experiment with rats, a goal box which elicits both approach (because of a prior association with food) and avoidance (because of a prior association with shock). Likewise, some responses can be addressed to more than one stimulus (R3Sb versus R3Sc), as in the case of a lever-press response which may be elicited by either a left or a right lever (or both) depending on the prior history of reinforcement. Any stimulus (e.g. Sa) is held to activate a particular goal (G1) defined by the conjunction of that stimulus and a particular response (R1Sa). The strength of activation is determined by integration of the prior affectively positive (+) and affectively negative (-) associations of that goal. In many cases, the goal (say G1) will be the only one with sufficient net activation to produce a response; or, if another goal is activated, it will nonetheless be the clear winner. In this case the response (R1) is directed to the relevant stimulus (Sa). The hippocampal formation will receive an efference copy of the output from G1, but in this case will not react. Conflict is defined as the case when two or more goals (e.g. G1 and G2) are highly and nearly equally activated. The hippocampus as a comparator determines the degree of conflict; and, the greater this is, the greater will be the hippocampal output. This output has two effects. First, it blocks the output from the areas defining the goals (e.g. G1, G2) to the areas responsible for achieving them (R1Sa, R2Sb). Second, it increases the value of any affectively negative associations (including, in human beings, inferences) specific to these goals. In many cases this will allow resolution of the conflict in favour of that goal which has the lesser negative associations. Output from the hippocampus is increased, recursively, until conflict is resolved. At the same time, exploratory behaviour is commanded. This can add information (either devaluing existing negative information, or providing new negative information) to help in the process of conflict resolution. From Gray and McNaughton (2000).

hippocampus needs to interact, not with the storage sites for episodic memories in the temporal lobes, but with motor programs run in the frontal cortex and basal ganglia. Fortunately, the hippocampus is equipped with connections to these regions, just as it is with connections to the temporal lobes, permitting it to do both jobs.

Indeed, our general hypothesis has the hippocampus interacting in this way with a number of other brain regions, to which it is again anatomically connected, in relation to a number of other psychological functions. Among these, we have paid particular attention to behaviour under conditions of conflict and threat and to the accompanying emotional state of anxiety. There is strong evidence that the hippocampal system plays a key role in this emotion, and in mediating the anti-anxiety effects of drugs such as Valium or Librium. Now, the neuronal architecture of the hippocampus is relatively simple and homogeneous throughout its extent. Given this anatomical simplicity, it would be unsatisfactory to attribute to the hippocampus three seemingly disparate psychological functions, spatial navigation, episodic memory and anxiety, in each of which it is clearly implicated by the experimental evidence. Thus we see it as a great advantage of our approach that we are able to account for this diversity of hippocampal psychological involvement in terms of one underlying computational function, as outlined in Fig. 14.5.

## 14.3   Hippocampal function and consciousness

The evidence reviewed in the previous section strongly implicates the hippo-campus in the encoding and retrieval of conscious, context-rich (episodic) memories. But the comparator hypothesis of consciousness goes further than this. It claims that, in addition to its role in episodic memory, the hippocampal system acts to select the contents of consciousness in the first place. This stronger hypothesis can draw upon a number of arguments in its favour.

First, as noted above, the firing repertoires of neurons recorded in the hippo-campus are sensitive to all sensory modalities and combinations thereof; and they are flexibly allocated to different fields in different environments. In this respect, hippocampal neurons mirror the rapidly changing and flexible contents of consciousness. I know of no other brain structure of which this can be said.

Second, the role played by the hippocampus in the construction of a 'map' of allocentric space may have a deeper significance than our discussion has yet revealed. Conscious experience is almost invariably situated in a stable three-dimensional spatial frame. It would not be surprising, then, if the final touch to each multimodal scene that enters conscious awareness were to come from a system capable of placing its varied components into a unified and unifying allo-centric spatial frame. This is just what the hippocampus appears to do. Recall, also, the suggestion (Section 7.3) that conscious perception differs from unconscious sensorimotor action in that it models the semi-permanent features of the external world. The appropriate spatial framework, since it too is relatively permanent, into which to slot such features is clearly allo- rather than ego-centric. The use by conscious experience of an allocentric spatial frame has yet another potential significance, pointed out by Chris Frith. 'Of all the representations held in the brain, that which is coded in non-egocentric coordinates will most closely resemble that held in the brain of another. It is these representations that will best enable prediction of the behaviour of another creature in the current situation' (Frith, 1995, p. 683). Representations which, in this way, are shared between human beings provide an essential basis for the development of language (see the earlier discussion in Section 9.2). (Frith would like to take this argument further and—echoing a hypothesis proposed earlier by Nicholas Humphrey in his book *Consciousness Regained*—infer that conscious experience and its underlying neural machinery evolved *because* it provides these social advantages; but this does not follow.)

Third, the hippocampus is equipped with anatomical connections to the critical sensory systems of the posterior neocortex whose outputs make up the contents of consciousness. These connections would allow it to interact with sensory systems in the same general way in which it interacts with memory storage sites in the temporal lobe and motor programming circuits in the basal ganglia and

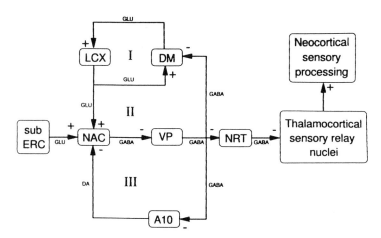

**Fig. 14.6** Connections from the subiculum (sub) and entorhinal cortex (ERC) to the nucleus accumbens (NAC) component of the motor system, and from that system to the nucleus reticularis thalami (NRT) and thalamocortical sensory pathways. LCX: limbic cortex, including prefrontal and cingulate areas. DM: dorsomedial thalamic nucleus. VP: ventral pallidum. A10: dopaminergic nucleus A10 in the ventral tegmental area. GLU, GABA and DA: the neurotransmitters glutamate, gamma-aminobutyric acid and dopamine. +, –: excitation and inhibition. I, II, III: feedback loops, the first two positive, the third negative. From Gray (1995).

frontal cortex. As noted above, the hippocampus receives input from all sensory modalities by way of projections from the entorhinal cortex in the temporal lobes (Fig. 14.2). There are at least two routes which might then be used for the reverse traffic. One is by way of return projections to the regions in the temporal lobe which send sensory information to the hippocampus. A second, more indirect, route is illustrated and described in Fig. 14.6.

Fourth, as noted above, there is good evidence that the hippocampus is responsible for the retrieval into conscious recall of episodic memories. Almost certainly, these can be recalled consciously only if they entered consciousness in the first place. It would be a parsimonious use of brain systems if the same structure that controls the storage and subsequent reactivation of a conscious scene into memory also played a role in the initial conscious perception of the scene. Consistent with this view, David Gaffan has demonstrated in monkeys that damage to the hippocampal system produces marked impairments in learning to pick out an object located in a particular place within a complex visual scene. However, it is impossible from these experiments to determine whether these impairments are due to a failure of learning, memory or the initial perception of the scene.

Fifth, conscious experience has temporal as well as spatial structure. To be sure, it is impossible to state just when one 'moment' of conscious experience ends and another begins. But events in consciousness nonetheless appear to occur in a definite temporal sequence. Within a brief time interval, however, temporal succession breaks down, and it becomes impossible to detect the order in which two events occur. The minimum inter-event interval over which temporal succession can be reliably detected is, broadly, of the order of a tenth of a second. Thus we might expect a system responsible for the final 'delivery' of the contents of consciousness to show signs of periodicity of functioning over time intervals of this duration. Note that oscillations in the firing rates of neurons in the 'gamma' range of frequencies (the famous '40-Hz' rhythm emphasised by Wolf Singer and others), and the similar waves that can be recorded in the human EEG, recur at intervals of approximately 25 milliseconds (see Section 16.5). Thus, despite their popularity in contemporary discussions of the neural basis of consciousness, gamma waves are too fast to parse successive moments of conscious experience.

In contrast, in both neuronal firing repertoires and the hippocampal EEG, there are prominent oscillations in the 'theta' range, that is, around 6–12 Hz (cycles per second) in the rat and 3–8 Hz in human beings. These waves appear to play a functional role in the gating of the passage of neuronal messages around the hippocampal circuitry: messages pass through more easily when the theta wave is in one phase rather than another. Such an arrangement implies a temporal parsing of successive outputs from the hippocampus at intervals of approximately 100–200 milliseconds, consistent with the apparent temporal structure of conscious experience. Theta waves are present also in other brain structures. However, in these structures they occur when the structure is relatively inactive. Only in the hippocampal system do they occur when, as shown by other experimental evidence, the structure is actively performing its normal functions. Other evidence that the hippocampus plays a role in temporal sequencing comes from a study by Andrew Mayes and his colleagues of a single patient ('Y. R.') with extensive loss of the hippocampus but little other brain damage. Y. R. was able to learn two lists of words as well as normal controls, but was severely impaired at discriminating the order in which the lists had occurred.

I am much taken by these arguments. This is not surprising. After all, the hypothesis that the hippocampus acts as a comparator, and that the contents of consciousness consist in its outputs, is my own. However, I am not fully persuaded. Here are some reasons for scepticism.

After damage to the hippocampal system severe enough to give rise to dense amnesia—complete loss of episodic memory plus much else besides—patients do not, as my hypothesis might predict, give the impression of a consciousness without contents. The most striking evidence against this prediction comes from a study, by Robert Stickgold and his colleagues in Boston, of hypnagogic imagery in a group of amnesic patients with hippocampal damage.

Stickgold had these patients and normal controls play a computer game called *Tetris*. This involves the rapid manipulation into desired arrays of 'play pieces' as these fall continuously and at increasing speed from the top to the bottom of the computer screen. The heroic subjects played this game for a couple of hours each day, slept wearing a kind of elaborate metal hair-net through which the EEG could be recorded to determine when they fell asleep, were repeatedly woken up as they were on the verge of falling asleep and throughout the first hour of actual sleep, and were asked to report any imagery they were then experiencing. By the second night the majority (3 out of 5 patients as compared to 9/12 controls) reported strong imagery of seeing *Tetris* pieces 'kind of float down and fit into the other pieces', as one subject put it. This is the expected hypnagogic imagery. The amnesic subjects improved their game, although much more slowly than the controls, but on each occasion denied ever having seen it before—the standard amnesic dissociation between unconscious procedural learning (intact) and conscious episodic memory (lost). The striking new finding was that the amnesics reported just as much *Tetris* imagery, and of the same kind, as the controls. Hypnagogic imagery is, by any standards, a conscious experience. So here we have people with no hippocampus and the dense amnesia that goes along with its loss, but conscious experience that in no way appears to differ from that of controls. The most likely site of the neural correlate of this imagery is in one or other of the modules of the ventral stream of the visual system. So the result of this experiment fits alongside the other work, reviewed in Chapter 13, suggesting that activity in these modules is by itself sufficient for the occurrence of conscious visual experience. On this view, there is no need for a further structure to select the contents of consciousness, and the comparator hypothesis would be supererogatory.

There is, however, an alternative prediction that can be derived from the comparator hypothesis: that damage to the hippocampus would not eliminate the contents of consciousness as such, but rather give rise to a consciousness that staggers chaotically from one randomly selected content to the next. Oddly, this second outcome does occur, but in acutely ill schizophrenics. These patients too have damage to the hippocampus (but to many other brain regions as well), and they suffer from memory deficits. Their hippocampal damage falls far short of the degree needed totally to destroy episodic memory. Nonetheless, it is possible to apply the comparator model to schizophrenia.

The resulting theory proposes that the comparator is present in the schizophrenic brain but that it malfunctions, owing to anatomical disconnections between some of its components. In particular, the theory proposes that the malfunctioning system tends to compute 'novelty' when in fact the relevant stimuli are familiar. Because novel stimuli capture attention, one can account in this way for many of the bizarre symptoms displayed by schizophrenic patients, including for example their tendency to move disjointedly from one fragmentary, disconnected thought or percept to the next. We have tested this model in an extensive programme of experimental research and verified many of its predictions (see my review in *Schizophrenia Bulletin*, 1998). In the light of this evidence, it is reasonable to retain the hypothesis, at least for heuristic purposes, that the hippocampus discharges the functions of a comparator system, and that partial damage to this system is able to disrupt selection of the contents of consciousness. But it remains the case that, in patients with much greater damage to the hippocampus and with total loss of episodic memory, conscious experience seems to persist and to remain orderly (despite its no doubt being impoverished). This fact inclines me to accept that there must be additional areas responsible for the selection of the contents of consciousness, besides the hippocampus.

It may be, however, that the additional areas are closely linked with the hippocampus. Inclusion of such areas would not necessarily constitute a change in the comparator model, as McNaughton and I have in any case defined the hippocampal system as all those regions that display the hippocampal theta rhythm. This definition includes a quite wide range of additional structures, though all are closely related anatomically to the hippocampus. The possibility that our model might be saved in this way is suggested by Barbara Wilson's detailed study of a dramatic single patient: Clive Wearing.

Clive was a highly talented and successful professional musician who contracted herpex simplex encephalitis. As a result, he suffered massive damage not only to the hippocampus, but also to a whole series of other structures in the temporal lobes (there was bilateral damage to the hippocampal formation, the amygdala, the substantia innominata and the temporal pole; and, in the left hemisphere, to the fornix, the inferior temporal gyrus, the anterior portion of the superior temporal gyrus and the insula). Clive has extremely severe amnesia for both events that preceded the onset of his illness and those that came after. However, his musical skills remain extraordinarily intact, and he is still capable of reading and playing music and conducting a choir. He has fluent, well-articulated speech and writing, and is even still able to translate from Latin to English. So far, then, his condition fits the usual pattern of impaired memory (especially episodic memory) but preserved intelligence after temporal lobe lesions.

It is Clive's own description of his condition that is remarkable. He feels constantly that he has 'just woken up' and keeps a diary in which this feeling is repeatedly recorded, at intervals of hours or even minutes. Upon so 'waking up', he regularly remarks upon the absence of conscious experience in the preceding period, and the sudden re-emergence of conscious experience in the present moment. 'I have been blind, deaf, and dumb for so long'; 'suddenly, I can see in colour'; 'I can hear traffic sounds now'; 'today is the first time I've actually been conscious of anything at all'; 'none of my senses are working at all'; 'I have no sense of taste'; 'I have no sense of touch or smell'; 'it's like being dead' (this particular remark is repeated many times). Clearly, Clive has consciousness in the sense that he's not in a coma. Clearly, too, he retains enough normal consciousness to be able, from time to time and fleetingly, to comment upon the loss of the contents of his consciousness during the periods between his 'wakings up'. But, if we take him at his word, he has suffered a remarkable encroachment upon the normal continuous richness of conscious experience. In Wilson's words:

> Clive was not able to retain impressions for more than the briefest moment. The effect was of course that the environment appeared to be in a state of flux. On many occasions he would comment, 'You weren't wearing blue just now. No, no, it was yellow or pink but it certainly wasn't blue'. In response to the constantly new appearance of the room Clive would keep asking, 'How do they do that?'. One day he put this phenomenon to the test. He held a chocolate in one hand and repeatedly covered and uncovered it with the other. He could feel that the chocolate never moved, yet each time he uncovered it, it appeared to be a new chocolate, however quickly he looked.

These phenomena fit remarkably well with what one would expect from the loss of the comparator system. Either nothing is selected for the contents of consciousness, or what is selected remains determinedly novel and out of context. So perhaps the comparator hypothesis is, after all, on the right lines, but the system takes up a great deal more neuronal space than just the hippocampus.

# CHAPTER 15

# Egocentric space and the parietal lobes

In the previous chapter I emphasised the importance of an allocentric, or world-centred, spatial frame for conscious experience; and this was one reason for concentrating so heavily on the hippocampus. However, there is another kind of spatial frame—egocentric, or body-centred, space—that is also intimately related to conscious experience. This frame is computed, not in the hippocampus, but in a neocortical region—the parietal lobes (Fig. 15.1).

## 15.1   Spatial neglect

We have come across this region before. It is lesions in the parietal cortex, most often right-sided, that give rise to the syndrome of unilateral spatial neglect. We have also come across the neglect syndrome before, as well as its significance for discussions of consciousness. Zeki's hypothesis (Chapter 13), for example, that activity in a specialised visual perception module is both necessary and sufficient for conscious experience, needs to be stated carefully in the light of studies of neglect patients who failed consciously to see stimuli (houses or faces) presented to their left field of view, despite the fact that fMRI detected activity in the appropriate visual modules on the damaged right side of the brain.

In the neglect syndrome, the patient lacks awareness for sensory stimuli in the region of space contralateral (usually the left) to the lesion. Neglect patients often behave as if only the right half of their world exists. They may shave only the right side of the face, eat from only the right side of the plate, dress only the right side of the body, read only the right side of the page, and so on. In formal tests, given a straight line to bisect, they mark the middle at a point three-quarters of the way over to the right, as though the left half of the line is missing (Fig. 15.2); or they copy only the right side of a drawing (Fig. 15.3). Their problems affect all the senses: vision, hearing, touch, proprioception (that is, perception 'from the inside' of the position and state of one's own limbs), even smell. Imagery, too, is affected in the same way. When asked to imagine a familiar scene, the patient may for example report only details to the right of the imagined point of view. The neglect syndrome has been the object of considerable clinical and experimental investigation. The details of these studies and their results are highly complex. But they give

(a)

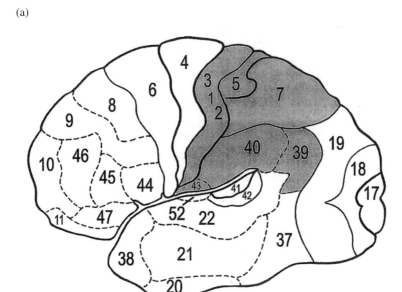

(b)

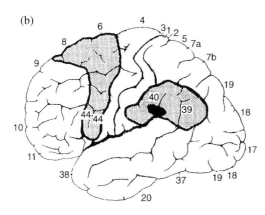

**Fig. 15.1 (a)** Left lateral view of the human brain showing Brodmann's cortical areas. The parietal areas are shaded. (b) The syndrome of spatial hemineglect: anatomical correlates (grey areas). In the majority of patients the lesion involves the supramarginal gyrus in the inferior parietal lobule, at the temporoparietal junction (black area). Neglect after frontal damage is much less frequent and is usually associated with dorsolateral lesions of the premotor cortex. From Burgess *et al.* (1999).

rise to a reasonably clear and consistent understanding of the nature of the fundamental cognitive impairment that affects these patients.

The common site of damage that gives rise to the neglect syndrome lies in the supramarginal gyrus within the inferior parietal lobule, usually in the right hemisphere, at the junction between the temporal and parietal lobes (Fig. 15.1). And the common cognitive impairment that underlies the diverse symptoms of neglect consists in a disruption of the brain's ability to form a map of egocentric space. Since the sensory and motor systems of the brain are predominantly 'crossed'— that is, the left side of the brain deals with the right side of the world and *vice versa*—a right-sided disruption in the brain's map of egocentric space affects the left

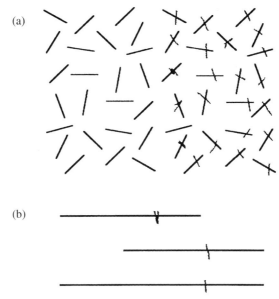

**Fig. 15.2** Examples of deficits found in patients with left spatial neglect on typical clinical tasks. (a) Line cancellation task. Patients have to mark each of many small lines that are spread out on a sheet of paper presented in front of them. Typically the patient fails to detect some lines on the contra-lesional side, even when given considerable time to complete the task. (b) Line bisection task. The patient is asked to mark the mid-point of long horizontal lines but deviates towards the right ipsi-lesional side, as if neglecting the left contra-lesional extent. Such an ipsi-lesional bias is often greater when the lines are positioned more to the left side. It can be partly alleviated when the patient is cued to the contra-lesional end of the line, for instance, by reporting a letter there. From Driver and Vuilleumier (2001).

side of the patient's world. The 'left' side of your world is, of course, 'egocentric' by definition: it changes as you change position.

In fact the brain computes many kinds of egocentric space. These include space relative to the position of the trunk, the limbs, the head, and even the eyeballs within their orbits. Each of these various 'spaces' is essential for one or other kind of action: reaching out, grasping, fixing the eyes on a moving target, and so on. Recordings from neurons in the monkey brain indicate that various regions within the parietal lobe play critical roles in the computation of these different kinds of space. The different spaces need also to be placed in register with one another. Consider, for example, the spatial computations required if you are leaning down towards the left, with your head and eyes swivelled upwards and to the right, trying to make a back-hand return of a tennis ball coming in fast across the court. Co-registration of this kind appears also to be achieved by communication from region to region within the parietal lobes. As in the tennis example, these kinds of computation are essential for the visual guidance of rapid action (but not only visual guidance: important additional contributions come from the vestibular sense of balance, proprioception, and so on). However, as we saw in Chapter 2, this kind of action is carried out with little contribution from, and results in still less entry into, conscious experience. Furthermore, the computations of each of these relatively specific egocentric spaces are conducted, not in the inferior parietal lobule in which damage causes neglect, but in the adjacent superior parietal lobule (see Fig. 15.1).

The correct co-registration of the various forms of egocentric space is not merely important in the guidance of sensorimotor action, it is almost certainly established and effected by way of such action. Cells in monkey parietal cortex are jointly sensitive, not only to a particular region of egocentric space (specified in one or more sets of coordinates centred on one body part or another), but also to the animal's next intended action (reaching here or looking there and so on). They show, in addition, effects of attention. If the experimenter instructs the animal to expect a cue stimulus in a particular region of space that will require a particular

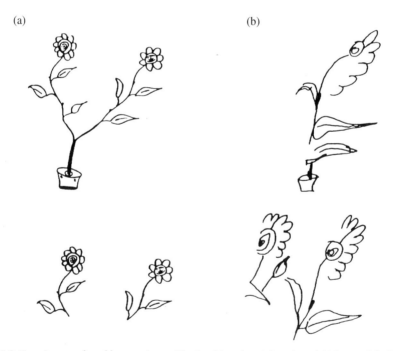

(a)  (b)

**Fig. 15.3** Drawings produced by a patient with visual hemispatial neglect. (a) The models that the patient was asked to copy. (b) The patient's copies: they show that he omitted left-sided parts of both flowers when they were seen as separate objects, but the whole left-side flower when both were seen as forming a single whole plant. (c) Copying performance of a right-hemisphere patient with severe left neglect. *Top*: the original to be copied. *Bottom*: the patient's free-vision copy. (a, b) from Milner and Goodale (1995); (c) from Burgess *et al.* (1999).

(c)

**Fig. 15.3** (*continued*)

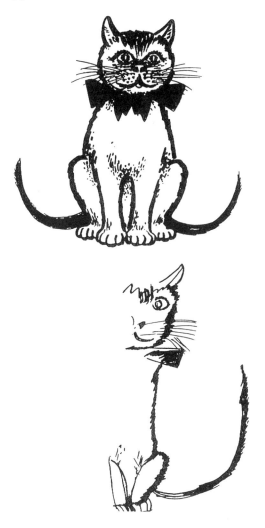

response (grasping, foveating, etc.) for a reward of fruit juice, then the appropriate cells will begin to fire in advance of the appearance of the cue. These 'attentional' effects are hard to distinguish from 'intentional' effects. That is to say, they are usually associated equally with the region to which the animal must attend and the response that it will be required to make. Thus the construction and utilisation of the co-registered egocentric maps are intimately bound up with activation of the kinds of sensorimotor feedback loops which we considered in Chapter 3. A co-registered sensorimotor map is, in effect, a map of goals for action (or controlled variables), rather than a map of either places or movements considered separately. (As noted in the previous chapter, a 'map' refers to a 'mapping' of one set of neuronal firings onto another. Co-registration can be said to occur when a set of neurons fires only when each member of the set receives appropriate inputs from neurons in both, or all, the mappings that are so co-registered.)

The kind of egocentric space that is disrupted in neglect operates at a still higher level of cognitive abstraction than these more specific spaces, even after their co-registration. This is best made clear by a famous clinical experiment carried out by Bisiach and Luzzatti in 1978. They asked neglect patients to *imagine* themselves standing in the Piazza del Duomo, a well-known square in Milan, first on one side of the square and then on the other, and to describe what they saw. In each case, the patient was able to report only what they would have seen on the right-hand side of the square, given the point at which they imagined themselves to be standing. If they could put together the two view-points, of course, a representation of the whole square would be potentially available to these patients. But the particular view-point adopted determined access to only half of the representation. This space, therefore, is best described as 'representational egocentric space'.

The loss of the left side of this representational space in the syndrome of unilateral neglect is not absolute, as demonstrated by a number of observations. (For the sake of simplicity, I shall confine myself to vision in describing these observations; but essentially the same things happen if, e.g. instead of being shown something on the left the patient is touched on the left arm.) To begin with, there is the phenomenon of extinction, which we have encountered before. The patient may be able to see and report an object presented in the left visual field, contralateral to the lesion, provided that this is the only object presented. But if another object is simultaneously presented in the right visual field, the one on the left is not seen—it is 'extinguished' by the competing stimulation on the right. These observations have led to the view that neglect reflects an attentional failure. In this respect, neglect contrasts sharply with the loss of vision that occurs after damage, e.g. to V1. No amount of attention can bring conscious vision back to the region of the scotoma.

Marcel Kinsbourne has demonstrated, furthermore, that these attentional effects do not respect an absolute distinction between the left and right halves of visual space. Rather, there appears to be a gradient of attention (see Fig. 15.4). For any part of the visual field, whether predominantly in the left or the right halves of egocentric space, items that are further to the right are attended to and consciously seen more readily than items further to the left. Furthermore, the effects of this attentional gradient depend upon what counts for the patient at the time as 'an item'. So, in the example of 'object-centred neglect' illustrated in Fig. 15.3, the patient copied only the right-hand side of each of two flowers, if he saw the drawing as consisting of two flowers, but only the right-hand side of a single plant with two blooms if he saw it that way.

Now, clearly, if representational egocentric space manifests itself, among other things, in the ability to imagine a city square in Milan and describe what you see

(a)

(b)

(c)

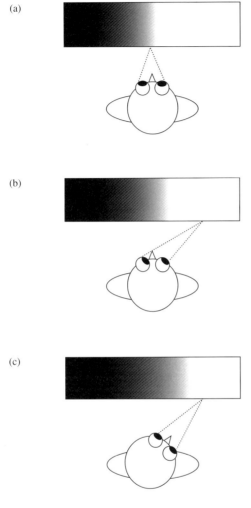

**Fig. 15.4** Schematic illustration of varying spatial coordinates in unilateral neglect and effects of posture. A hypothetical patient with right brain damage and left spatial neglect is depicted as seen from above the head when facing a visual scene. Perception of visual stimuli generally improves as a gradient from the contra-lesional side (black area, complete unawareness) to the ipsi-lesional side (white area, normal aware-ness). This spatial gradient could in principle be defined with respect to the retina (line of gaze, depicted by dashed lines), head, or body, which are often aligned in experi-ments. If the patient keeps his gaze straight ahead (a), he may fail to detect stimuli falling on the contra-lesional hemi-retina. But, if the patient directs his gaze to the right while keeping the head straight (b), or if he turns both gaze and head to the right (c), stimuli falling on the contralateral hemi-retina may now be perceived. Such effects indicate that neglect is partly determined by the head and/or trunk position in addition to the primary retinal afferents, and that posture signals can modulate awareness of contra-lesional stimuli. From Driver and Vuilleumier (2001).

there, it must in some way be related to conscious experience. This, then, is a crucial distinction between the kinds of egocentric space computed in the superior parietal lobule (unconscious and concerned with visuomotor action) and the inferior parietal lobule (conscious and concerned with visual perception). It would be neat if one could relate these two divisions of the parietal lobe to the cor-responding two divisions of the visual system (the dorsal stream, subserving unconscious action, and the ventral stream, subserving conscious perception; see Chapter 2). Unfortunately, this may not be possible, as both divisions of the parietal lobe appear to belong to the dorsal stream. However, there is psychological evidence for interactions between the computations performed in the ventral visual stream and the inferior parietal lobule.

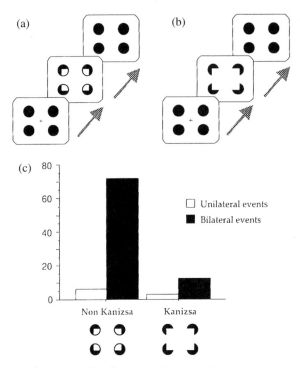

**Fig. 15.5** Reduction of extinction by illusory surface completion in Kanizsa figures. Example sequence of events in one trial when bilateral events did not form (a) or did form (b) a single object bounded by illusory contours (bright white rectangle in b). Arrows depict time between successive frames. In each trial, four black circles were first presented around a central fixation cross; then quarter segments could be briefly removed from all four black circles (bilateral trials), as shown here, or just from two circles on one side (right or left), or not at all. These displays were used to test a patient with right hemisphere damage and left extinction. Her task was to detect and report the side(s) of the brief offsets. The percentage of contra-lesional (left) events missed in each condition is shown below (c). The patient exhibited little extinction when removals from both sides produced a subjective Kanizsa rectangle (as in b), although there was a marked extinction when small arcs remained on the circles so as to prevent the formation of an illusory surface (as in a). Unilateral left events were correctly detected on most trials in both situations. From Driver and Vuilleumier (2001).

A first example of these interactions comes from an elegant study of a patient with unilateral neglect carried out by Jon Driver in London. His experiment used a Kanizsa square (see Fig. 13.3), with two of the pacmen presented on the left and two on the right. These are conditions, of course, in which one would expect the stimuli on the right to extinguish those on the left. This indeed is what happened when the patient was shown stimuli modified to prevent perception of the illusory square. However, when she was presented with pacmen able to sustain the illusion, she saw a complete square (Fig. 15.5). This result demonstrates two things.

First, if the stimuli presented to left and right visual fields can be combined into a figure with good Gestalt properties, then rather than inhibiting the damaged hemisphere, the intact side works with it to create the figure. Second, as we saw in Chapter 13, the illusory contours that make up the Kanizsa square depend upon activity in area V2 (which sends output to both the dorsal and ventral visual pathways). It follows that the construction of the square performed there must be communicated to the inferior parietal lobules in a manner that permits this interhemispheric cooperation to take place. More generally (and as supported by a number of other observations in Driver's laboratory), object segmentation (e.g. combining the left and right sides of a Kanizsa figure into a unified square) first takes place in the ventral visual pathway and then undergoes further processing in the inferior parietal lobule—processing that is in some way required for entry into consciousness.

## 15.2   Balint's syndrome

Damage to the inferior parietal lobule on the right causes unilateral spatial neglect. This is a disabling and distressing syndrome. But it is dramatically outclassed by what happens when the parietal damage affects both sides of the brain (fortunately a rare occurrence). This gives rise to a condition known as 'Balint's syndrome', after the German neurologist who first described it in 1909. This consists of optic apraxia and optic ataxia (see Fig. 2.2 and the accompanying discussion), as well as 'simultanagnosia'—a marked difficulty in seeing more than one thing at a time. Anne Treisman and Lynn Robertson have recently published a detailed clinical and experimental account of one such patient, 'R. M.' (see Friedman-Hill *et al.* 1995, and Robertson's 2003 review). Their observations are of great significance for our theme, as is the interpretation they give to them. I am sufficiently persuaded by this interpretation that I shall follow it closely here. Since it will then form the basis for some quite far-reaching conclusions, bear in mind that it is, after all, drawn from a single case study (although Treisman and her colleagues show that it also applies well to previous accounts of Balint's syndrome).

A key part of the experimental findings reported by Friedman-Hill *et al.* is that R. M. has great difficulty in binding together into one coherent percept the different features that make up a single visual object. R. M. was shown some simple displays consisting of just two coloured letters, selected from among T, X and O, and either red, blue or yellow. His task was to report which letter he saw first and what colour it was. In some sessions, even with displays lasting as long as 10 seconds, he made binding errors, reporting one letter in the colour of the other, on as many as 35% of trials. Now, normal subjects can also be tricked into reporting this kind of illusory feature conjunction, but for this to happen the display has to be much shorter (around 200 milliseconds) and three or more stimuli have to be presented together. Note that, if the same coloured letters were presented singly for 3 seconds, R. M. made no binding errors—he correctly reported both the letter and its colour. So he has no difficulty in seeing a single visual object. It is only when each such object can be made up of alternative feature conjunctions that his problem sets in. Lynn Robertson and her colleagues describe a still more striking case (presented at the 2001 Annual Meeting of the Cognitive Neuroscience Society), in which the afflicted patient makes binding errors in putting together faces. Her impairment is so severe that she sometimes sees a human face with the eyes of an adjacent cat, or a human body topped with a dog's head!

The same conclusions emerge from experiments with R. M. on what is known as visual search. Here the subject's task is to search for visual targets in a display containing many distractor items. The target may be defined by a single feature or by a conjunction of features. Treisman and Robertson tested R. M. with both kinds of display. In the first, he had to search for a red X among red Os (so the distinguishing feature was just the letter) or for a red X among blue Xs (the distinguishing feature now being just colour). R. M. had no difficulty in performing these tasks. In the second, feature conjunction, task, R. M. had to search for a red X among red Os and blue Xs. To perform this task it is necessary to pick out a target defined by two features, both the letter (X not O) and the colour (red not blue). Even with displays containing only 3 to 5 items R. M. took up to 5 seconds to perform this conjunction search, and even then he made errors on a quarter of the trials.

So here we have a person with damage to a region of the brain responsible for the computation of egocentric representational space, as considered above, and who has great difficulty in binding together into a unified percept even the simplest of conjunctions of visual features. Are these two facts connected? Treisman's answer is: yes, intimately so. Indeed, a theoretical model of feature integration that she proposed in 1980 (see her more recent overview in 1998) predicts just such a connection. The central postulate of the model is that the binding together of features into a coherent and unified object requires that the different features each be attributed to the same location in space. Thus space is the glue that does the binding. (Elsewhere— see Fig. 4.3—we have considered the hypothesis that neuronal synchrony is the mechanism by which binding is achieved. The two hypotheses are not necessarily incompatible, as synchronous firing could be the means by which the brain identifies information derived from the same point in space.) The data gathered with R. M. offer strong support for this model. In addition, they indicate that the region of the brain in which the relevant spatial frame is computed—and binding achieved—lies in the parietal lobes. Direct evidence that R. M. does indeed suffer from an impairment in the construction of egocentric space was provided by a further experiment. R. M. was asked whether an X was at the top, bottom, left or right of a visual display screen; or whether it was above, below, to the left or to the right of a simultaneously displayed O. He performed at chance on the second of these tasks and was only slightly better on the first. It is, of course, possible that these two impairments—in spatial localisation and feature binding—are independent outcomes of the damage to R. M.'s brain. But given the coherence of both sets of findings with Treisman's theoretical model, it makes more sense to suppose that they are each manifestations of the same underlying disruption in a single cognitive function.

## 15.3 Putting space together

We have reached several disparate conclusions concerning spatial frames during this and the previous chapter. The time has come to put them all together—if we can.

Let's start by trying to put together allocentric and egocentric space. Phenomenologically, *together* is after all where they belong. As I contemplate my place in the world, I find it hard, if not impossible, to draw a perceptual line between three of its aspects:

(1) the enduring, allocentric, three-dimensional frame in which objects are located irrespective of where I happen myself to be;
(2) the mobile, egocentric three-dimensional frame which moves about with me as I traverse this allocentric space; and
(3) the point of view from which I behold, and which is situated within, both of them. (I leave this third aspect, the point of view, for consideration in Chapter 17.)

Neuroanatomically, to achieve this seemingly indissoluble mix, one would look naturally to a projection from the inferior parietal lobule to the hippocampal system. I put it this way round, rather than the reverse, because it seems more likely that allocentric is derived from egocentric space than *vice versa*. Indeed, one analysis of allocentric space, argued forcefully by Rick Grush (see his website, *http://mind.ucsd.edu/*), is that this is tantamount to the ability temporarily to adopt, in relation to a particular region of space, a range of points of view, each centred upon a selected point in that space in essentially the same way that egocentric space is centred upon the observing subject. This direction of flow—from egocentric to allocentric space—is consistent also with the general flow from unconscious to conscious processing that characterises the operations of the brain. Thus, as we have seen, within the superior parietal lobule there are many unconsciously processed egocentric spaces. These, in some as yet unknown manner, give rise to the consciously perceived representational egocentric space computed in the inferior parietal lobule. For the allocentric case, in contrast, I know of no evidence suggestive of an unconscious space alongside the conscious variety.

There is indeed evidence of projections from the parietal lobes to the hippocampus. Mortimer Mishkin, whose pioneering work gave rise to the division of the visual pathways into a ventral stream (dealing with 'what?' is out there) and a dorsal stream ('where is it?'), has suggested that this distinction is maintained right up the level of

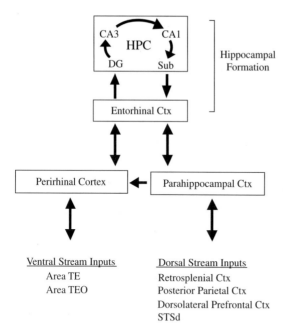

**Fig. 15.6** Schematic diagram of the connections of the medial temporal hippocampal system, depicting its hierarchical organisation. The areas listed under ventral and dorsal streams are those providing the strongest inputs to the perirhinal and parahippocampal cortices, respectively. Abbreviations: CA1 and CA3, pyramidal-cell subfields of the hippocampus; Ctx, cortex; DG, dentate gyrus; HPC, hippocampus; STSd, dorsal bank of the superior temporal sulcus; Sub, subicular complex, including the subiculum, presubiculum and parasubiculum. TE and TEO, cortical subdivisions. Compare with Figs 14.1 and 14.2. From Mishkin *et al.* (1999).

the hippocampus. According to his model (Fig. 15.6), the ventral stream is funnelled into the hippocampus by way of the perirhinal cortex, and the dorsal stream (including components originating in the posterior parietal cortex) by way of the parahippocampal cortex. This hypothesis is consistent with a great deal of research, including both experiments on monkeys and neuroimaging studies of human subjects. Little if anything is known, however, about how, or even whether, these projections mediate the knitting together of egocentric and allocentric space.

Does this lack of knowledge affect the argument we are pursuing? Perhaps not. But one should take nothing for granted in relation to consciousness, no matter how compelling one's introspections or intuitions. Yes, most normal conscious experience suggests that a combined allocentric and egocentric spatial frame is its *sine qua non*. But it does not take long to uncover counter-examples to this seeming necessity. One of them, we have just seen. R. M., Treisman's patient with Balint's syndrome, has a striking impairment in egocentric representational space and cannot, presumably in consequence, properly bind features into coherent objects. Since he can see only one object at a time, we must suppose that his allocentric spatial frame is also severely compromised. Indeed, if the general arguments pursued above are correct, loss of egocentric representational space would be expected normally, perhaps even necessarily, to be accompanied by loss of allocentric space. But R. M. does see objects, albeit one at a time and sometimes with features bound together in strange ways. We have no reason to suppose that he lacks all conscious visual experience. In the previous chapter we reached a similar conclusion in respect of patients who, after damage to the hippocampus, have lost their allocentric spatial frame. These patients too have serious impairments in finding their way about in the world and in forming or retrieving conscious episodic memories. But we have no reason to suppose that they lack all conscious experience. So neither egocentric nor allocentric spatial frames, alone or in combination, are *necessary* for conscious experience.

Once one is alerted to such pathological examples of conscious experience without a clear spatial frame it is not difficult to find counterparts in normal experience. If you listen to music through headphones, to the extent that it has any location at all, this is 'inside the head between the ears'. Only by major conceptual massage can this count as a location within a spatial frame. There is certainly no allocentric frame. Equally clearly, there is nothing that can count as an egocentric frame in the normal sense. For such frames are computed in the light of outcomes from sensorimotor action patterns that are centred upon the torso, head (its outside, not its inside!), eyes and so on. Listening to music is delightfully free of such action patterns, especially for someone like me who does not play a musical instrument. Other examples that seem free of spatial frames are thinking, in the form of hearing your own voice, and the feeling of drowsiness (more about this in Chapter 18).

What, then, if anything, might be necessary for conscious experience other than the particular qualia themselves? The answer to this question given by Zeki's hypothesis—that sufficient activity in a specialised module of the ventral stream is both necessary and sufficient for conscious visual experience—is: 'nothing'. Could he be right? As we saw, much of the neuroimaging evidence is consistent with his hypothesis. And the fact that other brain regions besides the specialised modules are also normally active is not evidence against it, since conscious events enter into many forms of processing, requiring attention, working memory, episodic memory, and so on. The only evidence against the hypothesis comes from studies in which neuroimaging detected clear activity in the specialised modules in the absence of concurrent conscious experience. And this evidence can perhaps be accommodated by the *caveat* that the 'sufficiency' of activity in a feature-specialised module lies in its not requiring activity in other brain regions, rather than the claim that *any* degree of activity in the module is sufficient.

As noted in Chapter 13, there are two kinds of study that have obtained this kind of result. The first looked at patients with unilateral spatial neglect. In these experiments conscious awareness of visual stimuli (faces or houses) on the side contralateral to the lesion was, as is normal in such patients, extinguished by simultaneous presentation of other stimuli on the opposite side. Thus one can think of these findings as demonstrating, not the simple absence of conscious experience, but rather its suppression when attention is captured by stimuli being simultaneously processed in the other, intact hemisphere. As we have seen, such an analysis of the neglect syndrome in terms of attentional effects is supported by many findings. Driver, indeed, has argued that the syndrome lies on a continuum with normal selective attention—that is, the process that allows you, for example, to cut out from your conscious awareness all other voices at a party while you concentrate on just one conversation. On this analysis, the *caveat* which saves Zeki's hypothesis may be phrased as follows: activity in the specialised visual modules is necessary and sufficient for conscious experience of the qualia they produce *unless these are suppressed by attentional competition from others.*

The other findings that appear to contradict Zeki's hypothesis (Chapter 13) were obtained in two patients with V1 lesions in whom visual motion and coloured pictures of objects caused activity in V5 and V4, respectively, with no reported awareness. Given the evidence reviewed earlier that activity in V1 is not itself necessary for conscious visual experience, the existence of damage in this region ought not to be relevant. So these findings constitute a definite obstacle to Zeki's hypothesis. Furthermore, the evidence that supports the hypothesis relies upon a combination of positive observations (activity in the specialised modules) and negative observations (no activity elsewhere), of which the negative ones may well be overthrown as neuroimaging methods become more sensitive. So the safest conclusion for the moment is that Zeki's hypothesis remains a contender, but no more than that.

What does seem clear is that activity in the specialised modules of the ventral stream, and the associated qualia of contours, colours, motion, etc., lie at the heart of conscious visual experience. The different modes of conscious visual experience then seem to depend upon just what else is concurrently activated. Veridical perception of stimuli projected out onto the world (not just experienced 'in the head') appears to require activity in V1, the inferior parietal lobule (egocentric space) and the hippocampus (allocentric space); imagined stimuli require top-down processing from frontal cortex; and remembered events require activation from the hippocampus. Illusory visual experience and after-images (the home ground for Zeki's hypothesis), however, may require nothing more than activity in the modules themselves. The hippocampus, together with other structures in the temporal lobe system that were severely damaged in the case of Clive Wearing (Section 14.3), may also play a more general role in the selection of the contents of consciousness (by way of a comparator system) for perception as well as for episodic memory.

## 15.4   The role of V1 in veridical perception

The evidence justifying these conclusions has been recounted above and in previous chapters. The special role played by V1 activity in veridical perception, however, calls for further comment.

Why should activity in V1 be (as current data suggest) necessary to perceive a visual object as being 'out there' but not to perceive after-images or illusions of colour, motion, etc.? A likely answer to this question is that veridical visual perception is normally (pathology apart) much more tightly located in space than are these other forms of visual experience. For such localisation to be possible, the visual system needs a fine-grained topographical record of where visual stimuli are present in the visual field, a requirement that is met in V1. This area has small visual fields and is thus able to relate its inputs to the precise retinal cells that are stimulated by light. In contrast, visual fields get progressively larger (so losing fine-grained spatial resolution) as messages pass further up the visual pathways. Thus the information contained in V1 is almost certainly essential for the computation of the different forms of egocentric space conducted in the parietal lobes; and therefore also essential for the binding of visual features into objects on the basis of a common location in this egocentric space. The scotomata (regions of the visual field in which one is blind) caused by damage to V1 can, in this light, be construed literally as losses of visual space. The much coarser parsing of space sustainable by the larger

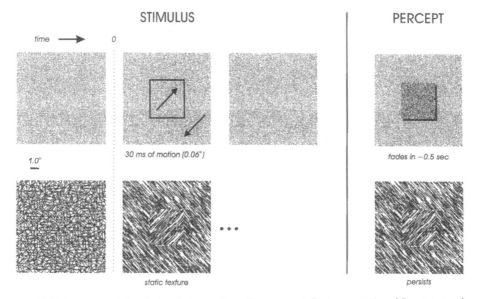

**Fig. 15.7** Sequence of visual stimulation and resulting percepts for two varieties of figure-ground displays. (*Upper*) Structure from motion defines a square figure region of $4^0$ width. Initially, the display is covered with a random dot pattern; 300 ms after fixation, a brief period of motion (30 ms) occurs in which dots inside and outside of a square region move in opposite directions, each dot moving $0.06^0$. After the motion, the random dot pattern remains stationary and contains no physical trace of the figure. The percept obtained from this sequence of stimulation is of a square figure that persists against the static random dot pattern for approximately half a second after the motion, if fixation is maintained. (*Lower*) Orientation contrast defines a square figure region. Initially, the display is covered with randomly oriented line segments; 300 ms after fixation onset, these are replaced by oriented texture in which line segments inside and outside of the $4^0$ square region are orthogonal; this remains for 500 ms. The percept obtained from this sequence of stimulation is of a square figure that persists for the duration of the presentation. From Lamme *et al.* (1998).

visual fields found in V4 or V5 are sufficient, however, for the experience of illusory and imaginary colour or motion. These are generally (as you can confirm by intro-spection) much less clearly localised in space than are veridical percepts.

The interactions of V1 with regions further up the visual processing stream are not one way. As is normally the case in the nervous system, it also receives messages back from areas to which it projects. There is evidence that these recur-rent interactions permit V1 to participate in the construction of conscious visual percepts beyond the mere passing forward of spatially precise information. This point is well illustrated in an experiment by Victor Lamme and his colleagues. They presented to monkeys displays of the kind illustrated in Fig. 15.7. Human beings who watch these displays see a square emerge from different patterns of motion (upper part of the figure) or texture (lower part). Perception of the squares requires integration over too wide a region of visual space for the cells of V1 (with their small fields) to be able to extract the requisite information on their own. Nonetheless, Lamme was able to demonstrate by recording from neurons in V1 that these cells do in fact acquire this information. Cells whose visual fields fell either on the 'edges' (derived from the patterns of motion or texture) of the square, or within the square, fired at a higher rate than cells whose fields fell onto the background to the square. This kind of segregation of figure from ground is almost diagnostic of a conscious percept. Notice that the directions of motion or orienta-tions of line were balanced across trials in their allocation to figure or ground. Thus the observed sensitivity of neuronal firing in V1 to figure-ground segregation occurred despite the fact that the local features of the displays (which were of a size appropriate to the small visual fields in V1) were identical between figure and ground.

So how does V1 do this trick? Almost certainly, because of feedback from other visual modules (perhaps V2, which as we saw in Chapter 13 plays a key role in the construction of such illusory contours). A role for such feedback is strongly suggested by a further observation: that, after the initial neuronal response to the displays, it took an additional 60–100 milliseconds for the differential rates of firing to figure and ground to appear. In a final important manoeuvre Lamme showed that anaesthesia eliminated these differential firing rates but not the initial response to the onset of the displays. The sensitivity of the figure-ground differentiation to anaesthesia provides, of course, good (though by no means conclusive) evidence that in the waking state the monkeys perceived the squares consciously.

Lamme's findings demonstrate clearly that V1 receives information regarding visual features characteristic of conscious percepts. But we should not let this demonstration override our earlier conclusion (Chapter 13) that activity in V1 is neither necessary nor sufficient for visual awareness. That conclusion is supported by too much other evidence. Rather, it seems likely that recurrent interactions between V1 and regions higher up the ventral processing stream enable it the better to fulfil the role of maintaining a stable spatial location for consciously perceived visual objects.

## 15.5   Consciousness in a brain slice?

Since Chapter 10 we have been searching for an alternative to functionalism. Global workspace, explored in Chapters 11 and 12, does not offer one—it is just functionalism again in another guise. What about the proposals for the neural correlate of consciousness that have occupied us in this and the previous two chapters? Do they offer a real alternative to functionalism?

Insofar as they go beyond the mere search for correlations (between activity in a particular brain region and the occurrence of conscious experience), all the proposals we have considered are—yet again—essentially functionalist in tone. They are based on the notion that executive function (or attention, or allocentric space, or a comparator system, and so on) is the vital ingredient that turns unconscious brain activity into conscious experience. The underlying assumption appears always to be that the specific properties of the brain tissue concerned or of the neural activity that it sustains are irrelevant: only the cognitive function discharged links the activity to consciousness. There are no explicit claims to the contrary; and the closest to an implicit claim I have come across is Christof Koch's plan to search for genes that might do special things in whatever brain tissue turns out to be the NCC.

But suppose Zeki's hypothesis turns out to be correct, and the necessary and sufficient conditions for experiences of colour consist in activity in V4, with no additional role at all required for any executive manipulative function (use in voluntary action, working memory, and so on). And suppose that, as indicated by the experiments on synaesthesia (Chapter 10), there is no need for the colour experience sparked off by activity in V4 to be linked to any kind of visual function at all. Then a natural question arises: do the *cells* in V4, or the *neural* activity that they sustain (as distinct from the functions that they discharge) have any special properties that give rise to just those qualia that we call colour, rather than qualia of other kinds (or no qualia at all)?

One can push this line of enquiry further. The great nineteenth-century Russian physiologist, Ivan Sechenov, spoke of the brain as an organ that secretes thought as the gall-bladder secretes bile. Now, you can cut a slice of gall-bladder, keep it alive in a dish and it still secretes bile. It has become routine in neuroscience to cut slices of brain and keep them alive in a dish too. Might it be the case that, if one put a slice of V4 in a dish in this way, it could continue to sustain colour qualia? Functionalists have a clear answer to this question: no, because a slice of V4, disconnected from its normal visual inputs and motor outputs, cannot discharge the functions associated with the experience of colour. But, if we had a theory that started, not from function, but from brain tissue, maybe it would give a different answer. Alas, no such theory is to hand. Worse, even if one had been proposed, there is no known way of detecting qualia in a brain slice!

Natural as these questions appear (at least to me), no neuroscientist has ever asked them, let alone proposed an answer. The only scientists who have come close are the physicists. We turn to their proposals in the next chapter.

# CHAPTER 16

# Taking physics seriously

Our starting point in this chapter remains the brain, but now it is the brain conceived as a physical system. Even more fundamental than the question, 'how does the brain create conscious experience?' is another: 'how does conscious experience fit into the world of physics?'. Physics strives to produce a unified account of everything in the universe, and in particular of all the fundamental forces that shape it. It has not yet completed GUT, its long sought-for Grand Universal Theory of everything, but it is well on the way. Leaving aside consciousness, the main outstanding obstacle to GUT is that it has not yet proved possible to unify the theory of gravity with quantum mechanical theory. But consciousness, too, will eventually need to be fitted somehow into GUT.

There are two ways in principle in which this might be done.

The first is to demonstrate that conscious experiences are a product of the brain's special features as a biological system that has evolved by way of Darwinian selection. These special features might require no new physics. If functionalism were correct, this indeed would be the case, as functions fit comfortably into the original contract between physics and biology (Chapter 3): they merely supplement standard physicochemical processes with cybernetic engineering. But, if brain tissue as such, not the functions it discharges, is endowed with properties that give rise to conscious experience, then potentially we have a problem. The problem might be solved in a relatively undramatic manner. That is to say, the special features of brain tissue might turn out to arise from some new arrangement of familiar physicochemical properties. In that case, once one has understood the new arrangement, no adjustment of the fundamental laws of physics or chemistry would be required. This is the case for the theories we look at in Section 16.1.

Alternatively, however, no such new arrangement of the existing laws of physics and chemistry will turn out to be possible. The fundamental laws of physics themselves will need supplementation in some way. It is difficult to see how new fundamental laws could come into play only at a stage, whether early or late, in biological evolution, or they would not be fundamental. So it may be inevitable that any theory which seeks to account for consciousness in terms of fundamental physical processes is 'panpsychic': that is, it must suppose that there is a degree of consciousness present in *any* physical system (in or out of brains) in which these processes occur. And, precisely because they are fundamental processes, it is likely that they will occur in many systems that are not neural, nor even biological. The Penrose–Hameroff theory, presented in detail below, is one such example.

One important feature of such a panpsychic approach is that it can in principle block the question: 'how does consciousness get into our universe?'. For, once it is postulated that an entity forms part of the set of fundamental physical laws, physicists do not ask further: how did that entity get into the set? The entity (e.g. the force of gravity, the strong and weak forces of quantum mechanics) is a given, and the physics then lies in working out its consequences. So, if a theory of consciousness were in some way to form part of the fundamental laws of physics, we would no longer need to ask how consciousness first came about, any more than physicists generally ask how the 'Big Bang' came about. Whether you see this as an advantage or a disadvantage of the panpsychic approach is perhaps a matter of taste.

Panpsychism is about as unpalatable to normal intuition as are conscious computers. They differ in that the conscious computer starts from the systemic aspects of brain function, and panpsychism from the components that mediate these functions. These starting points are, of course, the two sides of the 'contract' (Chapter 3) between biology and physics: feedback systems that respect physical laws made out of components that obey them. Start with the system only, and you may conclude that computers or robots can be conscious; start with the components only, and you may conclude (depending on the physical properties emphasised) that almost anything can be conscious. But there may be no solution to the Hard Problem which does not, one way or another, deeply offend our intuitions. The giving of such offense is insufficient ground to dismiss an otherwise coherent theory.

## 16.1   The Gestalt principles

In the absence of any proposal as to how brain tissue might create qualia in virtue of its specifically biological or neural properties, we need to look to its purely physicochemical properties. Over the years there have been a number of attempts to uncover a material basis for consciousness along these lines. Most have never gone beyond very broad speculation, closer to philosophy than to physics. Some have been frankly daft, like Eccles' conjecture that free will, not to mention the promptings of the Holy Ghost, could find somewhere to act within the indeterministic crannies of quantum mechanical events in the brain.

Several of the more serious attempts have taken as their springboard the holistic properties of perception so beautifully demonstrated by the group of German 'Gestalt' psychologists in the first half of the twentieth century. (The English for 'Gestalt' is 'shape' or 'form'.) We have seen many instances of these phenomena throughout the book. They include, for example, bistable percepts, such as those that flip between a duck or a rabbit (Fig. 4.1), a vase and two profiles (Fig. 10.1), or two gratings that slide over one another diagonally as against a single plaid moving vertically (Fig. 4.3); Titchener's illusion (Fig. 2.4), in which the apparent size of a circle depends upon the diameters of a ring of other circles that surround it; apparent motion ('phi'), in which two seen flickering stationary dots create the illusion of a single dot moving between their two positions, changing colour in mid-flight if necessary to do so, or the equivalent illusion in the tactile sense known affectionately as the 'cutaneous rabbit' (both described in Section 11.1); and the Kanizsa triangles or squares that emerge from an arrangement of 'pacmen' where no triangle or square is in fact to be found (Figs 13.1 and 13.3). In each of these cases (and many others like them) perception is determined by features that belong to the display as a whole, not just the local features initially analysed at the sensory surface, in the cells of the retina for example. Here, one finds cells that are exquisitely sensitive to what happens at just one point in visual (or tactile, auditory, etc.) space, but whose interaction with cells sensitive to other points in space is limited to very close neighbours. And, as the pathways responsible for sensory analysis have been traced in ever-increasing detail from the periphery to the centre, a conventional neural basis for these holistic properties of perception has remained elusive. Computational approaches, using for example neural networks, also find that modelling these properties presents great difficulty.

Gestalt properties seem to influence conscious perception to a much greater extent than unconscious sensory processing, as shown for example by Mel Goodale's study of the Titchener illusion in a patient with brain damage (Chapter 2). This fact, coupled with the lack of a ready account for the Gestalt effects in the conventional terms of point-to-point neural processing, has prompted the creation of a number of alternative accounts of conscious experience that depart radically from the conventional picture. The model for each has lain in the field effects which, though at one time fiercely resisted, are now commonplace throughout physics, like the gravitational field, electromagnetic fields or that most mysterious of all fields, quantum mechanical entanglement (see Plate 16.1). For such fields display exactly that action-at-a-distance which point-to-point neural processing lacks, but Gestalt properties appear to possess in abundance.

The first such alternative was proposed in 1947 by Wolfgang Köhler, himself a leader of the Gestalt school of psychology. He suggested that the totality of the electrical properties of individual nerve cells and their interactions with one another might give rise to electromagnetic fields spanning the entire brain and capable therefore of underlying the Gestalt properties of perception. This proposal is not entirely wrong, since integrated fields of this kind can indeed be detected via electrodes placed on the scalp, where they form the basis of the method of electro-encephalogrphy (EEG), already well established by the time of Köhler's proposal. More recently, the EEG has been supplemented by magnetoencephalography (MEG), which similarly picks up fluctuating magnetic fields in the brain. But the notion that cells in the brain, acting in ways already fairly well understood, *generate and broadcast* electromagnetic fields is one thing, and entirely compatible with conventional neurophysiology. It is quite another thing to suppose that these fields *have effects on brain function of their own*, over and above those of the neurons that broadcast them (effects, that is, besides affording experimenters a window of detection upon the collective action of large numbers of cells in the brain). And efforts to test that proposition, by way of stratagems intended to distort the postulated field effects in experimental animals, were universally negative in their results, so consigning Köhler's hypothesis to the footnotes of history.

A much more thorough-going alternative to conventional neurophysiology has been proposed very recently by Steven Lehar, who describes himself on his website as 'an independent researcher with a radical new theory of mind'. In his book, *The World in Your Head*, Lehar explicitly draws the inspiration for his 'harmonic resonance theory' from the Gestalt psychologists, and his theory aims at just the same issues targetted by Köhler. He starts with a lucid analysis of the major Gestalt principles of perception, describing them under four categories: emergence, reification, multistability and invariance.

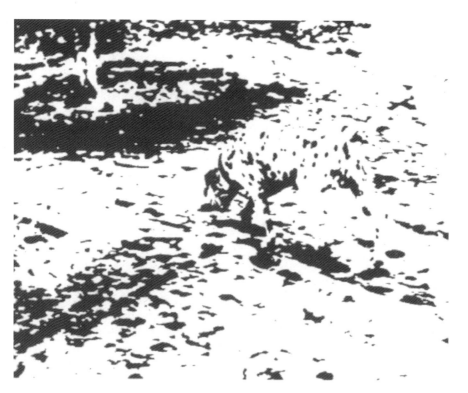

**Fig. 16.1** This picture of a Dalmatian is familiar in vision circles for its demonstration of the principle of emergence in perception. The local regions of this image do not contain sufficient information to distinguish significant form contours from insignificant noisy edges. As soon as the picture is recognised as that of a dog in the dappled sunshine under trees, the contours of the dog pop out perceptually, filling in visual edges in regions where no edges are present in the input. From Lehar (in press).

The principle of emergence is well illustrated in Fig. 16.1. If you haven't seen this display before, it will seem like a random pattern of dots and irregular shapes. But after a while, if you keep looking, you may see a coherent picture emerge. And, if I tell you what to look for, you will almost certainly see it: it is the picture of a Dalmatian dog sniffing at the ground in patchy sunlight under overhanging trees. Furthermore, once you have seen this picture, it will emerge almost at once every time you look at it.

As an analogy of the way in which emergence works, another leading Gestalt psychologist, Kurt Koffka, suggested the homely soap bubble. The form of the bubble (to quote from the relevant section in Lehar's paper in press in *Behavioral and Brain Sciences*) 'emerges from the parallel action of innumerable local forces of surface tension acting in unison. The characteristic feature of emergence is that the final global form is not computed in a single pass, but continuously, like a relaxation to equilibrium in a dynamic system model'. If this analogy is apt, we shall need to seek in the brain for a dynamic system with similar interactions between local forces that lead to the emergence of the global properties of perception.

We have already seen the second Gestalt principle, that of reification, at work, for example in the Kanizsa triangle (Fig. 13.1). Here, again, is what Lehar (*loc. cit.*) has to say about this:

> In this figure the triangular configuration is not only recognised as being present in the image, but that triangle is filled in perceptually, producing visual edges in places where no edges are present in the input, and those edges in turn are observed to bound a uniform triangular region that is brighter than the white background of the figure.... These figures demonstrate that the visual system performs a perceptual *reification*, i.e. a filling-in of a more complete and explicit perceptual entity based on a less complete visual input.

We are also already familiar with the third principle, multistability, as in the duck/rabbit (Fig. 4.1) or vase/profiles (Fig. 10.1) figures. Lehar again:

> The significance for theories of visual processing is that perception cannot be considered as simply a feed-forward processing performed on the visual input to produce a perceptual output... but rather perception must involve some kind of dynamic process whose stable states represent the final percept.

The fourth principle—of invariance—refers to the fact that 'an object, like a square or a triangle, can be recognised regardless of its rotation, translation, or scale, or whatever its contrast polarity against the background, or whether it is depicted solid or in outline form, or whether it is defined in terms of texture, motion, or binocular disparity'. This invariance is not restricted to the two-dimensional plane, but is also observed despite rotation in depth or perspectival transformation. So, for example, the rectangular shape of a table top is recognised when its projection on the retina takes the form of a trapezoid. 'The ease with which these invariances are handled in biological vision suggests that invariance is fundamental to the visual representation' (Lehar, *loc. cit.*).

Lehar (like the Gestalt psychologists before him) makes a strong case that these remarkable and all-pervasive features of visual perception simply aren't explained by standard existing theories, psychological, computational or neuroscientific. These assume an atomistic, bottom-up form of processing in which feature detectors first break up the stimulus display into localised fragments that are later combined into the eventual global percept. It is Lehar's contention that perception starts out exactly the other way around: with the global properties themselves. His

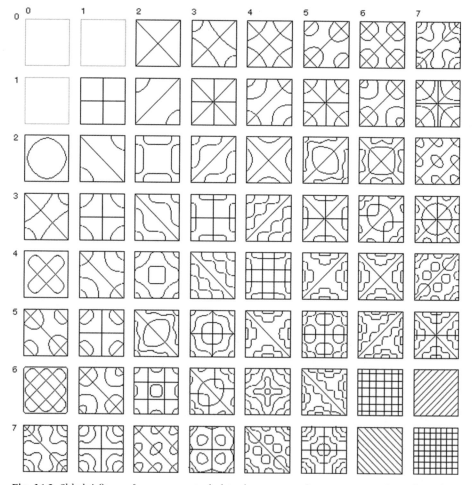

**Fig. 16.2** Chladni figures for a square steel plate demonstrate the enormous variety of standing wave patterns that can arise from a simple resonating system. A square steel plate is clamped at its midpoint and sprinkled with sand. It is then set into vibration, either by bowing with a violin bow or by pressing dry ice against it. The resultant standing wave patterns are revealed by the sand that collects at the nodes of the oscillation where the vibration is minimal. From Steve Lehar's website: *http://cns-alumni.bu.edu/~slehar/webstuff/hr1/hr1.pdf*

own model does just this. It depends on a detailed parallel between the Gestalt
features of perception and the patterns of standing waves that can be produced by
a harmonic resonator. Figure 16.2 shows some examples of these patterns, made
for example by sprinkling sand on a steel plate and then setting the plate vibrating
by bowing it with a violin bow. The patterns arise because the sand gathers at the
points on the plate which remain relatively stationary. Some further examples,
made by vibrating a vessel containing a fluid surface, are shown in Fig. 16.3. The
same mechanism underlies the tones and timbres produced when you blow into a
trumpet or a flute. Such patterns have an array of properties that map well on to
the Gestalt principles of perception. Most fundamentally, they affect the resonance
system globally, as the result of relatively simple local interactions at every point
at the molecular level. Lehar follows up on this basic analogy with a detailed ex-

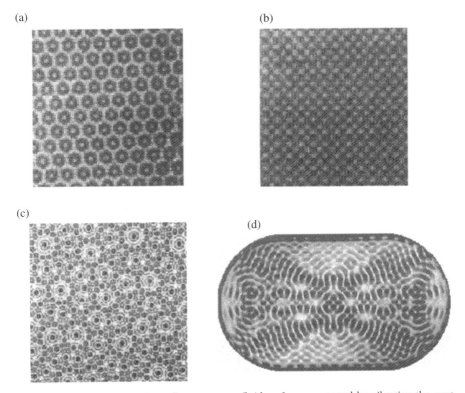

(a)

(b)

(c)

(d)

**Fig. 16.3** Various patterns of standing waves on fluid surfaces generated by vibrating the containing vessels with various driving frequencies, producing hexagonal (a) or rectangular (b) lattices
or quasi-crystal patterns (c), among many more. (d) This pattern is defined more by the shape of
the walls of the container than by the driving waveform, showing how interference patterns in the
resonating system tend to subdivide it into periodic and symmetric sub-patterns in an essentially
Gestalt manner. From Steve Lehar's website: *http://cns-alumni.bu.edu/~slehar/webstuff/hr1/hr1.pdf*

position of how, in principle, a system of damped oscillating harmonic resonators could reproduce all the Gestalt principles; but we shall not follow him into these details (to do so, read his book The *World In Your Head* or his article in *The Behavioral and Brain Sciences,* or consult his website at *http://cns-alumni.bu.edu/~slehar/*).

This *could* be a very promising new approach—but certain rather troublesome conditions need to be satisfied first.

On the positive side, Lehar makes an impressive case that harmonic resonators could in principle handle many of the problems posed by the Gestalt features of perception. He also does what many writers have recently been urging us all to do: he takes the facts of phenomenology seriously. Reduction of one scientific field to another is a lot easier if there is already a satisfactory theory of each field in its own right. The pre-existing theories circumscribe the number of entities that have to be related one to another and indicate the theoretical nodes at which successful reduction will have the most widespread effects. This was the situation, for example, when chemistry was reduced to physics, or Mendelian to molecular genetics. So one might hope that reduction of perception to brain function will be easier if perception is properly based upon theory in its own back yard. This was what the Gestalt psychologists tried to do; and Lehar has done sterling service in reviving that tradition.

On the negative side, beyond faint nods in the direction of electrochemical standing waves or the known oscillatory fluctuations in the electric potentials of neuronal membranes, Lehar gives little indication of what medium there might be in the brain that could sustain the harmonic resonance deemed to underlie perception. To give him credit, he fully acknowledges this deficiency. Thus he writes:

> The harmonic resonance theory is not a fully specified theory of neurocomputation, but a paradigm, i.e. a set of assumptions as to the fundamental principles behind biological computation.... Whether or not this principle is actually operational in the brain is a subject for future investigation.

Clearly, then, judgement will have to wait—perhaps for a long time. It would be premature to take Lehar's theory too seriously until there is experimental evidence that the brain indeed contains a medium capable of sustaining the requisite harmonic resonance, and that this gives rise to perceptual experience. The omens are not good. Three decades before Lehar's paper, Karl Pribram proposed an analogous approach based upon holography, then a sparkling new scientific discovery and now commonplace on the back of credit cards. Holograms have many of the same advantages as harmonic resonators for modelling the holistic properties of perception. But, three decades later, we still await any kind of experimental evidence that the brain contains a medium able to make holography work.

Suppose, however, that evidence supporting Lehar's proposal accumulates? Would we be in any better position with regard to the Hard Problem? At its most fundamental level, the answer to this question must be 'no'; as it would be also in relation to Köhler's electrical or Pribram's holographic fields, should these theories prove to be correct. Why would we be any closer to understanding how the material structure of the brain gives rise to conscious experience if its key features were specified in terms of electrical fields or harmonic resonance rather than the current favourite, neuronal spike trains? Lehar offers no account of harmonic resonance that would offer a clue as to why this should give rise to conscious experience of any kind. Nonetheless, if his theory were to prove correct, it would radically revise current notions of the neural correlates of conscious experience. And having a well-founded data base and understanding of those correlates would be bound to aid the future construction of an adequate explanatory framework into which to fit consciousness.

## 16.2   The Penrose–Hameroff theory

At present, the most fully worked out theory starting from the physics is the one developed by the Oxford mathematician, Roger Penrose (see his two books, *The Emperor's New Mind* and *Shadows of the Mind*), and the anaesthesiologist, Stuart Hameroff (see his 2001 paper), who works in Tucson, Arizona. It is an elaborate theory, incorporating many detailed concepts from both fundamental physics and molecular neurobiology. Penrose and Hameroff are thorough-going in their panpsychism. Here is a quote from an e-mail sent to me by Stuart Hameroff:

> We address the hard problem through a philosophical approach known as pan-experientialism, dating to Whitehead, who saw consciousness as 'occasions of experience' in a wider, basic field of proto-conscious experience. In our view the 'wider field' is fundamental space/time geometry—the fabric of the universe which is everywhere at the Planck scale. Consciousness is a series of events—quantum state reductions—in quantum space/time.

The 'quantum state reductions' of this quote are the fundamental tool in the theory. As well as the Hard Problem of consciousness, Penrose and Hameroff address two major outstanding problems in fundamental physics: the manner in which the strange sub-microscopic world of quantum mechanics 'collapses' to give rise to the macroscopic world of everyday life; and the unification of quantum mechanics with quantum gravity. The theory is nothing if not ambitious—it proposes an interlinked solution to all three of these problems.

Quantum, as the term is used in physics, means the smallest amount of something it is possible to have. The quantum world is the microworld of quarks and leptons, which appear to be the fundamental building blocks of reality. For readers unfamiliar with quantum theory, I attempt here a brief primer on quantum physics. Since I am barely more familiar with it myself, the primer—indeed, much of the chapter—is based upon papers by Hameroff himself. Although what follows has been modified (with permission) from Hameroff's text, it is largely he who is speaking—and he, of course, is a keen advocate of the quantum theory. I shall hold back my own views (except for a couple of stray interruptions) until later parts of the chapter.

The quantum realm is the foundation of our reality, yet it is a strange and mysterious place. In our everyday world (as described by classical physics), things are definite and fairly predictable. Yet at its quantum base the universe seems to be governed by different laws. This dichotomy haunts physics, for there is no obvious boundary between the quantum and classical realms.

The most bizarre quantum feature is 'superposition'. Quantum particles somehow exist in multiple locations or states—in superposition, in fact, of all possible states—simultaneously. Objects, at least small objects, can be literally beside themselves, existing in two places at once. When such quantum superpositions end, each multiplicity of possibilities chooses one definite state or location in our familiar world of classical physics. Because quantum systems are governed mathematically by an equation called the quantum wave function, and because: quantum systems seem to disappear abruptly, the transition from quantum to classical states is often termed 'collapse' (or sometimes 'reduction') of the quantum wave function.

Experiments in the early twentieth century seemed to show that quantum superpositions persist until humanly observed or measured. If a machine measured a quantum system, the results appeared to remain in superposition within the machine until actually looked at by experimenters. Therefore the prevalent view in physics at that time (the 'Copenhagen interpretation', after the home city of its chief proponent, the Danish physicist Niels Bohr) was that conscious observation led to collapse of the wave function. The Copenhagen interpretation, if it were correct, would be the ultimate riposte to epiphenomenalism. For, far from having no causal effects, consciousness would be responsible for the actual making of the furniture of the macroscopic world. This would go far beyond the stance taken in this book: that the unconscious brain is responsible for the construction of the conscious percepts that we *take* to be the furniture of the macroscopic world.

To illustrate the apparent absurdity of this notion, Erwin Schrödinger in 1935 described his now famous thought experiment: Schrödinger's cat. Place a cat in a box with a vial of poison. Outside the box, a quantum event—for instance, the passage/not passage of a single photon through a half-silvered mirror—is causally connected to the release of the poison inside the box. Since the photon both passes and does not pass through the mirror, the poison is both triggered and not triggered. Therefore, by Bohr's logic, the cat must be both dead and alive until the box is opened and the cat observed. At that moment (according to the Copenhagen interpretation) the system chooses either dead cat or live cat; thus, the conscious observation essentially selects reality. The precise choice or resolution in any given collapse (for example, dead cat versus live cat) was believed to be random and probabilistic, a prospect Einstein found unsettling. 'God does not play dice with the universe', he famously proclaimed.

Schrödinger intended his cat to be a burlesque example of the consequences of the Copenhagen interpretation, and indeed it turns out that conscious observation is not necessary for the collapse of the wave function. The prevalent view today is that any interaction of a quantum superposition state with the classical environment will be disruptive, causing 'decoherence'. But what happens to quantum superpositions when they neither are observed nor interact with the classical world? Do they collapse? We don't know, so Schrödinger's cat continues to pose (and have!) a problem.

This paradox suggests that quantum theory must be incomplete and that other approaches to the problem of collapse or reduction of the quantum wave function are needed. One suggestion is the 'multiple worlds' view put forward by Hugh Everett, which holds that each apparent collapse is a branching of reality. A dead cat in this universe corresponds to a live cat in a newly formed parallel universe. If so, there must exist an infinity of worlds. Other views hold out for an objective factor causing collapse or reduction. These are called objective reduction (OR) theories. For example, Ghirardi, Rimini, and Weber predicted that OR would occur at a critical number of superpositioned particles ($\sim10^{17}$). This theory has not held up to experimental evidence. However, another OR theory, proposed by Penrose and based on quantum gravity, is still in contention. It is this theory which Penrose and Hameroff apply to the problem of consciousness.

Quantum gravity is an approach to understanding the fundamental make-up of reality, a proposed geometry of space/time. Penrose begins by considering superposition. What does it mean to be in two places at once? The answer, he decides, is that underlying reality itself—fundamental space/time geometry—actually separates during the superposition. This is very much like the multiple worlds view, but with a catch. The difference is that, in the Penrose view, these separa-

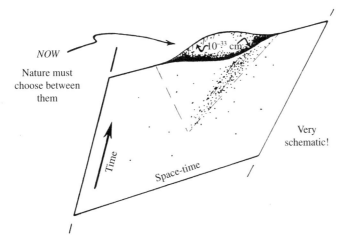

**Fig. 16.4** What is the relevance of the Planck scale of $10^{-13}$ cm to quantum state reduction? Rough idea: when there is sufficient mass movement between the two states under superposition such that the two resulting space-times differ by something of the order of $10^{-33}$ cm. From Penrose (1994).

still, by applying it to emotional and so-called paranormal connections between separate conscious individuals. For the author of this book, that is one step too far. Theories based upon physics (or is it the physicists themselves?) drift into mysticism with worrying ease.

The implication of these speculations is that evolution may have created biological mechanisms that exploit organised quantum processes. One of these may be quantum computation in the brain. There is a fairly long list of proposed quantum structures in the brain at the level of the neuron or smaller: receptor proteins, membrane lipids, presynaptic vesicle release structures, gap junctions, neurotransmitter molecules, calcium ions, DNA, RNA, and microtubules. The Penrose–Hameroff model of consciousness is based specifically on quantum computation in microtubules (which we shall come to soon) within the brain's neurons.

## 16.4   Objective reduction of the quantum wave function

The line of thought that led to the Penrose–Hameroff theory of consciousness started out as Penrose's proposal for objective reduction (OR) of the quantum wave function at the quantum-classical interface, illustrated in Fig. 16.4. This proposal is potentially of great importance in its own right. If it is correct, it hits with one arrow two bulls-eyes in physics. It unifies Einstein's theory of relativity and gravity with the theory of quantum mechanics; and it explains how quantum superposition of multiple possibilities gives rise to the world of macroscopic objects described by classical phsyics. This is not a book about physics. However, in order to understand how the Penrose–Hameroff theory is applied to the Hard Problem of consciousness, we need to get a little more closely to grips with this first step.

Penrose starts by asking what 'superposition' in the quantum wave function might really mean. His answer supposes that what separates into multiple states is reality itself, not just the possibilities for the next state of reality, as is the case if the basic equations of quantum mechanics are treated merely as probability density functions. But how can a particle be in two or more states or locations simultaneously? Following Einstein's theory of relativity and gravity, in which mass is a curvature in the fabric of space/time, Penrose treats each superpositioned particle or particle state as a minute and evanescent change in local curvature (Fig. 16.4). These changes are minute, because they take place on the smallest scale known to physics, the Planck scale. Take a volume of vacuum, with no atoms in it whatsoever. Go down and down in scale. It stays smooth until you reach the Planck scale at $10^{-33}$ cm, 25 orders of magnitude smaller than atoms. At this scale, physicists find an ultimate graininess. So, a particle being in two places at once means, according to Penrose, that at this Planck scale the local region of the universe separates and the particle exists in both separated versions. Penrose illustrates this idea as a kind of bubble or blister on the imaginary surface of space/time (Fig. 16.4).

tions are unstable and, before leading to anything so drastic as a new universe, will reduce or collapse to a single, unseparated reality (Fig. 16.4).

Can the phenomenon of quantum collapse explain the features of consciousness? In his books, *The Emperor's New Mind* and *Shadows of the Mind*, Penrose suggests that it can, that indeed quantum gravity *self*-collapse (a concept explained below) is an essential feature of consciousness. He argues, in essence, that 'choices' (the resolution of multiple possibilities into one definite state) made during this type of collapse are what distinguish our thought processes from the behaviour of completely deterministic classical computers. He suggests further that preconscious processing corresponds with quantum superposition, and that instantaneous quantum gravity self-collapse corresponds with a moment of conscious experience. According to this theory, consciousness would involve a series of such quantum state reductions.

## 16.3   Quantum computation

Penrose's stunningly strange idea begins to seem more connected to the world we live in when we consider that quantum theory is being applied successfully to a novel kind of computing. The collapse of multiple quantum possibilities to definite classical states is the key to a burgeoning new information technology known as quantum computation.

In conventional computation, as discussed in Section 10.2, elementary information exists in discrete 'bit states', the basic digital *1* or *0*. In what is called quantum computation, however, elementary information can exist in quantum superposition, as 'qubits' of both *1* and *0* simultaneously. While in this state, qubits interact (or compute) with each other; they each then reduce or collapse to a particular set of states. This provides the solution or answer to the computation. Quantum computers offer enormous potential advantages for certain applications, and prototype devices have already been constructed. Comparisons between brain, mind, and quantum computers are inevitable, though it remains to be seen whether they will take us usefully beyond the similar comparisons made with conventional computers.

Other quantum features lend themselves to possible explanations of other aspects of consciousness. Here are two examples (see also Plate 16.1).

In '*quantum coherence*' particles lose their individual identity and become part of a common unit (governed by one wave function, as is the light from a laser). This type of quantum coherence has been suggested as an explanation for the unitary nature of self, the 'one-ness' of conscious experience.

In *non-local quantum 'entanglement'* particles once unified in a common quantum state remain somehow connected or 'associated' at a distance. When one particle is then measured, its quantum partner reacts instantaneously, regardless of its location. This quantum coupling-over-distance has been proposed as a basis in the brain for some kinds of memory. Dana Zohar and Ian Marshall have gone further

How long does this separation last? Penrose's answer—his 'objective reduction' of the wave function—is summarised in a simple equation, similar in form to Einstein's famous $E = mc^2$ and which may yet become as well known: $E = \hbar/T$. In Penrose's equation $\hbar$ is Planck's constant, h, divided by $2\pi$. This reflects the operation of the fundamental principle of indeterminacy, introduced into physics by Werner Heisenberg, and provides a scaling factor. T gives the time before the separations in the local curvature of space/time recombine by choosing a final state—this is the collapse of the quantum wave function. E is the gravitational self energy from the totality of superpositioned states that make up the wave function. In the previous paragraph I spoke, for simplicity, of a particle being in only two states or locations at once, but in fact quantum mechanics allows for a much greater number of superpositions than this. They all summate to give the value of E. Inspection of the equation shows that T will be shorter, the higher the value of E. This value depends upon the number and nature of the particle states that enter into the wave function and upon their degree of separation. Crudely, the more states there are, the greater their mass, and the less the distance that separates them, the faster will the quantum wave function collapse.

Notice that the collapse of the wave function, in this formulation, depends upon the components of the wave function themselves. This is what is meant by '*self-collapse*'. In addition, any interaction of a quantum superposition with the macroscopic environment causes reduction or 'decoherence'. However, decoherence differs from self-collapse in that the outcome of the reduction is to a random classical state. Self-collapse, in contrast, gives rise to a state that is a predictable consequence of the superposition, as in quantum computing. Notice also that, in OR, the collapse is not induced by an act of human measurement or observation (as in the Copenhagen interpretation, discussed above). It is in this sense that there is an 'objective' reduction of the wave function. Notice, finally that the inverse dependence of time to collapse upon the gravitational energy of the totality of possible states of the wave function achieves one of Penrose's goals: to unify quantum mechanics with Einstein's theory of gravity and relativity.

It will be up to the physicists to judge just how successful this is as a theory within physics. So far as I am aware, the jury is still out. Should it be rejected within physics, it will presumably also fail in its further application to the problem of consciousness. Here, however, we assume its viability as a theory within physics, and move on to consider how Hameroff and Penrose apply it to answer our overriding question: how does the brain create qualia?

## 16.5 Descending into the quantum brain

The Penrose–Hameroff theory is applied to the problem of consciousness at two very different levels: the Planck scale and the level of brain function. I shall start at this second level, saving the scandal of panpsychism (the Planck scale) for later. The essential postulate of the theory, as applied to consciousness in the human (but not exclusively human) brain, is that a given instant of conscious experience occurs as the result of the objective, self-collapse of a quantum wave function. It is argued that there is a system in the brain that provides the physical conditions in which quantum superpositions can build up and undergo objective reduction according to Penrose's equation outlined in the previous section.

The key brain system underlying the creation of qualia in the Penrose–Hameroff theory consists in small structures called 'microtubules' that are located within each neuron. Hameroff rests the case for these organelles on several propositions:

(1) microtubules have the right biophysical properties to sustain quantum super-position and self-collapse;

(2) microtubules are able to interact across populations of neurons, so increasing gravitational self-energy (E) in Penrose's equation;

(3) in consequence the calculated time to collapse (T in the same equation) is consistent with the temporal features of conscious experience;

(4) microtubules have properties that would enable them to process information, acting as a quantum computer;

(5) microtubules are able to interact with the neuronal level of brain function at which normal, non-conscious information processing is generally thought to occur.

The interiors of neurons and other cells are organised networks of inter-connected protein polymers. Among them are the microtubules that make up the cytoskeleton (see Plate 16.1). As the name implies, the cytoskeleton is thought to provide the cell's structural support. Hameroff, however, endows them with much more interesting properties. He proposes that they process information, so acting in effect as a nervous system within each individual nerve cell. This hypothesis provides the link that Penrose and Hameroff need to cross between neural- and quantum-level processes. Situated in scale between neural- and quantum-level activities, microtubules seem well positioned for such a role.

To act as such a link, microtubules must be able to act in and upon both levels, quantum and neural. Here is how the Hameroff–Penrose proposal achieves this.

There are well-known ways in which highly ordered systems of mutually inter-acting components that, therefore, *potentially* have a computational function can organise themselves in nature. Information scientists call these 'lattice systems', meaning that the state of each lattice component depends on the states of its neigh-boring components, according to some rules. This mutual rule-following is a kind of natural or 'self' organisation. Simple rules in simple lattices can lead to complex self-organised information patterns. One example is the growth of crystals, but self-organising activities may occur at any level, from protein dynamics to the formation of galaxies.

In the case in point, the repeating elements are sub-units of the protein, tubulin, whose alignment in columns forms the microtubules. As illustrated in Plate 16.1, these molecules form a hexagonal lattice. The Hameroff–Penrose hypothesis is that each tubulin molecule can switch between two (or more) conformational states (different arrangements of physicochemical forces and three-dimensional shapes) on a nanosecond time scale. Such conformational transitions are well-known in chemistry and have equally well-known effects on the activities of neurons, including, for example, the opening of ion channels or changes in receptor sensitivity, both important for transmission across synapses. The factors that give rise to conformational change include some that operate at the quantum mechanical level. These are called (after the twentieth-century physicist Fritz Wolfgang London, whose work gave rise to quantum chemistry) 'quantum mechanical London forces'. Such London forces could provide the basis for interaction between separate tubulin molecules in the lattice array. So far, this account stays within accepted anatomical and chemical knowledge. It is at the next two steps that the Hameroff-Penrose hypothesis takes us into uncharted waters.

The first of these proposes that the lattice array of interacting tubulin molecules is not just potentially a computational system, but that it *actually* functions as one. If this is indeed the case, it provides an enormous increase in the brain's computing power. Conventional approaches consider the brain's $10^{13}$ neurons, each with thousands of synapses switching thousands of time per second, to yield roughly $10^{16}$ or 10 000 trillion operations per second. But this gigantic number may only scratch the surface of the brain's power. At the cytoskeletal level we have been discussing, roughly $10^7$ microtubule protein subunits in each neuron, switching on the order of nanoseconds, would give roughly $10^{16}$ operations per second per neuron (and roughly $10^{27}$ operations per second in an entire brain).

The second step takes us to the quantum mechanical heart of the theory. It proposes that the separate conformational states of each tubulin molecule may co-exist in quantum superposition (Plate 16.1) for a time long enough to reach self-collapse according to the Penrose equation. Furthermore, these quantum superpositions are given information-processing functions, adding yet another layer of computation—quantum computation—on top of the already enormous layer described in the previous paragraph.

For this hypothesis to be taken at all seriously, Penrose and Hameroff have to show how the parameters E and T in the equation can achieve values in the real brain that are in the right range for self-collapse to occur. This requires, first, that the quantum wave superposition taking place in the microtubule system be protected from interactions with the macroscopic environment in which the system is embedded. Any such interaction would cause decoherence, so self-collapse (objective reduction) would not take place, nor would any computation undertaken by the quantum superposition reach fruition. In some way, therefore, the tubulin molecules in which the putative quantum wave superpositions take place have to be isolated from their macroscopic environment. Probably the most frequent criticism levelled by physicists at the Penrose–Hameroff position is that, given the heat of the brain, this isolation simply cannot be achieved. Quantum computers in today's technology require isolation and near absolute zero temperatures. But the brain operates at body temperature, is 60% water, and is electromagnetically noisy. Large-scale quantum states are thought by most physicists to be impossible in the brain, because a single ion, photon, or thermal vibration can cause decoherence and random reduction to classical states.

The solution proposed by Hameroff to the isolation problem runs as follows. For ease of exposition I state it as though it were fact. It isn't. But it *is* experimentally testable. We are still in the realm of science, not philosophy (but wait!).

Quantum superpositions occur in microtubules during isolated quantum state phases, which alternate with classical phases, depending on the state of the neuron's cytoplasm. (The cytoplasm is the watery medium that occupies the interior of every biological cell. It contains a host of intra-cellular components of which the cytoskeleton is just one.) The cytoplasm can exist in two phases: solution (Sol) and gelation (Gel), states that are coupled to the polymerisation of actin. This protein acts as a bridge between the microtubules and the cell's membrane (see Plate 16.2). Sol is a liquid phase in which cytoplasmic actin is depolymerised, thereby enabling microtubules to receive input from, and send output to, the environment (i.e., to communicate with the neuronal membrane). Gel is a solid state phase in which actin densely encases microtubules. In the Gel phase, water on microtubular and actin surfaces becomes ordered, so that it is coupled to the cytoskeleton and acts, not as environment, but as a shield or part of the quantum system. Based on these (and other) mechanisms, decoherence times for microtubule bundles in actin gel have been calculated to lie in the range of hundreds of milliseconds, compatible with both physiological processes and the temporal properties of conscious experience.

In this way, then, Hameroff arrives at a range of values for T in the Penrose equation that fit the general bill. He next needs to obtain a corresponding set of values for E which will be sufficiently great to cause self-collapse before decoherence takes place. Recall that E depends upon the totality of superpositioned states and the distance over which they extend. Recall also that in 'quantum coherence' individual particles yield their identity to a collective, unifying wave function. Collectives of this kind were originally proposed in 1924 as an exercise in pure theory by Bose and Einstein. Today, barely a month goes by without *Nature* or *Science* carrying a description of a new method for demonstrating 'Bose–Einstein condensates' in the laboratory. It is not known, and generally doubted, that such phenomena occur in the brain. However, for E to reach a sufficiently large value, Hameroff and Penrose need to suppose that they do. Quantum coherence, indeed, must extend beyond even the array of tubulin molecules that go to make up the microtubules in one cell (as illustrated in Plate 16.1). There needs also to be quantum coherence stretching across *different* neurons.

To provide this additional, massive (literally—E is *gravitational* energy) support, Hameroff calls upon yet another quantum mechanical process: quantum tunnelling. In this, a wave/particle (e.g. an electron) is able to 'tunnel under' an energy barrier and be, not just in two different locations at once, but within two different macroscopic structures at once. Like the rest of quantum mechanics, quantum tunnelling is bizarre, yet regularly demonstrated in the laboratory. Conveniently, there are certain known kinds of connections between neurons which might support quantum tunnelling. These are called 'gap junctions'. Unlike the much more common synaptic junction, in which transmission from one neuron to the next is accomplished by a chemical messenger released into the space between them, gap junctions link neurons by direct electrical transmission. In consequence, unlike synaptic connections, gap junctions ensure that electrical changes in the membranes of the cell they link are perfectly synchronous, so that they may be said to behave as one giant neuron.

The gaps in gap junctions are typically about 4 nanometres wide, small enough that, theoretically, quantum tunnelling might cross them. And that is just what Hameroff supposes to take place. In this way, he is able to obtain sufficiently large values for E, summed over superpositions, first, within each tubulin molecule, then across tubulin molecules within a single neuron, and finally across tubulin molecules within all the neurons temporarily linked by electrical transmission and quantum tunnelling across gap junctions. He and Nancy Woolf have illustrated how this might work to produce the conscious perception of a visual stimulus that has both shape, colour and motion. Their diagram is presented here as Fig. 16.5, with their calculations in the legend.

There are two important temporal and one spatial assumption built into this figure.

First, you can see that there are a number of successive increments in E (vertical axis), each lasting 25 milliseconds (ms) or so (horizontal axis). This time is chosen to fit with much current work in electrophysiology on so-called 'gamma' or '40-Hz oscillations'. It has been proposed that these may provide a solution to the 'binding' problem (Section 4.1). We have already encountered this idea indirectly in our discussion of Wolf Singer's experiment on binding in the cat's visual cortex of separate parts of the visual field, depending on whether the cat was likely to perceive them or not as belonging to the same object (a plaid vs a grating; see Fig. 4.3). When, and only when, binding occurred, there was synchronous firing in neurons responsive to the different and separated parts of the visual field forming part of the same visual object. Synchronous firing of this kind is enhanced when the overall pattern of neuronal firing oscillates at a frequency in the gamma range, 30–70 Hz, with frequencies around 40 Hz (i.e., every 25 ms) being the most common. We shall come back to the binding issue several times in this chapter.

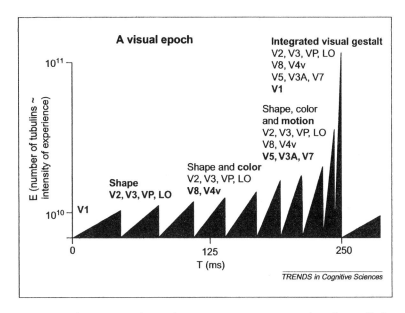

**Fig. 16.5** A crescendo sequence of several ~ 25-ms quantum computations (i.e. oscillating near to 40 Hz) constitutes a visual epoch lasting 250–700 ms. Woolf and Hameroff propose that a visual gestalt occurs at the end of the epoch as a cumulative function of Orch OR in all the contributing visual areas, including V1. The time until Orch OR (threshold for conscious event) is given by the indeterminacy principle: $E = \hbar/T$ (where E is related to the magnitude of the superposition, $\hbar$ is Planck's constant over $2\pi$, and T is the time until self-collapse). Thus, the larger the isolated superpositions (higher intensity, more vivid experience), the more quickly will they reduce. Calculations suggest that, for $T = 25$ ms (i.e. time intervals at 40 Hz), E is equivalent to $2 \times 10^{10}$ tubulins (subunits of microtubules), which occupy roughly 20 000 neurons. For $T = 500$ ms, E is about $10^9$ tubulins, or about 1000 neurons. This implies a spectrum of conscious events of varying intensity and content. Phenomenal consciousness is suggested to correspond to putative and known functional roles of visual areas of cortex (cf. Plates 2.1 and 4.1, and Fig. 2.1). Abbreviations: LO, large-scale object visual cortex; V1-V8, visual areas of cortex; VP, ventral posterior visual cortex. From Woolf and Hameroff (2001).

Here, note simply that the Hameroff model has borrowed the concept that information processing occurring with a roughly 40-Hz periodicity may contribute to a solution of the binding problem. In Fig. 16.5, this concept has been transmuted into the notion that there is a sequence of mini-events, in which E builds up and collapses, succeeding one another every 25 milliseconds or so.

   The second temporal assumption is that these mini-events gradually become larger (E gets bigger) and take place more and more rapidly, until there is a final crescendo to a large peak followed by complete collapse. The time to the final collapse is set at around 250 milliseconds. This is of the same general order of magnitude as the time it takes for a fully conscious percept to develop (see Chapter 2).

The spatial assumption is indicated in the labels (V1, V2, etc.) placed above each successive mini-event in Fig. 16.5. These refer to the separate and spatially separated (but interconnected) modules of the perceptual visual system (see Plate 4.1) responsible for computing the shape, colour, motion, etc., of visual objects. The known flow of information through these modules (V1 first, V2 next and so on) is mimicked in the sequence of labels. At the end of this flow, the outputs of the different modules have to be put together: a red colour patch, with an irregular shape and moving against a blue background has to be integrated into a flying red kite. How this integration is achieved is the substance of the intramodal binding problem for the visual system (Section 4.1). So the spatial assumption built into Fig. 16.5 is that the quantum superpositions whose gravitational self-collapse is supposed to cause conscious experiences gradually move through, and embrace more of, the tubulin molecules that lie within the neurons in each of the modules of the visual system which respond to the visual object (a flying red kite, for instance).

The flow-through and build-up of E in Fig. 16.5 reflect: (1) the inputs arriving at each visual module via the classical routes of electrophysiology (passage of impulses down axons from one neuron to another in the visual pathway); together with (2) the spread of the quantum wave superposition by quantum tunnelling. These alternate with one another as the Sol and Gel phases in the cytoplasm encasing microtubules also alternate (see above). In the Sol phase, microtubules are in contact with the cell membrane and can both affect and be affected by events at the classical, neurophysiological level; in the Gel phase, they are isolated from the membrane and E can again build up. The roughly 25-milliseconds duration of each mini-event in Fig. 16.5, therefore, requires that this also be the periodicity of the Sol/Gel alternation. Recall, also, that during the Gel phase, the quantum superpositions are supposedly acting as a quantum computer. Thus, in the Sol phase, the manner in which microtubules affect the functioning of the host cells at the classical level of neurophysiology is able in principle (and Hameroff gives some specific examples of how this might occur in practice) to reflect the outcome of these quantum computations. Also in the Sol phase, influences brought to bear upon the state of the microtubules from the rest of the cellular environment (Plate 16.2) are able to affect the next quantum computation in the Gel phase. In this way, objective reduction of the quantum superposition becomes, in Hameroff's terms, an 'orchestrated objective reduction' (Orch OR), orchestrated, that is, by the non-quantum computations that take place at the classical level and are observed, e.g. by intracranial electrodes.

On these assumptions, Hameroff is able to put the Penrose equation to work, with apparently satisfying results. Put together the right number of tubulin molecules from one or a set of visual modules and you can solve the equation with values of E and T (see the legend to Fig. 16.5) that correspond, more or less, to the time it takes both for visual binding to occur (on the further assumption, which we shall examine below, that the general 40-Hz account of binding holds good) and for a full visual percept to develop. You can also compute the increasing values of E generated by each successive mini-event in Fig. 16.5. The theory postulates that the intensity of a conscious experience is proportional to the magnitude of the self-collapse, and therefore to E at the time the collapse takes place. Thus the 'integrated visual gestalt' (in our example above, the complete percept of a flying red kite) to the right of the figure is said to have a greater conscious intensity than any of the component visual features (to the left) that have entered into it.

This is a remarkable theory, spanning and integrating many levels of science. Earlier I gave you a preview of its key claims. I repeat them here, so that you may judge the extent to which they have been justified by the additional detail presented since then. The claims are that:

(1) microtubules have the right biophysical properties to sustain quantum super-position and self-collapse;
(2) microtubules are able to interact across populations of neurons, so increasing gravitational self-energy (E in Penrose's equation);
(3) in consequence the calculated time (T in this equation) to collapse is consistent with the temporal features of conscious experience;
(4) microtubules have properties that would enable them to process information, acting as a quantum computer;
(5) microtubules are able to interact with the neuronal level of brain function at which normal, non-conscious information processing is generally thought to occur.

I think it fair to say that these claims stand up well. But that is to say only that the theory is internally consistent, not that it is correct.

## 16.6 Psychophysical isomorphism

A further line of argument used to buttress the theory points out that a variety of features of phenomenal consciousness have parallels in features of the processes postulated in the theory. As we saw earlier in the chapter, this general approach to the problem of consciousness was first employed by the Gestalt psychologists, who called it *psychophysical isomorphism*. Wolfgang Köhler (1969, p. 66) defines psycho-physical isomorphism as the hypothesis that 'psychological facts and the under-lying events in the brain resemble each other in their structural characteristics'. The Gestalt psychologists themselves took these underlying events to be electrical; Steven Lehar takes them to be harmonic resonances. For Penrose and Hameroff, and other theorists treading the same path, they are quantum mechanical.

Consider again, for example, the binding problem. To keep matters simple, let us stay with the example of the unified visual percept of a flying red kite. This percept (and all others like it, whether they involve just one, as here, or many sensory modalities) faces classical neurophysiology with a difficulty. The features that go to make up the percept (shape, colour, motion, etc.) are known each to be represented by the firings of neurons in a different region of the brain. Where, then, do they all get put together to construct the single, unified conscious percept? Initial attempts to solve this binding problem along classical lines looked to fixed anatomical convergence from the neurons in each region upon some further region. Thus somewhere there would be a single neuron, or a small set of locally connected neurons, which would fire only to the right combination of redness, kite-like shape, and kite-like movement, and so 'represent' a flying red kite (and presumably, though this was never said at the time as talk about consciousness was taboo, insert this percept into conscious experience). The example employed in this argument was usually that of one's grandmother; so such neurons have come to be called 'grandmother cells'. But it is now accepted that grandmother cells could not solve the binding problem, if only because of the huge combinatorial explosion caused by the need for neurons representing any and all of the combinations of features that each person is able to recognise over the course of a life-time.

Contemporary approaches, still at the classical level, therefore emphasise temporary alliances between neurons in the separate, feature-specific regions. An example of this approach that we have already met is Wolf Singer's work showing that distant neurons fire in synchrony with one another, if and only if they each represent part of the same, momentarily integrated, percept (Fig. 4.3). But, while these are very encouraging findings, they beg the question: how does synchrony (which occurs with a precision in the millisecond range) take place over a distance? Action at a distance, of course, is what quantum mechanics does best. Plate 16.1 will remind you of two relevant processes: quantum coherence and quantum entanglement, to which we can add quantum tunnelling, as discussed above.

In this way a quantum mechanical model of binding can provide just the kind of parallel between the phenomenal properties of consciousness and the structural features of the model that the Gestalt psychologists sought.

A second example of psychophysical isomorphism apparently lies in the temporal courses of the collapse of the wave function and the attainment of conscious perception, respectively, as illustrated in Fig. 16.5. However, there is an ambiguity in this figure, or rather in the concepts upon which it is based. According to the Penrose–Hameroff theory, a moment of consciousness occurs whenever there is orchestrated objective reduction of quantum superpositions. If this is the case, there is a separate moment of consciousness every 25 milliseconds or so, each adding successively new features to make up the eventually integrated percept. But conscious perception just does not work like that. It goes straight to the integrated percept, at the end of the time course displayed in the figure. So, to fit the facts of perception, some additional principle would be needed to distinguish between the final big collapse of the wave function at the end of the time course and the mini-events before that point. Psychophysical isomorphism can be a two-edged sword!

## 16.7   Whence qualia?

Figure 16.5 has another troubling aspect. Within the quantum-mechanical model, there is no justification whatsoever for the labels that link the model to the qualia whose entry into consciousness (when the quantum wave function collapses) it purports to explain. These labels jointly name types of qualia (shape, colour, etc.) together with corresponding anatomical regions of the visual system (V1, V2, etc.). It is then postulated that an orchestrated objective reduction of the quantum super-positions that take place in a given region gives rise to the corresponding type of qualia. But there is no reason within the quantum mechanical model to link a given type of qualia with a given region. The model gives an account of the event (orchestrated objective reduction of the wave function) that causes *something or other* to enter consciousness, but not of what. The determination of 'what' is smug-gled into the model by way of knowledge stolen from elsewhere. That might not matter much if the stolen knowledge itself provided an account of how it is that, e.g., V4 gives rise to the experience of colour. But, if we already had an account of how activity in the brain gives rise to qualia, we wouldn't need to look to quantum mechanics to provide it. All we do have is a series of brute correlations between, on the one hand, activity in this or that part of the brain and, on the other, the occurrence of this or that kind of qualia.

The standard this criticism sets for the quantum-mechanical model is a high one. It asks the model to give an account, not just of how qualia are created, but also of how specific qualia are allocated to particular roles. This, I think, is indeed the gold standard that, ultimately, a successful model of consciousness will need to meet. But we are so far away from that goal that judgements regarding current theory should surely apply more relaxed standards. So let us ask of the quantum-mechanical model: where does it find the qualia (*any* qualia) caused by self-collapse of the wave function to enter consciousness?

The answer the Hameroff and Penrose theory gives to this question is the hardest part to swallow. 'Protoconscious' qualia, they say, are embedded as quantum superpositions in the fundamental geometry of space/time at the Planck scale (see above). They are 'protoconscious' in a sense with which we are now familiar. When a superposition of quantum states self-collapses, it collapses into just one such state. That state, if the collapse is objective as defined by Penrose, becomes fully conscious. The others (into which the quantum function did not collapse) had the capacity to become conscious, but they did not: they were 'protoconscious'. So we should find protoconscious qualia wherever there are quantum superpositions.

It turns out, however, that this prospect is a lot less panpsychic than it seems. *Proto*consciousness may be everywhere you look, but not consciousness itself. For the conditions that allow for Penrose objective reduction are remarkably rare. Here is Hameroff in an e-mail to me on the subject:

> Only quantum superpositions which remain isolated long enough to reach threshold for objective reduction are conscious. And this is a fairly stringent requirement, met only in the brain and perhaps nowhere else. Why? Because you need a superposition large enough to reach threshold in a reasonably short time (to avoid decoherence). An isolated electron in superposition wouldn't reach threshold for 10 million years. But a large superposition is difficult to isolate. Proteins are fairly large mass-wise (compared to electrons) and have the unique property of having their mechanical conformational state sensitive to quantum level events like location of electrons, so they are the "levers", or amplifiers. They are large enough to exert action in our macroscopic physical world, but small enough to be in superposition and sensitive to quantum level events. Evolution (or God) is very clever.

So, might one say, are Penrose and Hameroff. By this argument they show that the system of microtubules in neurons is the *only* one in the natural world likely to provide conditions for objective reduction (and *a fortiori* orchestrated objective reduction) of quantum superpositions. In this way, the theory manages neatly to find protoconsciousness in the very fabric of space/time, while yet limiting full-blown qualia to just those systems—brains—where we know them to be housed.

What advantage, then, if any, does the theory derive from its having linked proto-qualia to the fundamental fabric of space/time?

To sharpen this question up, consider three different starting points that one might adopt in the search for a theory of the physical basis of qualia. These could be said to derive from function, from neurophysiological processes, or from quantum-mechanical processes. In each case, there would need to exist, in the first place, some kind of a systematic relationship between, on the one hand, qualia (red, green, high C on a violin, the hum of a bee, the smell of a rose, etc.) and, on the other, variation in the chosen process (functional, neurophysiological or quantum-mechanical). In the absence of such a systematic relationship, the starting point is a non-starter. For both function and neurophysiology rather well-established systematic relationships already exist. So, for example, colour sensations are well correlated with, on the one hand, the behaviour of allocating colour names to defined types of surfaces (function) and, on the other, activity in area V4 of the visual system (neurophysiology). (I ignore for the present the dents wrought in the functionalist set of relationships by the work on synaesthesia considered in Chapter 10.)

The quantum-mechanical approach, by contrast, lags far behind. No-one has yet even measured any quantum-mechanical process in a manner that would allow it to be correlated with sensation. The processes pointed to by Hameroff and Penrose are, in their application to brain tissue, almost entirely theoretical; and their relationship to any kind of sensation is asserted merely by proxy, as discussed above in relation to Fig. 16.5. Still, let us suppose that, as science marches on, such measurements become possible and, it is triumphantly revealed, quantum super-positions of the right kind, and their self-collapse at the right time, take place just as the theory says they should. We would now have the systematic relationship with sensation needed to lend plausibility to a quantum mechanical starting point. But the very nature of the Penrose–Hameroff theory entails that, if this were the case, the quantum-mechanical correlation with qualia would merely shadow the other two kinds of correlation. For the quantum computations putatively carried out within Gel-encased microtubules are closely coupled, in the Sol phase, to the non-quantum computations carried out by neurophysiological processes. That postulate is built into the theory. And so it must be, since function in the end has to be played through to those solidly macroscopic structures, muscles. All we would now have, therefore, is *three* sets of comparable relationships: between qualia and *each* of function, neurophysiology and quantum mechanics.

In any case, the presence of a systematic relationship, on its own, is no more than a 'brute correlation'. To advance to the status of a scientific theory, one needs an account of just *why* the systematic relationship takes the form that it does. No-one has yet achieved this for the brute correlations of either function or neuro-physiology with qualia, whether these are considered separately or jointly. Is there any reason to think that a brute correlation between quantum-mechanical processes and qualia would fare any better?

On the face of it, there is one reason that this might be so. Both functionalists and physiologists have so far been content to rest with their correlations as indeed brute. Neither have anything at all to say about the *nature* of qualia. These just *are*—either identified with function or, in Sechenov's graphic phrase, 'secreted' by the brain. The Penrose–Hameroff theory, in contrast, does say something about the nature of qualia. They are 'superpositioned patterns embedded in fundamental space/time (Planck scale) geometry'. To be more accurate, a quale is the particular one among these *proto*conscious patterns chosen at any given moment to achieve quale-hood due to orchestrated objective reduction in a microtubule system located in a sufficiently highly organised brain. To say something about the nature of qualia is already an advance—it at least recognises that something needs to be said. But one could forgive Dan Dennett if this particular something drew from him a scornful 'wonder tissue!'

So just what might this formulation mean? Let's try to work through a possible argument. You see a red kite flying in a blue sky, and so do I. Figure 16.5 illustrates how, within the Penrose–Hameroff model, this might happen. Let's concentrate on the final self-collapse in this figure, giving rise to the 'integrated visual Gestalt'. Let's also assume that our brains are constructed in a sufficiently similar manner (due to evolution) that we experience the red flying kite in much the same way; that is, we experience the same qualia. (In making this assumption, I deliberately set aside millennia of philosophical argument purporting to show that we could never know this similarity of experience to be, or not to be, the case.) So, on the

Penrose–Hameroff theory, the self-collapse of the quantum superpositions in a set of tubulins in a set of microtubules in a set of neurons in the visual system in your brain has accessed a chosen state in fundamental space/time (chosen because of the state to which the superpositions collapsed). On the assumption that we both have the same qualia, then the same thing has happened in my brain. Since the theory states that qualia are embedded in space/time then, if you and I experience the same qualia, our brains must have both accessed the same state in fundamental space/time.

All the relevant events are taking place in two separate brains, yours and mine. In each brain, presumably, the only route of access to fundamental space/time is *within* that brain. (This step in the argument excludes Dana Zohar's speculations, wilder even than the already wild shores where we find ourselves, that quantum mechanical processes in one brain can get into superposition with such processes outside the confines of that brain and even within the confines of another.) If we put this line of thought together with Penrose's starting point for the nature of superpositioned quantum states—that they are multiple curvatures in space/time which exist until self-collapse, whereupon space/time takes up one final state of curvature—then, when you experience a red flying kite, somehow space/time in your brain adopts a state of curvature that it didn't have before. And, if we both experience the same qualia, the same thing happens in my brain.

I have used the term 'curvature in space/time' in the previous paragraph some-what simplistically. There are roughly $10^{107}$ Planck volumes in a human brain and each of them can, theoretically, be in one of a very large number of states, depending upon such factors as the edge length and the 'spins' of the edges. So, according to Hameroff, one quale might be one pattern (superposition of curvatures and separations between states) and another, a different such pattern, and so on; and these might all be integrated or combined in various ways. So, when self-collapse occurs, only one pattern is chosen, but that pattern is a very complex entity. In this way, the theory attempts to provide a physical basis for both the simplicity of relatively isolated qualia (the sound of a high C played on a flute) and the complexity of a total conscious multimodal 'scene'.

If we are to take the account further, we need to answer three questions. (I shall ask them in relation to the same example as before, the flying, red kite, so sticking within the confines of one sensory system, vision. However, they can readily be generalised to an example involving multiple modalities, e.g. hearing a melody vs seeing the violinist play it.) How does the final state of self-collapse in e.g. V4 deter-mine the colour quale of red? How does this determination differ from the deter-mination of the motion quale of 'flying' in V5? Why does the access of the relevant protoconscious qualia and the choice of the final conscious qualia take place in the same way in the two separate regions of space/time bounded by our two skulls?

The Hameroff–Penrose theory gives partial answers to these questions as follows. Specific patterns in space/time give rise to specific qualia. So the qualia accessed by V4 (colour) must differ from those accessed by V5 (motion) because the corresponding patterns of space/time superposition differ. These patterns depend on the possible types of conformational arrangement of the microtubules that might be superpositioned in each region. And these, in turn, it might be argued, depend on at least the following two factors. First, there are local differences in the neuronal organisation in V4 and V5; second, there are differences in the neuronal connections to V4 and V5 from other regions, including e.g. V1 and V2 lower down the visual system. (These arguments become stronger if one considers the differences between different sensory systems, sound and vision for example; but if this type of theory is to work at all, it must also be applicable to the harder case of intramodal differences in qualia.) But these factors are—once again—*functional*, not themselves quantum mechanical or even physical at any level.

## Conclusions

Despite its magisterial complexity, then, we see that, in the end, the Hameroff–Penrose theory of how different quantum superpositions in microtubules in different brain areas give rise to different qualia must rely for the origin of these differences on arguments taken from neuroanatomy and neurophysiology. And, despite its intricate Gothic architecture, the theory is incomplete. It offers no account of how differences at the Planck scale might relate to differences between qualia; nor of how differences in space/time in one brain might relate to differences in another brain observing the same scene at the same time. Nonetheless, the theory does offer an account *in principle* of the origin of differences in qualia. Whether even this is testable in practice is another matter. But quantum mechanics has a habit of taking the absurd, putting it into a laboratory experiment and showing the absurd to be reality. So we should not write the Penrose–Hameroff position off too lightly. And even an account in principle of how qualia might arise is better than no account at all.

# CHAPTER 17

# Consciousness of self: the point of view

The feverish modernity, in the last few chapters, of neuroscience and quantum mechanics has perhaps obscured the hoary antiquity of the problems we are dealing with: the nature of consciousness, the reality of the external world, and so on. The questions tackled in this chapter are no less hoary. They keep steady company with the Hard Problem. Whose consciousness is it anyway? What is this mysterious 'self' to which conscious experiences are automatically attributed? (Automatically, but sometimes erroneously, as we saw when we looked at 'illusions of the will' in Chapter 2.)

As in earlier chapters, I make no attempt to grapple directly with the huge philosophical literature on the self and related concepts, like 'free will' (for a thorough if daunting survey, see *Models of the Self*, edited by Gallagher and Shear). But, also as before, we shall keep a weather eye out for philosophical issues. They may (dare I say?) end up looking usefully changed in the light of empirical science.

The central theme of this book is consciousness, so what concerns us is not the issue that has most bedevilled the philosophy: what, if anything, is the nature of the self as such? Rather, it is to understand what it is that gives rise to the *sense* of self: the feeling that there is in each one of us a unified focus of conscious perception and conscious action. (This 'consciousness of self' should not be confused with the much narrower concept of 'self-consciousness', as when one feels embarrassed giving a speech in front of an audience.)

Considered from the vantage points of psychology and neuroscience, there are several different issues entangled in the skein of 'consciousness of self'. This and the next two chapters deal with each in turn. Some of the time we run over ground already covered. Why this should be so will become clear in the next section.

## 17.1 The point of view

It is universally agreed that conscious experience normally comes equipped with a point of view. This phenomenological fact is often made to bear a great deal of philosophical baggage. The very different facts of physics and chemistry, it is argued, are independent of point of view. The speed of light, $c$, is what it is, wherever it is and whoever is measuring it (aside from recent speculations that it may undergo evolutionary change during the history of the universe). Even the Copenhagen interpretation of quantum mechanics, which (as we saw in the last chapter) holds that the act of observation collapses the wave function into a macroscopic object, gives no role to the individuality of the person making the observation. Conscious experience is different. It is irredeemably relative to the observer. If you and I attend to exactly the same segment of the external world, we each see (and hear, smell, and so on) our own version, interpreted in our own way. As Tom Nagel puts it in *The View from Nowhere* (p. 7):

> There are things about the world and life and ourselves that cannot be adequately understood from a maximally objective standpoint.... A great deal is essentially connected to a particular point of view, and the attempt to give a complete account of the world in objective terms detached from these perspectives inevitably leads to false reductions.

As in this quotation from Nagel, this contrast in regard to point of view is often stated as one between the 'objective' world of physics (this is what Nagel means by 'the view from nowhere') and the 'subjective' world of consciousness. But, before considering how subjectivity might enter into the conscious realm, we should first ask whether it is perhaps already present in the unconscious biological world. As we saw in Chapter 3, biology grafts selection by consequences (Darwinian evolution plus cybernetic systems) onto the objective laws of physics and chemistry. That alone is not sufficient to bring in consciousness. But is it perhaps sufficient to endow a creature with a point of view?

To help us answer this question let's look at a specific instance of complex behaviour governed by a series of feedback loops.

Termites build highly elaborate nests. The construction is carried out by a whole collective of the insects. An essential feature of the building programme is the construction of arches from balls of mud (Andy Clark, *Being There*, p. 75; see Fig. 17.1).

> Here is how it works: All the termites make mudballs, which at first they deposit at random. But each ball carries a chemical trace added by the termite. Termites prefer to drop their mudballs where the chemical trace is strongest. It thus becomes likely that new mudballs will be deposited on top of old ones, which then generate an even stronger attractive force.... Columns thus form. When two columns are fairly proximal, the drift of chemical attractants from the neighbouring column influences the dropping behaviour by inclining the insects to preferentially add to the side of each column that faces the other. This process continues until the tops of the columns incline together and an arch is formed.

The insects go on in much the same way to make a complex structure of tunnels, cells and chambers.

This is a beautiful example of careful behavioural analysis of complex social behaviour. And the analysis shows that the entire process is accomplished by the knitting together of a series of feedback loops. Each of these embraces a termite, other termites, and the environment. The environment itself dynamically changes as the result of the termites' work, and so enters into successively different inter-

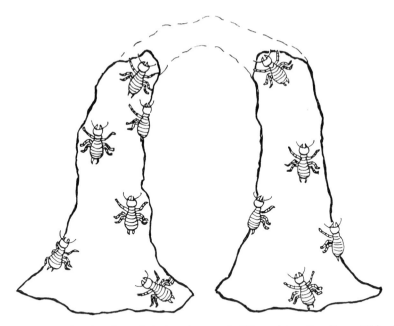

**Fig. 17.1** Pillars and arches formed during the nest building of termites. From Michaels and Carello (1981).

actions with the insects' feedback loops. The ultimate loop is Darwinian natural selection, which has favoured the survival of termites possessing the lower-order loops over those lacking them, as discussed in Chapter 3.

Does it make any sense to speak of a 'point of view' in relation to these feedback loops? Clearly not: neither an individual termite nor the collective has a representation or plan of the nest being built. It does not even make sense to think of the feedback loops as belonging exclusively to the termite. To be sure, the loop's machinery is specified in each insect's brain and nowhere else. But its operation extends out into the environment. Nor is this environmental extension an idiosyncratic feature of just termite feedback loops (though it is made particularly clear in this example). On the contrary: it is a ubiquitous feature of all behavioural feedback loops that their controlled variables are amalgams of effects due to sensors and control mechanisms in the nervous system together with other effects due to the environment. Such amalgams, inevitably, are jointly part of the animal and part of the outside world.

This type of analysis is equally applicable to the unconscious mechanisms which, in the human brain, underlie activities like turning the head and eyes to capture in central vision a fast moving peripheral stimulus, or maintaining your balance on a bicycle. In these activities, motor output and sensory input combine to operate feedback loops and to control essential variables. There is no division of self from the world—and, consequently, *no point of view*. Points of view come into being only in the territory of consciousness. (But, like everything else that enters consciousness, points of view are constructed unconsciously.)

That conscious experiences should necessarily be bound to a point of view is a direct consequence of the machinery for their making. As we saw in Chapter 15, a key role in that machinery is played by neurons in the inferior parietal lobe that are responsible for the construction of a model of egocentric space. A map of this space is essential for the binding together of features into a perceived object. Thus the self (as the centre of the map of egocentric space, i.e. as a point of view) separates itself from the object of conscious perception in that very act of perception.

This statement goes deeper than the obvious fact that we each stand at a spatially different point in the physical world and so with a corresponding spatially different point of view. For the very manner in which the brain creates conscious experience entails that the point of view and the perceived world are two sides of the same coin. Furthermore, each person experiencing the same scene necessarily gets both sides of a different (though closely related) coin, since each brain constructs its own world with its own corresponding point of view. There remains, of course, the mystery of how the brain creates conscious percepts. But there does not seem to be an *additional* mystery about how or why there is an observing self who has a particular point of view on the percepts.

The separation of the self from the external world that comes with conscious perception allows, for the first time, contemplation of (as distinct from interaction with) that world, as when for example one simply gazes at a sunset. This kind of standing back from interaction cannot be achieved by feedback systems that loop continuously into and back out from the environment. Contemplation is made possible also by the fact that conscious perception models the semi-permanent features of the world (Chapter 8), extending by many orders of magnitude the brief time scale of cybernetic interaction. These powers of contemplation may, however, be blocked off during periods of intense, vigorous and continuous rapid action. At such times the sense of self may become much weaker. This is what many people experience while for example dancing or skiing: bodily movement seems to become automatic, to take on a life of its own.

A final point to note about the point of view is that the same conscious processes that model the external world also model the observing self within it. As we saw in Chapters 2 and 15, in discussing the 'alien hand' and 'spatial neglect' syndromes, the image of our own body is as much a construct of the brain as is any other part of conscious experience. And this includes the head, ears, nose, eyes etc through which we experience ourselves experiencing the world (Plate 17.1).

## 17.2 Belongingness

The self thus enters into perception by providing and being a point of view in the literal spatial sense; that was our concern in the previous section. But there is another sense in which one perceives the world 'from a point of view'. The objects we perceive, and the framework we perceive them in, are endowed with personal meaning—they 'belong' to us and to our personal history.

There are two ways in which this 'belongingness' manifests itself.

First, objects and events are almost invariably perceived *as* something or other. This fact is part of what is meant when philosophers talk of 'intentionality' (see Chapter 4). The exceptions to the rule lie either in the consequences of certain kinds of damage to higher regions of the brain (leading to one or other of the 'agnosias', in which objects lose their normal meaning); or are of a kind we come to in the next chapter. An excellent example of the intentionality of visual experience is given in John Searle's book *Intentionality* (p. 54), as illustrated in Fig. 17.2:

> This can be seen as the word 'TOOT', as a table with two large balloons underneath, as the numeral 1001 with a line over the top, as a bridge with two pipelines crossing underneath, as the eyes of a man wearing a hat with a string hanging down each side, and so on. In each case, we have a different experience even though the purely physical visual stimuli, the lines on the paper in front of us and the light reflected from them, are constant.

The particular way in which one perceives 'TOOT' (or any other pattern of sensory inputs) is determined by our 'set': that is, the mixture of concerns, expectations, direction of attention, plans for action and so on which dominate the behaviour of the moment.

Second, objects are almost always perceived as part of a process with a preceding and future-embracing personal history. This is the process of 'autobiographical memory'. Autobiographical memory comes closest to the everyday meaning of 'self'. The self is the person I remember being last year and yesterday, and the one I expect to become next week or next year, as well as the person who is experiencing the here and now. And the experiencing of the here and now takes the form it does, just because it is imbued with these past and potential histories.

As we saw in Chapter 14, this mode of constructing the sense of self is discharged by a brain system separate from the one that constructs the map of egocentric space. The additional system is centred on the hippocampus. This structure plays a key role in the encoding and retrieval of episodic memories—memories capable of being consciously recalled, and which have an associated time, place, and relationship to personal history. The spatial framework for such memories is typically allocentric, rather than egocentric, although it is also possible to recall the egocentric point of view one had at the time the memory was encoded. A key role in

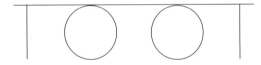

**Fig. 17.2** An example of the intentionality of visual experience (see text for futher explanation). From Searle (1983).

this construction of allocentric space is again played by the hippocampus. If my 'comparator' hypothesis of the selection of the contents of consciousness (Chapter 8) is correct, this structure is equally central to the process that gives conscious percepts their intentionality. This hypothesis does not have as much empirical support as those that attribute episodic memory and allocentric spatial cognition to the hippocampus. However, it has the advantage that it unifies all three of these processes into a single underlying computational function (Fig. 14.5).

This analysis places heavy emphasis upon the intentional nature of the contents of consciousness. That emphasis works well in relation to the cognitive conscious-ness of the external world. But, as pointed out in Chapter 1, conscious experience occupies an additional 'space': that of the inner bodily senses. This space is much less amenable to analysis in terms of either intentionality or the comparator hypothesis. It is also, as we shall see in the next chapter, a form of conscious experience with special importance for the sense of self.

# CHAPTER 18

# The bodily senses

In the previous chapter we considered the sense of self as being made up of a point of view (computed in the parietal lobes) and belongingness (computed in the hippocampal system). These processes both require the construction in consciousness of a model of the *external* world. Furthermore, they are both strongly *cognitive*. The point of view requires the construction of a map of egocentric space; and the sense of belonging requires semantic and associative interpretation of current sensory input. In both these respects, the aspect of the sense of self we consider in this chapter offers a sharp contrast. It is concerned, not with the external world, but with states of the body; and it largely lacks that hallmark of cognitive processing, intentionality.

## 18.1   Intentionality revisited

The kinds of state I have in mind are quite varied. Here are some examples: itches, tingles, pins and needles, pain, giddiness, feelings of tiredness, drowsiness, tension or alertness, feeling relaxed, sexually aroused, jittery, depressed, anxious or panicky. None of these feelings is *about* anything other than themselves. You cannot interpret an itch as anything other than an itch, nor change your mind and decide that it isn't after all an itch but something else (unlike the changeable interpretations of Searle's TOOT in Fig. 17.2, or the duck that suddenly becomes a rabbit in Fig. 4.1). Nor can you be mistaken. The menacing figure you see in the dark can be a complete mistake, as when you realise that it is in fact a bush. But you cannot be mistaken about a pain or a tingle. The feeling of pins and needles can vanish quite quickly, but you do not then conclude that, when you were feeling it, it was an illusion. In all these ways, these varied bodily sensations lack all the marks of intentionality. And, in this respect, they differ radically from conscious percepts that relate to the construction of the external world.

Interestingly, when one does make a mistake in relation to bodily sensations, the mistake affects not the sensation itself but its significance in relation to the external world as constructed in the public space of consciousness. So, for example, in a series of ingenious experiments young men rated the attractiveness of women or their photographs. If they were first made to feel physiologically aroused (e.g. by the threat of electric shock) or merely given false physiological feedback (of an elevated heart rate), then they rated the women as more attractive than otherwise. Or take another example (put to me by Max Velmans in criticism of the view that bodily sensations are not normally intentional): the pain one experiences in one's head may turn out to be in the eyes. In cases such as these, however, one is not mistaken about the experienced qualia—physiological arousal (heart pounding) or pain—but about their significance in relation to the external world simultaneously constructed by cognitive consciousness of the external world (not the woman, but the impending shock; not one location in the body, but another). Such 'causal attributions' are separate from the qualia to which they are attributed. But no such separation is possible between qualia and their intentional interpretation in the seeing of Fig. 4.1 *as* a duck (or a rabbit).

This completes a double dissociation between conscious experience and intentionality. For we saw earlier that unconscious processing (within domains capable of achieving consciousness) can display all the hallmarks of semantic interpretation and intentionality (consider, as an example, the discussion of Groeger's experiment in Section 4.4). So one can have intentionality without conscious experience *and* conscious experience without intentionality. In the terms established in Chapter 1, whereas intentionality attaches to both the public and private spaces of cognitive consciousness, it does not attach to the private space of inner bodily sensations (Fig. 18.1).

Bodily sensations differ radically from percepts of the external world also in not being located within an egocentric (let alone allocentric) spatial framework. To be sure, some of these states can readily be located within bodily space. The pain may seem to be clearly localised in a tooth. And in *this* respect, as just noted, one may be mistaken: probing the tooth may fail to make the pain worse, while probing the ear does. Such mistakes of spatial localisation may even be enduring, as in the case of pain in a phantom limb. But this space is different from the egocentric space marked out by sensorimotor interaction beyond the body. The egocentric space computed in the inferior parietal lobes is, as we saw in Chapter 15, critical for the correct conjunction of the different features that bind objects perceived as being in the external world. But, consistent with the absence of such a space for bodily sensations, these never (so far as I can see) require feature conjunction. A pain and an itch together, even if they are located in the same region of body space, do not combine to form a single object of perception in the way that colour and form or heard words and seen moving lips do when they are located in the same region of egocentric space.

Despite these differences from percepts of the external world, there can be no question that bodily sensations are experienced consciously. Indeed, pain, vertigo or nausea often dominate conscious experience to the exclusion of everything else. Thus great significance attaches to the fact that bodily sensations lack both intentionality and dependence upon spatial maps computed in the parietal lobes or hippocampus. For this provides decisive evidence against any hypothesis postulating that intentionality, feature binding, the construction of egocentric or allocentric spatial maps, or the brain regions that mediate these cognitive powers play any *necessary* role in the creation of qualia. And, indeed, bodily sensations are largely the responsibility of quite other brain regions with quite other anatomical arrangements.

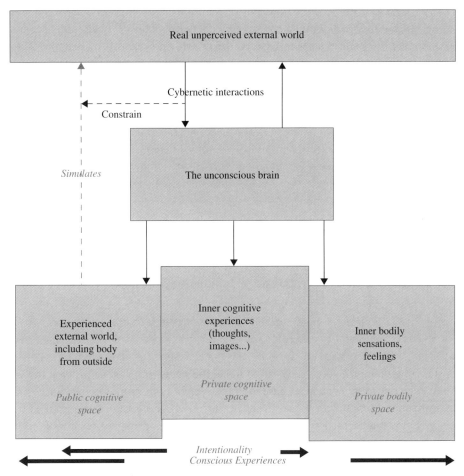

**Fig. 18.1** As noted in Fig. 1.1, of which this figure is a modification, the constructed world of consciousness can usefully be divided into three 'spaces': the 'public cognitive space', containing the experienced external world in all its visible and tangible glory, including the body as perceived from the outside; the 'private cognitive space', containing inner cognitive experiences, such as thoughts, memories and images; and the 'private bodily space', containing inner bodily sensations and feelings. Intentionality is a property of most conscious experiences in the former two spaces, but is not normally a property of those in private bodily space.

## 18.2   The approach from the brain stem

Antonio Damasio's book, *The Feeling of What Happens*, describes these brain regions in great detail. They form a series of interlinked structures ascending from the base of the brain (the 'brain stem'), largely clustered around the cerebral ventricles in the midline. This location next to the ventricles permits the receipt of strong influences from chemical messages travelling in the circulation (from blood to

the cerebrospinal fluid) and providing direct information regarding the states of
bodily tissues and fluids, metabolic processes, hormonal levels, indicators of illness
or infection, and so on. Particularly vital roles in the overall functioning of the
brain (vital indeed for life itself) are played by structures located at the level of the
brain stem (Fig. 18.2). Damage in this region has devastating effects. The nature of
these effects differs dramatically depending on whether the lesion is at the front
(anterior) or the back (posterior) of the brain stem (Fig. 18.3). A lesion to the anterior brain stem gives rise to a syndrome termed 'locked in'; a posterior lesion, to
coma. At first sight the contrast between these two syndromes looks as though it
may offer a simple key with which to unlock the riddle of the brain basis of

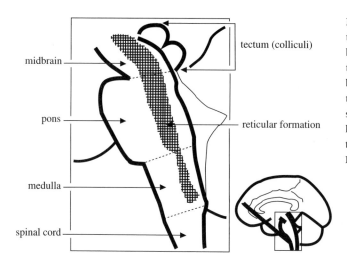

**Fig. 18.2** The main anatomical divisions of the
brain stem, seen in a sagittal section through the
brain's midline. The ana-
tomical orientation is
shown in the inset panel
located to the right of
the main panel. From
Damasio (1999).

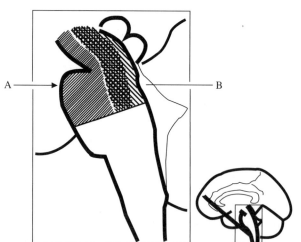

**Fig. 18.3** Location of brain-
stem damage in cases of locked-
in syndrome (A) and in cases
of coma (B). The anatomical
orientation is as in Fig. 18.2.
The damage which causes the
locked-in syndrome is located
in the anterior (front) part of the
brain stem. The damage which
causes coma is located in the
posterior (back) part of the brain
stem. From Damasio (1999).

consciousness. For consciousness is lost after the posterior lesion but retained after the anterior one.

The retention of consciousness after damage to the anterior brain stem is remarkable, given the other devastating consequences of the lesion. As Damasio (*loc. cit.* p. 292) describes it:

> The motor pathways which convey signals to the skeletal muscles are destroyed, and only one pathway for vertical movement of the eyes is spared, sometimes not completely. The lesions that cause locked-in are placed directly in front of the area whose lesions cause coma or persistent vegetative state, yet locked-in patients have an intact consciousness. They cannot move any muscle in their face, limbs, or trunk, and their communication ability is usually limited to vertical movements of the eyes, sometimes one eye only. But they remain awake, alert, and conscious of their mental activity.

Once again we see, in these terrible cases, the lack of relationship between the systems that mediate action (here, the final common pathway to all skeletal movements) and consciousness.

It is the posterior region of the brain stem (Fig. 18.3) which at first sight offers a royal road to the understanding of the neural basis of consciousness. For damage here produces coma. Surely this, then, is our long-sought Cartesian Theatre, the place where conscious experience all comes together? Alas, it's not so simple, for two reasons.

First, someone in a coma has lost, not only all consciousness, but also all waking behaviour. Before it became clear how much of waking behaviour is accomplished by *unconscious* mechanisms—as seen over and over again in this book—this co-incidence of loss of consciousness and loss of wakefulness would not have posed an interpretive problem. But now we must reckon with the possibility that the loss of consciousness during coma is not a primary consequence of damage to the posterior brain stem, but a secondary consequence of disruption to the normal waking state and to the unconscious processes that go on during that state. Put simply: if your eyes are closed you cannot have conscious visual experience. But that does not tell us anything about the difference (when your eyes are open) between those activities in the visual system of which one is or is not consciously aware.

Much is known, by the way, of the neural mechanisms that control the differences between the waking and sleeping states, and of the manner in which lesions in the brain stem disrupt these states. But, for the same reason as before, we cannot necessarily deduce anything from this knowledge to elucidate the nature of the neural machinery that controls conscious experience. For the difference between conscious and unconscious processing cuts right across the one between waking and sleeping. Much waking behaviour is performed unconsciously; and dreaming, during sleep, is of course a conscious experience. I shall not, therefore, spend time describing the neural mechanisms that control sleeping and waking.

There is a second reason why the coma that follows lesions to the posterior brain stem does not necessarily indicate that this region is a critical 'neural correlate' of consciousness. Such lesions inevitably damage, not only the neural cells that reside in this region, but also the many fibre pathways that criss-cross it on the way to or from higher centres in the brain. So the loss of conscious experience after lesions to the brain stem may well reflect the role in conscious experience played by one or more of such higher centres.

Nonetheless, both Damasio and Jaak Panksepp (in his book, *Affective Neuroscience*) have strongly argued that the brain stem plays a key role in consciousness. They see this phylogenetically ancient region of the brain as creating a correspondingly ancient form of consciousness, one more fundamental than the neocortical variety that hosts the model of the external world constructed by vision, audition and the other distance senses. They both argue, also, that this more fundamental form of consciousness provides us with the core feeling of 'self'. This feeling of self is made up of the conscious appreciation of our momentary bodily states. A further point of agreement between Panksepp and Damasio lies in their analysis of the concept of 'emotion'. Essentially, they identify 'emotional state' with 'bodily state'. Thus it is the awareness of the different and fluctuating bodily states which provides the conscious feelings that constitute one emotion (fear, anger, depression, elation, and so on) rather than another. So this more fundamental form of consciousness and of the feeling of self is quintessentially emotional, as distinct from the more cognitive form of consciousness associated with activity in neocortical sensory systems like vision or audition. For the sake of brevity, I shall call these two putative forms of consciousness 'core' and 'cognitive', respectively.

On all this, Panksepp and Damasio agree. They differ, however, in what they see as the key brain stem activities underpinning core consciousness. Panksepp emphasises that the brain stem contains a cluster of motor output systems, *controlling* bodily states. For Damasio, in contrast, the key function exerted by the brain stem is that of receiving *feedback* from these states. Both are right in the sense that this general region of the brain houses both neurons which control a wide variety of bodily activities and neurons which receive input from a wide variety of bodily sensors. But, when it comes to relating these two complementary functions to consciousness, it will come as no surprise to anyone who has read the earlier chapters of this book that there are strong reasons to prefer Damasio's position to Panksepp's.

First and overridingly, there is the general fact that conscious experience is, to the best of my judgement, only ever perceptual in nature. And, if there *are* any counter-examples to this rule, they belong to the realm of cognitive, not core, consciousness.

The nearest thing I know to such a counter-example is the familiar 'tip of the tongue' phenomenon. This happens most commonly when you are attempting, but failing, to retrieve from memory a word, for example, someone's name. Under these circumstances you may have a 'feeling' for the 'shape' of the missing word but you can't bring the actual word into sharp focus. It is rather like knowing the shape of the missing piece in a jig-saw puzzle and casting around for one that might fit. (Of course, as in all such cases where one tries to describe an elusive content of consciousness, I am not really relying upon my clumsy words to get the point across, but upon your experience of the same phenomenon. Had you never experienced 'tip of the tongue' yourself, you wouldn't know what I am talking about.) So, is 'tip of the tongue' a perceptual experience or not? To me, it feels like a perception (of the phonemes that go to make up the missing word) striving to be born. But I suppose one might equally say that it feels like an action system (engaged in top-down processing, as described in Chapter 14) striving to create the missing phonemes. Rather than pursue this line of introspection further, let us choose here to be guided by theory. In Chapter 14 I developed the idea of a comparator system, which selects items to become the contents of consciousness. The items so selected are each an amalgam of top-down processing (specifying what is predicted) and bottom-up processing (describing current inputs to thalamo-cortical sensory processing systems). Viewed in this light, 'tip of the tongue' feels like a top-down prediction searching for the bottom-up sensory input that will make the best match. And, since this is a case of memory, not actual perception, the top-down prediction must itself assume responsibility for selecting from memory stores the best matching, 'bottom-up', quasi-sensory input.

I have dealt at length with 'tip of the tongue' because, if this is indeed the furthest from perception that conscious experience ever gets, it lies at the extreme cognitive pole of the putative distinction between core and cognitive consciousness. The pains, itches, drowsiness, giddiness, etc. that make up the various bodily states of core consciousness just don't partake of characteristics that might make one think in terms of top-down processing or comparator systems at all. (And, in this way, they threaten the generality of the comparator hypothesis as an account of conscious experience, just as they threaten other hypotheses derived from the study of cognitive consciousness.)

We have already noted, as does Damasio himself, a second reason to prefer his position to Panksepp's: the 'locked-in' syndrome (motor output blocked, but conscious experience preserved) that occurs after lesions to the anterior brain stem. A less dramatic example of the same essential dissociation occurs every night when you dream. At the time dreaming is most intense (in so-called 'rapid eye-movement sleep'), there is a strong and general inhibition of all neural output to the muscles. It seems safe to conclude from these facts that conscious experience is not related at all closely to movement or the systems that control movement.

## 18.3   Emotion

A third reason to prefer Damasio's position to Panksepp's lies in the nature of emotional experience itself. Introspectively, there are, in the context of this discussion, two compelling features of this experience. First, the feeling components of one's being in a given emotional state consist, in accordance with Damasio's hypothesis, of *feedback* from bodily states. And, second, these feelings occur, relative to the behaviour with which they are associated, even *later* than the lateness of conscious experience of the external world with which we are already familiar.

Here is an example of what I mean. You may readily check it against your own experience.

First, imagine yourself driving at speed and having a near-miss collision with another car. If you are like me, it will be quite some seconds after you have successfully steered your car away from the collision that you will 'feel afraid'. And when you have this feeling, it will consist of one or more of the following: heart pounding; hands clammy with sweat; feeling hot, cold or one followed by the other; nausea in the pit of your stomach; tension in the limbs. This list is not exhaustive, but it will do for our purposes. The interesting thing about these feelings is that they all represent feedback from changes that the brain has instructed to occur in the body. And, as always where consciousness is concerned, we are *not* conscious of the issuing of the instructions. It seems, indeed, as though the body just does its own thing. But the bodily changes that occur during states of fear are in fact all orchestrated by outputs from the brain.

As it happens, we have a very good understanding of the functions served by each such bodily change. They are all aimed (as the result of Darwinian selection) at increasing your chances of winning out in a vigorous physical competition, archetypically one in which you fight with or run away from a predator or another human being. So, the sweat on your hands increases your capacity to grip; the tension in your muscles is in readiness to run, hit or kick; your heart pounds in readiness to supply your limbs and brain with the extra oxygen they are going to need; and so on. Even the odder symptoms can be understood along these lines. The feeling of nausea arises because blood is withdrawn from the stomach to be pumped to the muscles and brain, thus serving the more immediate needs of 'fight or flight' rather than digestion. As to hot and cold flushes, these arise because the body is vainly trying to erect its hair to make you look bigger, just as a cat does when it faces up to a dog. Sadly, your body doesn't know that the human species has lost most of its body hair. All it achieves, in a follicular equivalent of the grin of the Cheshire cat, is goose pimples and the ensuing reflex changes in temperature control.

In sum: you are faced with a danger; you react appropriately with skilled motor action (steering the car, for example); along with that, your brain instructs your body to respond in a way that used to be appropriate for vigorous action but which, in our modern times, only rarely is; and detection of those bodily changes throughout the body is fed back to neurons in the brain stem. Only *after* that feedback arrives in the brain stem is there anything with which to create the qualia that make up the conscious appreciation that you are in a state of fear. (As we shall see in a moment, even now we may not have reached the last neural stop before fear

*based on "emotions" literature*
*— unconscious emotional states precede conscious awareness of consciousness*

'enters into consciousness'.) These processes take a long time. In particular, both the instructions out from brain to body and the return feedback from body to brain utilise phylogenetically old types of nerve fibre that conduct nervous impulses very slowly. So the conscious appreciation of one's emotional state follows on very late behind, not only the events that cause it, but even one's reactions to those events. So delayed is conscious experience in these cases that there is no need for sophisticated experimental designs to make it manifest. Each of us can literally feel the lateness of consciousness for ourselves.

I would rather not require you, however, to have a near-miss road accident to verify the truth of these assertions. So here is a second, less life-threatening example. Suppose yourself in a seemingly tranquil and innocuous conversation with the Dearly Beloved (as 'significant others' were once, more romantically, called). She (or he, to taste) says something wounding (or rejecting, or arousing your jealousy, also according to taste). At first, you merely notice the offending remark and carry on the conversation as before, perhaps calmly thinking 'I can ignore that', or 'it isn't all that important anyway'. But then—and again it takes some seconds to happen—you start to feel a knot in the stomach, a clenching in the jaws, a clamminess in the hands, a tremulousness in the voice. The wounding remark has after all hit home, it just took you some time to find out.

Damasio, then, is surely right to emphasise feedback from bodily changes to the brain (not the brain's instructions to make those changes) as the warp and weave of core or 'emotional' consciousness. So let's go on to consider his position in a little more detail.

Notice, first, how well his view fits with the general stance this book has taken towards the contents of consciousness (see Chapter 3 and Section 8.4): that they consist in a re-representation of variables (here, heart rate or the sweatiness of one's palms, etc.) initially controlled unconsciously by the brain's servomechanisms. This pattern is, indeed, nowhere clearer than in emotional experience.

Notice, too, how well the two examples, above, of the nature of emotional experience fit the hypothesis (see Chapters 7 and 8) that an important aspect of the survival value of conscious experience is to act as a late error detector. By the time the emotional disturbance is consciously felt, the peril that caused it may well be over (as in the driving example). Indeed, without such rapid-action mechanisms to respond behaviourally to the peril, our ancestors could not have survived. So we need to look for *additional* survival value from the specifically conscious appreciation of the feedback from the bodily adjustments to meet the peril. Such survival value can come only from benefit to future behaviour. Next time round, for example, one may adopt more cautious driving habits. But we must not be too Panglossian about this. Evolution falls far short of perfection. This is particularly so in the case of emotion. Many features of the phylogenetically ancient systems of emotional disturbance and alarm bring little benefit (often, indeed, great harm, in the shape of the so-called 'stress diseases') to coping with the perils of modern life.

*? or simply "deliberation"*

Notice, next, the way in which emotional experience so neatly fits Edelman's pithy description of conscious experience as being a 'remembered present'. This notion is implicit in the comparator hypothesis of conscious experience, since each content of consciousness has been selected only after current sensory input has been compared to predicted input. But the memorial nature of conscious experience of the external world is obscured both by the short time scale over which the comparison process operates (an 'instant' of approximately 100 milliseconds), and by the seamless merging of the cause of perception (a rose, say, standing in a vase of water) with the percept itself (merged because the brain, as we have seen, constructs the perceived rose). The long-drawn-out process of emotion eliminates these obscurities. The Dearly Beloved's wounding remark is sharply separate in time and form from the tension in the stomach muscles that it causes but in no way resembles. Rather, the conscious appreciation of the knot in the stomach is a 'remembered present' that reminds you of the emotional wound. (Pain, incidentally, is another such remembered present, occurring late after injury and reminding you, this time, of a physical wound.)

Notice, finally, that, just as there are two visual systems, one for action and one for perception (Chapter 2), so there are two emotion systems, one for action and one for feeling. We have so far discussed the one for feeling. The emotion action system—again like the visual action system—works faster. It is this system that deals with the immediate danger. It has been much studied, especially in experiments on how animals learn to avoid danger or find food. These experiments give rise to an understanding of the different emotions as states caused by 'reinforcing events'—that is, rewards, punishments and other events with the power, if their occurrence is made contingent upon behaviour, to cause animals (including, of course, human beings) to change their ways.

In a further parallel with vision, the brain contains not one, but several 'emotion action' systems. There is no universal agreement as to their number or nature. My own analysis (see Gray and McNaughton, *The Neuropsychology of Anxiety*) indicates that the mammalian brain contains several such systems, each of wide-ranging influence upon behaviour. The first corresponds to human panic; it organises behaviour in response to strongly threatening stimuli at close proximity. A second corresponds to human fear. This emotion consists of responses to stimuli that warn of potential but avoidable threats. A third corresponds to human anxiety. This consists of responses to stimuli that warn of threat under circumstances in which it is necessary nonetheless to remain in or even approach the threatening situation. A fourth corresponds to hopeful anticipation, and organises responses to stimuli that are associated with primary rewards, such as food, water, comfort, safety and so on. Each of these systems produces a set of characteristic behavioural outputs designed to optimise reward and/or minimise punishment. So, the output from the panic system is 'fight or flight'; from the fear system, it is withdrawal; from the anxiety system, it is inhibition of ongoing behaviour plus risk assessment; from the 'hope' system, it is 'approach' behaviour, designed to obtain access to the primary reward. In addition, there are other emotion systems of less general behavioural effect; disgust, for example, functions so as to minimise the ingestion of potentially toxic substances.

The behavioural outputs from these various systems occur, in response to the stimuli that trigger their activity, much more rapidly than the bodily disturbances whose feedback to the brain provides the qualia for consciously felt emotion. Each system is widely distributed throughout the brain, but with some regions playing a more commanding role than others. So, in the case of panic, the central peri- aqueductal grey of the brain stem (just that region emphasised by Panksepp in his theory of core consciousness) is the final output station for fight and flight behav- iour; in the case, of fear, critical roles are played by the hypothalamus and the amygdala; and for anxiety the hippocampal system takes centre stage, using the same basic computational processes as it does for spatial navigation and episodic memory (see Fig. 14.5).

Although each emotion action system has its own neurology, they also extens- ively interact one with another. A key feature of this interaction is the existence of a vertical hierarchy, in which systems located higher up the neuraxis can inhibit and/or excite those located lower down (e.g. hippocampus → amygdala → hypothalamus → central grey; Fig. 18.4). Functionally, this arrangement permits, for example, the hippocampal system to orchestrate cautious approach to a feared but desired object or place (paradigmatic cases of situations that evoke anxiety). For this to be possible, the hippocampal system must be able to inhibit the with- drawal primed in the amygdala and the fight/flight primed in the central grey, while at the same time maintaining the bodily readiness for vigorous action that is also programmed in these latter areas. This hierarchical arrangement will be important for some of the arguments deployed below.

## 18.4   Signals of error?

Just as in the parallel case of vision and the other senses by which we interact with the external world, the existence of a conscious set of emotions alongside a set of apparently self-sufficient emotion action systems prompts the question: what purpose is served by core consciousness, delayed as it is until after the action systems have already done their work?

When we asked this question in respect of consciousness of the external world (Chapter 7), the answer I gave was that conscious experience serves as a late detec- tor of error. At first sight the same answer can seamlessly be given for some— indeed, for the most prominent—contents of core consciousness: pain, vertigo, nausea, extreme heat or cold. These all tell us that something has gone wrong. So the apparently natural and easy move, within the overall comparator model, is to treat them as signals of error. But this move faces problems. So as not to prejudge

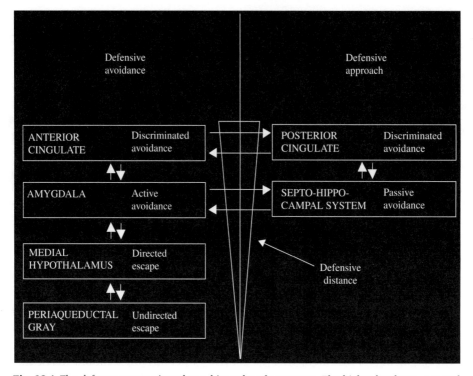

**Fig. 18.4** The defence system viewed as a hierarchy of structures. The higher levels are engaged by increasing defensive distance (i.e. distance from the threatened danger); and there are two parallel streams which control behaviour when danger is to be avoided or approached, respectively. Activity in the higher levels of the defence hierarchy can override behaviour that would otherwise result from activation of the lower levels alone. From Gray and McNaughton (2001).

whether or not they can be overcome, we need (at least for the moment) an alternative terminology for events of this nature. In the language of animal learning theory, they are termed 'punishments' or 'negative reinforcers'. Here I shall use the former term.

In terms of the comparator model, 'error' as applied to cognitive consciousness of the external world results directly from the operation of the comparison process. The comparator system, operating unconsciously, compares the predicted and actual states of the world, as represented in the thalamocortical sensory systems of the brain. 'Error' then consists in the discrepancy, or 'mismatch', between these two states, and is used to select some of the contents of the next instant of consciousness (typically, the most salient ones). The information that defines the nature of the error lies in the very contents so selected. These appear to consciousness simultaneously as the item constructed (e.g. a spider in a vase of water) and as being in some way unpredicted (the last time you looked at the vase, it contained a rose). The perceptual construct and its unexpectedness are tightly bound together, conforming to the general manner in which intentional perception works. Let us call this way of binding an error signal tightly to the information that defines the nature of the error, 'intrinsic error'.

Punishments don't seem to work in this way at all. To see the difference, consider nausea. The mode of entry into consciousness of this sensation fits with Damasio's model. What is sensed is feedback from a whirlwind of events, commanded by the brain, taking place in the gut as it goes into reverse (vomiting or 'emesis'), usually in order to expel noxious substances. The most common trigger for emesis is the detection by the brain of neural messages signalling the presence of toxins in the gut. These triggering messages do not themselves reach conscious awareness, they just set emesis going unconsciously. The conscious feeling of nausea arises when the brain receives feedback indicating that the gut is complying with its instructions. All these processes, both the commands to and the feedback from the gut, are coordinated at the level of the brain stem.

Where, in this process, lies the 'error'? Cybernetically speaking, there isn't any. On the contrary, the feedback from the gut tells the brain that emesis is going according to plan. Behaviourally (in the example I have given), the error lies in the ingestion of the toxic substance in the first place. However, the feeling of nausea conveys no information at all about the nature of this substance or the circumstances of its ingestion. Commonly, indeed, one has to wrack one's brain to think what on earth one has eaten, often to no avail. Worse still, one cannot even be sure that the nausea results from food poisoning at all—it might be due to illness or pregnancy. From this point of view, then, if one were to treat nausea as a signal of error, it is the very antithesis of the intrinsic error of cognitive consciousness. All that nausea tells you is that there is *something* unpleasantly wrong, not what that something is. (This, by the way, is another way of saying that nausea, like the other feelings that make up core consciousness but unlike the contents of cognitive consciousness, lacks intentionality. It is not about anything other than itself, it does not refer.) Let us call this kind of generalised signal, that *something's wrong*, 'extrinsic error'. Intrinsic and extrinsic error differ markedly, too much so perhaps for them both to count as discharging the same function.

Nausea has a second feature that is troubling for any treatment of core consciousness within the comparator model. Part of the justification for this model is that it offers a survival value for consciousness, despite the fact that this comes too late to affect the on-line behaviour with which particular contents of consciousness are associated. The putative survival value is that late error detection permits you to look back, in the 'remembered present', at what led to the error and thus, perhaps, to work out how to remediate it next time around. For this process to get off the ground, however, it must be possible to see the connection between what has just gone wrong and what happened just before that. These are not always both available in a single instant of the remembered present. But it is often then possible to retrieve from episodic memory the necessary information about what has just happened. It is for this reason, on the comparator model, that there is such a close alliance between conscious perception and the conscious recollection of episodic (time- and place-stamped) memory. But, as we have just seen, the feeling of nausea does not bring with it access to this information. In this respect, indeed, nausea provides a particularly telling example, for it commonly follows the ingestion of the toxic substance by many hours. Thus the event of ingestion is never available within the same moment of consciousness as the nausea; nor is there typically any consciously available link between the ingested substance and the feeling of sickness.

Our putative survival value, then, doesn't seem to apply at least to this content of core consciousness. Can we find any alternative? Why does natural selection bother to make us feel so wretched when we retch, if there is nothing we can do about the retching?

The issue is not whether it is possible to associate sickness as such with the circumstances that provoke it. To the contrary: there is a vast experimental litera-ture on 'conditioned taste aversion' demonstrating that animals form such associ-ations with enormous efficiency. Both the learning and the performance of these associations conform to the general principles of 'classical' or 'Pavlovian' con-ditioning. In this form of learning, an animal is presented with a 'conditioned stimulus' followed in time by an 'unconditioned stimulus'. The unconditioned stimulus is typically one of biological significance (food, for example), and this significance is not shared with the conditioned stimulus (a tone, say, or a light). After a number of 'pairings' in which the conditioned stimulus is regularly fol-lowed, shortly afterwards, by the unconditioned stimulus the animal learns the association between the two, as demonstrated most often by a response to the conditioned stimulus that is appropriate to the unconditioned stimulus. So, in Ivan Pavlov's classic experiments at the start of the twentieth century, dogs were exposed to the sequence tone → food and came to salivate in response to the tone alone.

In experiments on conditioned taste aversion this same Pavlovian design is used. The conditioned stimulus is typically food or water with a particular flavour added—that of vinegar, say, or sucrose. After consuming the food, the animal (most often a rat) is made sick. Subsequently, it is offered the flavoured food again, but now rejects it, so demonstrating that it has learnt the association between the flavour and the sickness. Conditioned taste aversion is a particularly efficient form of Pavlovian conditioning. Learning usually takes place with just one exposure to the flavour-sickness association (whereas other forms of conditioning often require many such pairings); it takes place even when many hours separate the flavour and the sickness (whereas the best conditioning is usually obtained when the conditioned and unconditioned stimuli overlap in time); and it needs no direct causal link between the food and the sickness. So, for example, the rat may drink a perfectly innocuous sugar solution and then, four hours later, it is made sick by an injection of lithium chloride. If it is offered the sugar solution next day, it resolutely refuses to drink it. Importantly, however, for the experiment to work, the sugary flavour has to be novel when it is first associated with sickness. The brain seems to come equipped with a special-purpose learning mechanism that associates sickness with the most unusual flavour the animal has recently experienced. The survival value of such a mechanism will be evident. Flavours you have frequently tasted in the past without untoward consequences are less likely to signal toxic substances than flavours never before encountered.

*good taste may betray toxicity*

So, given this efficient learning of taste aversions, what added survival value comes from the *conscious* awareness of nausea? A possible solution to this conundrum has been suggested by Tony Dickinson, in his account of how sickness transformed his feelings about water melons.

To remind you (see Section 8.4), Dickinson first tasted water melon as a young man one summer in Italy and thought it delightful. But shortly after eating the melon, and for unrelated reasons, he fell violently ill. Next day he once more came across a water melon and bit into it with gleeful anticipation—only to find that he at once felt extremely sick. Subsequently, he has avoided water melons. This is a clear case, then, of learned taste aversion. It is also, just as in the experiments with rats, a clear case of *spurious* learning: the innocent water melon played no role in making Dickinson sick, but got the blame anyway. Dickinson, of course, knew that the water melon was blameless, but that did not stop him forming an aversion to it. He now knows, indeed, as much as anyone in the world about the mechanisms underlying this spurious learning; but his aversion persists till this day. This imperviousness to consciously available intellectual knowledge is typical of classical conditioning. This makes it even more puzzling that the brain clothes both the initial nausea and its conditioned simulacrum in conscious qualia.

As a solution to this puzzle Dickinson and his colleague, Bernard Balleine, proposed the hypothesis that the function of conscious experience is to act as an interface at which emotional reactions (in the example, a conditioned taste aversion to the hitherto pleasant water melon) can interact with a cognitive and behavioural action program (buying, cutting into and eating water melons). This cannot be a general account of the function of consciousness. It has no natural application, for example, to the synaesthetic experiences described in Chapter 10 or to listening to music. But the hypothesis deserves serious consideration on its home territory—territory we have now reached.

## 18.5   *Core* consciousness?

Damasio and Panksepp take 'core' consciousness of bodily emotion to be, in some sense, more fundamental than cognitive consciousness of the external world. In what sense might this be?

Part of what is meant is that core consciousness evolved earlier than cognitive consciousness. This notion fits well with the anatomical facts: the region of the brain to which core consciousness is allotted—the brain stem—is a much earlier evolutionary development than the regions (neocortex, thalamus and limbic system) thought to play host to cognitive consciousness. But the notion of an 'earlier evolution' for core compared to cognitive consciousness itself raises problems. Might consciousness have evolved *twice* in the vertebrate brain—once when the brain stem commenced monitoring feedback from bodily change, and then again when the forebrain began to construct its model of the external world? This possibility cannot be excluded; and, indeed, there are possible precedents. Long before the elaboration of the mammalian visual system, for example, receptors sensitive to light evolved as a skin sense. However, there are reasons to doubt a similar scenario for consciousness.

First, there is the issue of survival value. As we have seen, it is hard enough to establish a survival value for cognitive consciousness. It is much more difficult to find one in mere awareness (after the fact, as always) of bodily change. Introspectively, this awareness seems to give no purchase for the control of bodily change. Such control as it may afford seems always to involve additional awareness emanating from cognitive consciousness. So, for example, I may well use the feeling of a growing nausea to get myself home and into bed as quickly as possible. But that requires a range of knowledge, both conscious and unconscious, that would surely not be available to the unaided brain stem.

The Dickinson and Balleine hypothesis explicitly acknowledges this need for both forms of consciousness to work together. Their experiments (described in detail in Section 8.4) demonstrate that, for a rat to develop a conditioned taste aversion, it must re-taste the flavour (of sucrose) that was earlier followed by sickness. It is as though the rat needs to discover that, when it drinks a sucrose solution, it no longer tastes so good (or even induces nausea), before it can use that information to devalue the reward of sucrose (and so give up the action—lever-pressing—for which sucrose had been the reward). Drawing upon his own experience with the water melon, Dickinson supposes, therefore, that the final step in the establishment of a conditioned taste aversion is the conscious experience within a small unit of time of both the conditioned stimulus (sucrose for the rat, water melon for him) and the conditioned response of nausea. This mechanism could be seen as an evolutionarily earlier version of conscious recollection (see Sections 14.2 and 14.3), which similarly allows the juxtaposition in conscious awareness of events that are initially separated in time. Unlike conscious recollection, however, conditioned taste aversion does not depend upon the integrity of the hippocampus. But it is highly unlikely that structures in the brain stem discharge this function. Rather, it appears to lie with another forebrain region, the insular cortex, which we shall shortly consider in more detail (see Fig. 18.6).

Dickinson's account is cogent and consistent with the general position adopted in this book (see Section 8.4), namely, that an important function of consciousness is to change the settings of controlled variables in feedback loops. But there is a weak link in his chain of argument. On the second occasion of tasting water melon

Dickinson had two conscious experiences, one shortly after the other: the taste, smell, sight, etc., of the water melon, followed by a feeling of sickness. The neural underpinnings of these two experiences lie, one largely in the forebrain, and the other largely in the brain stem. The weak link in the chain of argument is this: there is no evidence that the key juxtaposition, allowing the final establishment of the conditioned taste aversion, is between the two *conscious* experiences rather than simply the two sets of neural events that underpin them. (This, of course, is a specific version of the general epiphenomenalist problem already encountered many times throughout this book.) To be sure, Dickinson and Balleine showed (Section 8.4) that the anti-emetic drug, ondansetron, given at the time of re-exposure of rats to sucrose prevented the development of the conditioned taste aversion. But this blocks the systems responsible for emesis as well as the conscious feeling of nausea that accompanies emesis.

Nonetheless, the Dickinson–Balleine hypothesis of the survival value of core consciousness is the best we have. So let's assume it to be correct and go on to explore its implications.

These are, in fact, quite far-reaching. If the survival value of core consciousness depends upon further conscious experience of the external world mediated in the forebrain, this renders it very unlikely that there could have been any independent evolution of core consciousness prior to that of cognitive consciousness. So, if this inference is correct, 'core' consciousness may deserve the name only in the relatively trivial sense that it is consciousness of the body core. That is, 'core' consciousness would occupy a conceptual level equivalent to that of 'visual' or 'auditory' consciousness. In that case we need to ask, along lines made familiar by the Crick and Koch treatment of vision (Chapter 13): where within the systems that mediate bodily sensations is the neural correlate of core conscious experience? It is by no means clear that the answer to this question is 'in the brain stem'. Indeed, studies of pain perception strongly suggest a very different location: one in the neocortex.

The pathways that mediate pain (triggered by stimuli either to the skin or in the internal organs) travel in the spinal cord to the central grey of the brain stem and then onwards to the thalamus and neocortex. The neocortical regions most concerned with pain are the insula (Fig. 18.5) and the anterior cingulate cortex (Fig. 18.6). These two regions lie quite close to one another and are strongly interconnected.

It is in the insula that lesions (in the rat brain) eliminate conditioned taste aversion. This effect is not unexpected, since the insula serves as part of the primary cortical gustatory area (i.e. it is concerned with the analysis of tastes). It also receives inputs from stimulation of the oesophagus and is active during gastric disturbance and vomiting. In human beings, the role in disgust of the insular cortex extends well beyond these primary reactions to toxic substances and includes reactions to facial expressions of disgust in other people. We saw an example of this

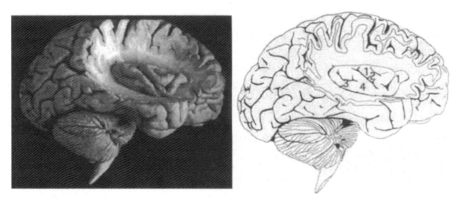

**Fig. 18.5** The insular cortex after removal of overlying cortical structures. 1: Short gyri of insula. 2: Central sulcus of insula. 3: Circular sulcus of insula. 4: Long gyrus of insula. The insula is a substantial portion of cerebral cortex that forms the floor of a fossa that can be opened up by removing the lips bounding the lateral sulcus and its rami. These lips are known as the frontal, parietal, and temporal opercula. After their excision, the insula appears as a triangular eminence that is marked by a number of sulci and gyri. The so-called circular sulcus surrounds the insula, except inferomedially where the cortex of the insula is continuous, at the limen insulae, with the cerebral cortex lateral to the anterior (rostral) perforated substance on the basal aspect of the brain. The insular cortex is indented by a number of sulci, one of which—the central sulcus of the insula—is deeper and more prominent than the rest. The central sulcus of the insula runs in an upwards and backwards direction, almost parallel to the cerebral central sulcus that delimits the frontal lobe from the parietal lobe. In front of the central sulcus of the insula, a few short gyri tend to radiate from the vicinity of the limen insulae. Behind the central sulcus one long gyrus of the insula is present in this specimen, partially divided by a shallow sulcus near its upper and posterior end. From Williams *et al. The Human Brain,* Chapter 5. *http://www.vh.org/adult/provider/anatomy/BrainAnatomy/TOC.html*

role in Chapter 11 (see Fig. 11.2). The insula reacts also to sexual arousal, heat, cold, feelings of hunger and thirst, vestibular stimulation (conveying information about balance or its loss, as in vertigo), and even during the emotional 'chills' people sometimes get from listening to music (a fascinating experiment reported by Anne Blood and Robert Zatorre in Montreal). This region appears, therefore, to constitute a general cortical centre for the analysis of bodily sensation, providing a higher-order re-representation of information that is initially detected in the brain stem. This, indeed, is the way Damasio treats the insula; thus the argument pursued here does not conflict with his overall model of core consciousness.

As well as participating in these other bodily senses, the human insula is also involved in pain, as shown by both neuroimaging studies and case reports of patients with damage in this region. Of particular interest is a striking syndrome— 'asymbolia for pain'—which occurs in people who, as the result of stroke, suffer destruction of the insular cortex. Such patients are able to detect a painful stimulus, e.g. a pin-prick applied to the skin, and have normal thresholds for the detec-

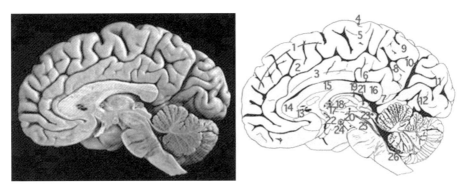

**Fig. 18.6** The cingulate cortex (3) on the medial surface of the brain. 1: Medial frontal gyrus.
2: Cingulate sulcus. 3: Cingulate gyrus (cingulate cortex). 4: Central sulcus. 5: Paracentral lobule.
6: Callosal sulcus. 7: Isthmus of cingulate gyrus. 8: Subparietal sulcus. 9: Precuneus. 10: Parieto-
occipital sulcus. 11: Cuneus. 12: Calcarine sulcus or fissure. 13: Rostrum of corpus callosum.
14: Genu of corpus callosum. 15: Trunk of corpus callosum. 16: Splenium of corpus callosum.
17: Choroid plexus in interventricular foramen. 18: Interthalamic adhesion. 19: Habenular
trigone. 20: Hypothalamic sulcus. 21: Pineal body. 22: Anterior (rostral) commissure. 23: Tectum
of midbrain. 24: Mammillary body. 25: Medial longitudinal fasciculus. 26: Choroid plexus of 4th
ventricle. The cingulate sulcus begins below the rostrum of the corpus callosum and arches in front
of the genu of the corpus callosum, about a finger's breadth distant from it. Above the splenium
of the corpus callosum, the cingulate sulcus turns abruptly upwards to reach the superior margin
of the hemisphere. Where the precentral and postcentral gyri come together, the central sulcus
cuts into the paracentral lobule. The cingulate gyrus is a long strip of cortex that curves around the
corpus callo-sum. Posteriorly, it becomes very narrow under the splenium of the corpus callosum
and is continuous with the isthmus, which separates the splenium from the calcarine sulcus or
fissure. The cingulate gyrus has profuse reciprocal connections with the anterior thalamic nuclei
and is an important constituent of the limbic system. From Williams *et al. The Human Brain*,
Chapter 5. *http://www.vh.org/adult/provider/anatomy/BrainAnatomy/Ch5Text/Section03.html*

tion of such stimuli. But the pin-prick fails to evoke normal avoidance behaviour
or emotional reactions. Here is a description of one such patient: 'He tolerated
prolonged pin-prick or soft-tissue pinching in all four limbs without adequate
grimacing or defensive movements of the limbs...On occasion, the patient willingly
offered his hands for pain testing and laughed during the stimulation' (Berthier,
Starkstein and Leiguarda, 1988, p. 42). In his book (with Sandra Blakeslee),
*Phantoms In The Brain* (p. 268), Ramachandran describes similar patients who
'actually start giggling, as if they were being tickled and not stabbed'.

These observations strongly implicate the insula as an essential link in the chain
of neural activity that leads to the conscious sensation of pain, with all its emotional sequelae. Given the view that these emotional feelings consist of consciously
appreciated feedback from bodily changes, this conclusion implies also that down-
stream impulses from the insula to the brain stem may be required to set such
emotional processes in motion. This hypothesis is supported by observations that

stimulation of the insula, or epileptic electrical activity which invades this region, can elicit vomiting and changes in heart rate and blood pressure. These and other outputs to the internal organs may pass by way of projections from the insula to the amygdala and the prefrontal cortex, both of which have extensive control over a wide range of bodily changes controlled by the autonomic nervous system. Thus the notion that core consciousness arises from activities in the brain stem that are then passed up to a cognitive consciousness higher up in the brain may be exactly the wrong way round. It is just as likely—perhaps more so—that emotional consciousness, just like cognitive consciousness, is linked directly to activity in higher cortical and limbic regions of the brain.

The insula is not the only cortical region with a claim to acting as the site of the neural correlate of the conscious experience of pain. To appreciate this, consider some experiments employing the 'thermal grill'.

A 1994 paper in *Science* by Craig and Bushnell described this intriguing new way to produce a sensation of burning pain. The subject places his hand over an array of 15 parallel horizontal silver bars, each of which can be set at a different temperature. If they are all set at 20°C, the subject reports a cool sensation; if they are all at 40°C, they are felt as warm. The trick is to set alternating bars at 20°C and 40°C. When that happens, the subject feels a sensation of pain akin to 'burning' cold. Two years later the same group of scientists used positron emission tomography (PET) to measure brain activity in response to the thermal grill. You will recall that neuroimaging methods require subtraction of the pattern of brain activity elicited by a control condition from the one elicited by the experimental condition of primary interest. The thermal grill is ideally suited to these requirements. Thus Craig and his colleagues were able to subtract from the pattern of activity elicited by the grill each of the patterns elicited by its component parts, that is, bars set only at 20°C or only at 40°C. The insula was the only cortical region that was activated by all thermal stimuli, innocuous or painful. But a different region—the anterior cingulate cortex—was selectively activated only by the grill and not by its component parts. Such activity was also elicited by bars set all at painfully cold (5°C) or painfully hot (47°C) temperatures.

There is therefore a slight tension between the data from brain damage, which indicate the insula as the key centre for the conscious appreciation of pain, and those from neuroimaging, which indicate the anterior cingulate cortex. However, since both these regions are in the neocortex, not the brain stem, this detail is not important for our general argument.

Alongside this positive evidence for neocortical representation of the conscious sensation of pain, there is negative evidence showing absence of activation of the central periaqueductal grey in response to a painful skin injection. In this study, by Hsieh and others in Martin Ingvar's laboratory in Stockholm, three conditions were compared: (1) a painful injection of ethanol, (2) a non-painful injection of saline under conditions where a painful injection was expected, and (3) a non-painful injection of saline with an explicit statement that this would not be painful. The central grey was activated in both of the first two conditions compared to the third; and there was no difference between the activations observed in the central grey in the first two conditions. Thus central grey activation did not reflect pain as such (which differentiated the first two conditions), but rather the anticipation of pain (which the first and second conditions shared but the third one lacked). This result is consistent with what is known about the functions of the central grey in animals. This region is concerned with active efforts to escape from pain or the close-up threat of pain. But Hsieh's result is inconsistent with the notion that there is a neural correlate in the central grey of the conscious perception of pain as such.

The anterior cingulate cortex plays a wider role in conscious experience than just the perception of pain. Bilateral damage to this region, due for example to stroke, can give rise to the severely disabling condition of 'akinetic mutism'. As the name implies, patients with this condition neither move nor speak, and they may remain this way for months. Damasio describes the residual behaviour of one such patient as follows (*The Feeling of What Happens*, p. 102):

> She would lie in bed, often with her eyes open but with a blank facial expression. On occasion she might catch an object in motion—me, for instance, moving around her bed—and track for a few instants, eyes and head moving along for a moment, but the quiet, non-focused staring would be resumed rapidly. The term *neutral* helps convey the equanimity of her expression, but once you concentrated on her eyes, the word *vacuous* gets closer to the mark. She was there but not there.

We know enough about the possibility of visual tracking in the absence of awareness not to take this residual behaviour as indicative of conscious experience. And indeed, in sharp contrast to patients with the locked-in syndrome considered earlier, upon eventual recovery from akinetic mutism patients report an almost total absence of conscious experience while they lay mute and unmoving. These reports, if accurate, add to the dissociation, noted earlier, between wakefulness and consciousness, since patients with akinetic mutism continue to cycle more or less normally between sleep and waking. However, the assumption of accurate report may be unwarranted. Self-reports *after recovery* from akinetic mutism—the only kind possible—may indicate absence, not of conscious experience, but of consciously available memory of experience. The latter possibility is supported by the very close anatomical connections between the cingulate cortex and the hippocampal system, which as we know (Section 14.2) mediates conscious episodic memory. These connections take the form of a loop (Fig. 18.7) described in 1937 by the anatomist Papez, after whom it is named.

Let us stick, however, to the view that akinetic mutism reflects loss of the conscious experience itself. Damasio then interprets these observations in the light of his general model of consciousness. This postulates that, for full conscious experience—what Damasio calls 'extended' consciousness—there has to be a conjunction between consciousness of the self (mediated by the system that ascends

# Papez Circuit

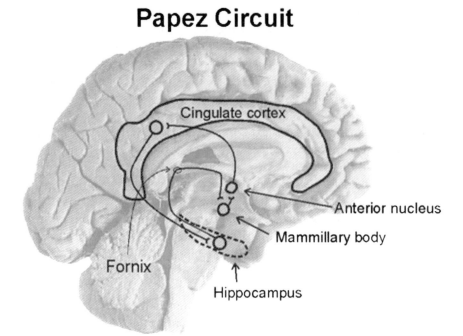

**Fig. 18.7** The Papez circuit, linking together the hippocampus, the cingulate cortex, the anterior nucleus (n) of the thalamus, and the mammillary bodies in the hypothalamus. From *http://w3.uokhsc.edu/human_physiology/EEG%20and%20Liimbic%20System/Papez.html*

from the brain stem to the insula and cingulate cortex) and cognitive consciousness of objects or events in the external world. Nor is this a *mere* conjunction between two aspects of conscious experience. For Damasio further holds that 'being conscious goes beyond being awake and attentive: it requires an inner sense of self in the act of knowing' (*op. cit.*, p. 250). That inner sense of self, moreover, is emotionally toned. This follows from Damasio's treatment of the conscious appreciation of emotional state as depending upon the same system (ascending from brain stem to neocortex) that constructs the conscious model of internal bodily states in general. Such views of the cingulate cortex as being central to emotional experience go back a long way. Papez, for example, inferred from the pattern of inputs to the cingulate cortex from the mammillary bodies (in the hypothalamus) and thalamus (Fig. 18.7) that it 'may be looked on as the receptive region for the experiencing of emotion', in much the same way that the ventral stream of the visual system (Chapter 13) is the receptive region for visual experience; and Neil McNaughton and I have incorporated this view of the functions of the cingulate cortex into our general model of the neuropsychology of anxiety.

Damasio's model of consciousness, then, places considerable explanatory burden upon the insular and cingulate cortices. His arguments tend, indeed, towards the conclusion that activity in the insular and/or cingulate cortex (by providing the 'inner sense of self in the act of knowing') must be a necessary feature of *all* conscious experience. Have we at last, then, found a site for the Cartesian theatre? There are reasons to doubt this.

First, this is not the only region of the brain in which lesions can give rise to akinetic mutism. The same syndrome also sometimes occurs for example after damage to the thalamus.

Second, the loss of conscious experience that characterises akinetic mutism, rather than being a direct effect of damage to the cingulate cortex, may be secondary to a reduction in the motivation to engage with the environment or with anything else (perhaps associated with additional damage to the adjacent supplementary motor area). Reduced motivation is, after all, just what you would expect after damage to a region that is critical to normal emotional experience; and Damasio's observations make it clear that this is indeed what happens. As he writes (*op. cit.*, p. 103), the patient 'during her long period of silence...had never felt fear, had never been anxious, had never wished to communicate.' These observations, of course, do not allow one to decide whether the loss of reported experience or of motivation is primary. But they do raise doubts about the strength of the case for allotting to the cingulate cortex a central role underpinning all conscious experience.

Third, ordinary introspection seems to reveal a fairly clear distinction between states of consciousness in which bodily sensations, whether indicative of emotional turmoil or not, figure prominently and states of consciousness in which they do not. I do not, for example, notice many such sensations as I write this book; and, when I do, they are an extraneous distraction—an aching back, for example— rather than intrinsic to the main contents of my consciousness while I am absorbed in the writing.

This does not necessarily imply that Damasio's insistence on the ubiquity of a 'sense of self' as part of conscious experience is wrong (though the emphasis upon the *inner* self may be too narrow). For there is more than one possible source of such a sense of self. As noted at the previous chapter, in its construction of the external world cognitive consciousness necessarily adopts a 'point of view'. This is as much a source of the sense of self as are bodily sensations. Furthermore, the objects that cognitive consciousness constructs in the external world include one's own body, but this is then seen, heard and felt from the outside rather than the inside. Consider, for example, what happens when you use a mirror to shave or put on lipstick. This gives you a distinct feeling of self, but it does not depend upon the kind of internal bodily sensations for whose analysis the insula and cingulate cortex are specialised. Rather, like the point of view, this kind of percept depends upon interactions between the appropriate sensory cortex (vision and touch if you are shaving) and the parietal cortex (for the construction of egocentric space; Chapter 15). Which kind of sense of self is conjoined with perception of the external world probably determines, at least in part, the degree to which one's feelings at any given moment are emotional. Given a self that is largely constructed from the outside, one is likely to feel relatively unemotional; but, as more bodily sensations get added to the mix, the experience is likely to become more emotionally toned.

## 18.6   An evolutionary scenario

I conclude, therefore, that core consciousness (consciousness of bodily states and the emotional reactions that reflect these states) does not differ radically from cognitive consciousness in terms of brain location. Both depend for their proximal neural correlates upon activity, not in the brain stem, but in the neocortex (however, core consciousness does differ sharply from cognitive consciousness in its general lack of intentionality).

This, at any rate, seems to be the state of affairs in human beings today. We should note, however, that the situation may have been different at an earlier time in evolution. Evolutionary development of the brain shows a steady trend towards 'encephalisation': that is, functions which, at an earlier point in evolution, are discharged by structures low in the neuraxis come to be taken over at a later point by structures higher up. Typically, when this happens, the newer, higher structures operate by acquiring the capacity to modulate (by excitation, inhibition or a mixture of the two) activity in the lower structures. We saw an example of this arrangement when we looked at the defensive hierarchy (Fig. 18.4). In this hierarchy, the amygdala modulates activity in the hypothalamus, and this in turn modulates activity in the central grey. Activity in the amygdala may itself also be modulated by structures higher still in the neuraxis, notably the hippocampus, temporal lobe and insula. These are the very structures with which we have been concerned. So one possibility is that core consciousness was at one time in evolution closely related to activity in one of these lower structure, but this arrangement later fell under control from higher centres. However, this hypothesis is both speculative and difficult to test. To be taken seriously it needs, at least, a great deal more evidence from comparative anatomy and comparative behavioural research than is currently available.

I suggested in Section 18.4 that the notion that the emotionally negative features of core consciousness (pain, nausea, vertigo and the like) function as error signals may run into certain problems. The error signals of cognitive consciousness are derived from the operations of a comparator system and thus carry *intrinsic* information as to the nature of the error. Core consciousness, in contrast, provides an *extrinsic* signal of error: one that says merely *something has gone wrong* without specifying what that something is. In the light of the evolutionary considerations sketched above, can we now make progress in integrating such extrinsic error with the intrinsic variety postulated for cognitive consciousness?

Our task is now indeed easier. We may suppose that there was a single time when the brain evolved the capacity to construct a semi-permanent model of the external world that could be used to facilitate the late detection of error and so provide the possibility of error-correction for application on a future occasion. For reasons that are not at present understood, this capacity required the use of qualia. Still less understood is the mechanism by which the brain was suddenly able to create and read qualia. Nonetheless, we are each of us here as proof that the brain did evolve these capacities. Having dismissed the idea that the evolution of core consciousness might have preceded that of cognitive consciousness, we may suppose further that the same basic mechanism that evolved for the construction of a model of the external world was applied, and at the same time, to the construction of consciously perceived inner bodily sensations.

The relevant feedback systems of the brain stem were already in place by the time this evolutionary leap occurred. Many of the variables controlled by these systems bear strong motivational valences. For some (those, for example, indicative of tissue damage), the desired setting of the variable is as low as possible; for others (those, for example, indicative of nutriment), the setting is rather high. I suggest that negatively valenced variables of the former kind (punishments) were co-opted by the newly evolving system of consciousness to act as extrinsic error signals. (Positively-valenced variables—rewards—provide signals confirming that motor programs are on the right track, and so might also be slotted into the same general kind of theory. But I shall not consider these further here.) The occurrence of extrinsic signals of error is used to reactivate the recent record of events in cognitive consciousness in order to facilitate identification of the faulty motor program that gave rise to them (cf. the discussion in Section 18.1 of the *kind* of mistakes that can affect consciousness of inner bodily sensations). This formulation implies a close relationship between the neural centres responsible for the conscious identification of extrinsic error and those responsible for episodic memory. This inference is supported by the anatomy. Both the insula and cingulate cortex project to the entorhinal cortex, which is the cortical gateway to the hippocampus; the insula also projects directly to the hippocampus; and the cingulate cortex projects to the subicular area, which is the main output pathway from the hippocampus (see Figs 14.2 and 18.7).

This theoretical perspective has the advantage that it offers a principled account of why the contents of cognitive consciousness possess intentionality, whereas those of core consciousness do not. The intentionality of cognitive consciousness reflects the computation of intrinsic error, derived from the operation of the comparator system and from the model of the external world upon which the comparator system operates. Intrinsic error signals thus refer to that model. In contrast, the extrinsic error signals of core consciousness do not emerge from or depend upon computations of this kind. That is why they refer to nothing beyond themselves.

There is one further aspect of the sense of self that we need to consider. But its implications for society are potentially so far-reaching that it deserves a chapter of its own.

# CHAPTER 19

# Responsibility

In the previous two chapters we looked at a number of different aspects of the sense of self: the point of view, the feeling of belongingness and the emotional self of the body. There remains one final aspect of the sense of self to consider—the sense of agency.

## 19.1   The sense of agency

The sense of agency is the 'I' of 'the archetypal narrative of consciousness', as I described it in Chapter 2, or what Daniel Dennett calls 'the centre of narrative gravity'. Chapter 2 went into this aspect of the sense of self in some detail, under a heading which can serve here also as a pretty good recapitulation: *illusions of the will*. As we saw in that chapter, the conscious awareness that one has taken a decision to act occurs after the brain has unconsciously already taken that decision. Furthermore, the conscious sense that one is or is not responsible for a given action can be in error in both possible directions: one can be responsible for an act but unaware of the responsibility; or consciously believe that one is responsible for an act which is not one's own. In short, in just the same way that the unconscious brain constructs a conscious model of the external world, so it constructs a model of the self as actor in that world. And, just like the model of the external world, the model of the self-as-agent comes after the event and is open to error. However, and again like the model of the external world, the model of the self-as-agent is more often right than wrong. Both models are guaranteed (by the pressures of evolutionary selection) to be sufficiently accurate guides to the reality of what actually happens 'out there' for them to be serviceable in the interests of action and survival.

The similarity between the models of the external world and the self goes still deeper. For the brain appears to use essentially the same methods to construct both models. The French neuroscientist, Marc Jeannerod, has reviewed the data gathered in a large number of neroimaging experiments, many from his own laboratory, and concludes that there is considerable overlap between the patterns of activation observed, on the one hand, when subjects execute or imagine executing actions of their own and, on the other, when they observe such actions performed by others. One of the regions to show this overlap is the inferior parietal lobule. As we saw in Chapter 15, this region plays a critical role in the construction of egocentric space and in feature binding for the model of the external world.

This same conclusion—that the brain uses the same machinery to model one's own actions and those of others—emerges from studies in which recordings have been made from single neurons in the brains of monkeys. The animals in these experiments either perform an action themselves or observe others (monkeys or human beings) performing the same action. In an experiment of this kind, Giacomo Rizzolatti and his colleagues described what they call 'mirror neurons' in an area that corresponds to part of the human prefrontal cortex. These neurons fire in response to a particular form of action (for example, grasping a piece of food) irrespective of who performs it, the observing monkey or an observed actor. Similar findings have subsequently been reported in human neuroimaging experiments.

Results such as these indicate, on a relatively microscopic scale, that the computation of what counts as one's own actions is performed by neural machinery that participates in the general computation of the external world. The self, as it were, observes its own actions from the outside and deduces its role as agent in the light of these observations. This conclusion is echoed in behavioural data at a much more complex level. Thus, for example, when patients receive behavioural treatment for anxiety disorders, improvement is first noted in measures of their behaviour. There is then a lag of many weeks before this improvement is reflected in the patient's self-ratings. The patient's view of his condition seems to be garnered from observations of his own behaviour, much as he would form a view of others from theirs.

The fact that the brain uses the same machinery to model action irrespective of the actor, oneself or another, raises the question: how does it then distinguish between the two? The short answer is: with difficulty. We saw some examples of this in Chapter 2.

Jeannerod's group has analysed the difficulty further. In one of their experiments the subject, wearing a glove, was asked on each trial to perform a given hand movement, such as to stretch a thumb or the first two fingers. The experimental arrangement illustrated in Fig. 19.1 was deployed so that what the subject then saw was, on some trials, his own gloved hand and, on others, someone else's making a corresponding movement. When it was someone else's, the 'alien' hand either made the same movement as the subject had been instructed to perform or a different one. After each trial, subjects were asked whether the hand they had seen was their own or someone else's. Accuracy in making this judgement was, as you might expect, very good when the subject saw his own hand or saw the alien hand making a movement different from the one he had executed. But on trials when the observed hand made the same movement as the subject, but it in fact belonged to someone else, accuracy plummeted: subjects took the alien hand to be their own 30% of the time.

Experiments such as these led Jeannerod to conclude that the judgement of agency depends upon the operation of a comparator system. This seeks to match the motor command 'stretch a thumb' with the perception of a thumb stretching. If there is a good match, the system concludes that the observed thumb is the subject's, even on occasions when it isn't. This, of course, is the same general

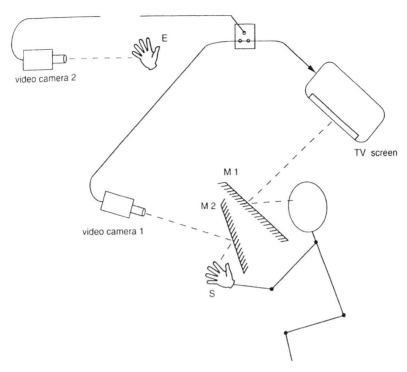

**Fig. 19.1** Schematic representation of experimental display used for presenting a subject with his own hand (Hand S, filmed by Videocamera 1 through Mirror M2) or an alien hand (Hand E, filmed by Videocamera 2). Either hand could be shown to the subject on a TV screen seen through Mirror M1. Hands were covered with the same glove. The subject and the experimenter were placed in different cabins. At the onset of each trial, both the subject and the experimenter received the instruction to perform a hand movement. On specific trials, however, the experimenter executed a movement different from that requested by the instruction. Hand exposure lasted throughout the movement. After the completion of each trial, a verbal response was requested from the subject about whether or not the hand seen during exposure was his. From Jeannerod (1999).

mechanism as the comparator which I have postulated as participating in the construction of the model of the external world. Thus Jeannerod's analysis is consistent with a view of the sense of agency which treats this as being on a par with the other contents of cognitive consciousness of the external world.

Ramachandran has used this aspect of brain function to come up with an ingenious treatment for patients who suffer from phantom limb. Here is his description of one such patient:

> Robert Townsend is an intelligent, fifty-five-year-old engineer whose cancer caused him to lose his left arm six inches above the elbow. When I saw him seven months after the amputation, he was experiencing a vivid phantom limb that would often go

into an involuntary clenching spasm. 'It's like my nails are digging into my phantom hand,' said Robert. 'The pain is unbearable.' Even if he concentrated all his attention on it, he could not open his invisible hand to relieve the spasm.

To treat Robert, Ramachandran used a 'mirror box'. This simple device is a box divided in two by a vertical mirror. On each side of the mirror there is a hole through which a hand can be inserted. Robert inserted his good right hand into the hole on the right and used the mirror to superimpose its reflection over where he felt the phantom hand on the left to be. He then made a fist with the good hand. In this way, Robert now had two simulacra of a left hand: the felt phantom and the seen reflection in the mirror of his real right hand. Ramachandran now asked Robert to try to unclench 'both' hands. Unclenching the good, right hand, of course, caused a visual impression in the mirror of an unclenching left hand. The very first time he did this 'Robert exclaimed that he could feel the phantom fist open along with his good fist'—something he had been completely unable to achieve before. 'Better yet, the pain disappeared' (*Phantoms in the Brain*, pp. 52–3).

## 19.2   The concept of responsibility

Clearly, this way of understanding the sense of agency as a fallible construction of the brain has potentially dangerous consequences for concepts of human responsibility. One cannot, of course, tailor the results of scientific enquiry so as to avoid such dangers. The world, and ourselves in it, are the way they are, and it is the business of science to find out what that is. In the long run, it will do no-one any good to get it wrong, whether by negligence or design. Nonetheless, there are today so many pressures to remove the concept of responsibility from the ethical landscape that we should not add to them unthinkingly.

Attacks upon concepts of responsibility usually stem from a determinist analysis of action. You may believe, so the argument runs, that you have freely decided to undertake a given action, but your decision was in fact fully determined by a preceding causal chain of some kind or another. One may not, in any particular case, be able to identify or describe the offending causal chain—indeed, one normally comes nowhere near doing so—but one can be sure that some such chain exists. The experimental facts reviewed here and in Chapter 2 appear greatly to strengthen this argument. For they reveal that the decision you apparently take consciously is in fact made unconsciously. The various rational pros and cons that you believe swayed your judgement may, despite appearance, have had nothing to do with your decision at all. This just emerged from the unconscious workings of the machinery of your brain.

Before we subject this attack upon responsibility to closer scrutiny, there is an obvious point to get out of the way.

Some actions do not fit the above analysis at all well. For in many cases one does go through a more or less prolonged period of soul-searching, consciously listing the reasons for and against undertaking a particular action. There is no reason, within the position adopted in this book, to suppose that, in these cases, conscious reflection upon the reasons for action has no effect upon the choice eventually taken. To the contrary: I have strenuously argued the case against regarding conscious experience as a mere epiphenomenon. Indeed, to accept the epiphenomenalist case is profoundly unbiological. But that, of course, is not to say that the influence of consciously entertained reasons upon choice and action is an influence independent of underlying neural mechanism. We don't yet know what that mechanism is—that is why there is a Hard Problem of consciousness—but it is highly unlikely that there isn't a neural mechanism at all. The alternatives to this view—dualism, free will and the like—always end up in hopeless contradiction and muddle.

There are, nonetheless, cases in which conscious reflection does appear to play a part in decision making. In these cases, the determinist attack upon the concept of responsibility cannot seek further strength in the lateness of conscious volition or its proneness to illusion. But, then, this attack is already strong. And there are anyway plenty of other cases in which decision and action occur with no soul-searching at all. A famous instance (for British readers) was when the then Deputy Prime Minister, John Prescott, struck out, in full camera view, at a heckler who had had the temerity to throw flour at him. Mr Prescott moved impressively fast—far too fast for any soul-searching. But if his punch had landed him in court, its rapidity would not have been a sufficient defence. He would have been held responsible for his action, soul-searching or none. However, the law does recognise the distinction I am making. *Premeditated* acts are punished more harshly than the ordinary variety. But the ordinary variety nonetheless attracts due punishment. So, if we are to ward off the determinist attach upon responsibility, this is where we should start. Any successful defence of the concept of responsibility in the case of unpremeditated decision and action is likely to succeed also for the premeditated kinds.

So, in the light of the analysis pursued in this book, what defence against the determinist attack might there be? Surprising as it may seem, there is, I think, a powerful one.

The defence turns on the distinction made in Chapter 3 between the two different kinds of lawful processes by which all biology is bound: on the one hand, the laws of physics and chemistry and, on the other, the properties of cybernetic systems. In their book *Mind, Meaning and Mental Disorder*, Derek Bolton and Jonathan Hill have elegantly traced the application of this distinction to psychopathology. As they point out, one can seek explanations for e.g. depression or anxiety by having recourse either to the *meaning* of events in the patient's life or to the *physicochemical* properties of his brain. And, as we saw in Chapter 4, 'meaning' can be seen in principle as arising from the workings of a cybernetic machine, in a manner well analysed by Stevan Harnad in his treatment of the problem of 'symbol grounding'.

Let us apply this type of analysis, then, to the trial of John Doe. John is accused of having killed Mary Smith in a fit of road rage. It is not in dispute that John killed Mary—there are witnesses and John has admitted it anyway. John's defence is that, given the causal chains that led up to his action, he could not have acted otherwise and so should be let off. In analysing this defence, we need to distinguish between the two types of possible cause—cybernetic and physicochemical.

A pretty pure example of a physicochemical line of defence would go like this. Just before the killing, John suffered a stroke (itself due to mechanical dysfunction in a blood vessel) which destroyed a part of the frontal lobes of the brain whose normal function is to restrain impulsive action. Had the stroke not occurred, no matter how murderous his impulses, John's intact brain would have blocked them from translation into action. But, unfortunately for Mary, the critical bit of John's impulse-restraining feedback system just wasn't in place.

Consider, in contrast, two types of 'cybernetic' defence. They both stem from established knowledge that adult personality depends upon a mixture between the influences of genetic factors (inherited in the fertilised egg) and the environment in which one grows up. The first emphasises the genetic factors. John Doe, it is argued, got a bad deal of the genetic cards, making him impervious to society's attempts to turn him into a good citizen. The second emphasises John's unfortunate upbringing by criminal parents in an underprivileged part of town—again leading to the 'impervious' outcome. John's smart lawyer combines the two causal chains (as indeed they are often combined in reality): John had both a bad set of genes and a terrible upbringing. So what else could he do but kill Mary?

Before letting this defense dissolve you into compassionate tears, you should ask: what does it actually mean for John to be 'impervious' to society's (or Mum and Dad's, for that matter, if it's bad genes that got him into trouble) 'attempts to turn him into a good citizen'?

To a first approximation, those attempts consist in the application of rewards (for good behaviour) and punishments (for bad), along with explanations of what it is that makes them good and bad. Rewards and punishments work by acting as feedback to cybernetic systems. Those systems are phylogenetically ancient, having evolved so as to enable us to learn what to do in order to find food and avoid predators and so on. But they are also enormously flexible. The basis for this flexibility is the principle of 'secondary reinforcement'. 'Primary' rewards and punishments (food, pain, sex and so on) work without our needing to learn that they are rewarding or punishing—evolution just built them into the system. Secondary reinforcement works by conferring the same rewarding (or punishing) properties on other things which initially lack them. The trick is association. If a rat finds food in my dustbin but a cat next door, it will haunt mine and avoid my neighbour's. The preferences and aversions you build up for different parts of town work in the same way—as does moral education. Over a lifetime of learning, this seeks to make you prefer actions that society (and a good home) favour and desist from those it wishes to prevent. The law is just one part of this process, called in when all else fails.

In sum, the distinction between the physicochemical and cybernetic defences is this. If John has had a stroke, the critical impulse-restraining feedback system is damaged. If he has received bad genes or a bad upbringing, the settings on this feedback system are insufficiently sensitive to the rewards and punishments his society metes out. If John were a thermostat, we would send it off to be mended in the first case, but change the temperature settings in the second.

In both cases, John asks the judge and jury to let him off. How should we respond?

Leniency seems both a compassionate and a sensible option for the John who had a stroke. But I suspect that many readers have a queasy feeling in the second, cybernetic case, as though leniency here might undermine the very fabric of civilised society. That feeling is well-founded. For judicial decisions form part of the very machinery by which society installs its desired settings into the feedback systems of reward and punishment that guide the behaviour of its citizens. To show leniency because a culprit hasn't got the settings right has effects that go far beyond the individual concerned: it changes the balance of influences that set the settings for everyone. Thus, rather than dispense with punishment on such grounds, one might instead set the tariff higher, so as to bring more such Johns into the net. This, of course, is the familiar argument from deterrence. It's too late for John: he's already committed murder. But we need to punish him *pour encourager les autres*. There are those—and they are many—who find the argument from deterrence morally repugnant. They tend to go for another, biblical, quotation: 'it is expedient that one man should die for the people', famously said by Caiaphas, High Priest of the Pharisees (John 11:50).

Whether it is morally repugnant to you or not, the argument from deterrence fits the facts of behaviour, viewed both biologically and socially. Responsibility for one's actions is essentially a social construct; but it is one whose smooth function-ing depends upon neural machinery which has the prime biological purpose of favouring survival. Society's general attitude—before liberalism and scientism combined to chip away at moral consensus—was to hold people responsible for just those kinds of action (called by psychologists 'instrumental behaviour') which, as a rule and under normal conditions, are influenced by rewards and punish-ments. Conversely one was not generally held to account for 'reflexes', which (like the kicking of your leg when the patellar tendon is struck) are immune to reward and punishment'; nor for behaviour traceable to brain damage, such as an action carried out automatically during an epileptic seizure. This seems to me just the right place to strike the balance. Given the wide range of differences between individuals, no fixing by society of rewards and punishments will work for every-one. So there will always be some individuals who fail to conform and who will therefore suffer punishment. That their failure to conform will always result from a causal chain of one kind or another is a truism. But, if the causal chain turns chiefly on the settings of the feedback systems that make us who we are, it does not serve to exculpate from responsibility: rather, it forms part of what responsibility is all about.

I am somewhat dismayed (though the reader may be relieved) that this chapter is so short—dismayed, because I believe it contains the essentials of a reconciliation of the long-time irreconcilable: determinism and individual responsibility. (Velmans, 2003, advocates a similar reconciliation.)

What has all of this got to do with consciousness? Not very much—but that is the point! Responsibility has to do with the correct functioning of the feedback systems that control an individual's interactions with environmental rewards and punishments. These operate largely unconsciously. The conscious recognition of a decision to act and the ensuing action as *my* decision and *my* action comes after the event; but they nonetheless *are* mine (save for the relatively rare case of illusion or experimental manipulation). Responsibility for instrumental behaviour lies with *the entire system that is 'me'*, its unconscious as much as its conscious part. The extra bits that come into conscious awareness—recognition of an act as mine, premeditated action, consciously taking on responsibility for action, and so on—do not change these essentials. At most, they ratchet the legal tariff up or down a little.

# CHAPTER 20

# Overview

We have travelled a long way since this book began, following what must have often seemed a pretty meandering path, and mostly uphill at that. In this final chapter we look back over our journey. Where have we reached? Have we indeed reached anywhere at all? After all, philosophers have been making the same journey for more than two millennia (and that's just the ones we know about), but generation after generation has seemed to require an entirely fresh start. Has the burgeoning high-tech instrumentation of modern science enabled us to do any better? For sure, whatever progress we may have made, there is much further to go. At best we have climbed to the top of one of those peaks that seem awfully high while you are on the way up, but then turn out to be just foot-hills, with the Himalayas proper still spread out endlessly before you.

Nonetheless, even from a foot-hill a look back at the way you have come can show the landscape in a new and revealing panoramic light. So you may find this final chapter as good a place to start as the beginning of the book. For this reason, I have written it as a relatively self-contained overview of the entire argument, not necessarily following the order in which particular ideas emerged earlier. Inevitably, as befits an overview, there will be some repetition of material that has gone before. But I have also introduced a small amount of new material, if it seems to fit best here.

## 20.1 The problem: qualia and only qualia

The Hard Problem of consciousness concerns *only* perceptual experience. The philosophical term 'quale' (plural, 'qualia') is a convenient way of referring to the elemental components of perceptual experience (the colour red, an itch, the smell of jasmine, and so on), and I use it here to mean just that, with no further philosophical baggage. Many writers have disputed the notion that conscious experience can be broken down into any such elemental components. However, we have considered many empirical discoveries that demonstrate its usefulness, ranging from synaesthesia (Chapter 10), through experiments on the compartmentalised nature of visual perception (Chapter 13), to the difficulties in feature binding encountered by patients suffering from Balint's syndrome (Chapter 15). From a scientific perspective, then, the Hard Problem of consciousness boils down at its simplest to just this: *how does the brain create qualia?* (There are some subsidiary questions, but we'll come to these later.) Mental processes that do not involve qualia do not pose any difficulty in principle for scientific analysis.

This conclusion is to some extent already widely accepted within both the scientific and philosophical communities. However, that acceptance usually takes qualia to be necessarily endowed with a range of properties that go well beyond their straightforward qualitative perceptual 'raw feel'. By the latter I mean simply that which, say, makes the experience of red different from that of green or of high C on the violin or an itch. But most views hold that qualia necessarily include also further properties like intentionality, or result from special processes like feature binding. (*Intentionality* is defined by John Searle, on the first page of his 1983 book of that name, as that property of 'mental states and events by which they are directed at or about or of objects and states of affairs in the world'; and 'binding' is that process by which, intramodally, the colour, shape and motion of a red kite flying in the sky are all put together into a single seen object, or by which, multi-modally, I hear the sound of your voice as issuing from between your moving lips.)

I am not convinced of the need for these surplus properties and processes. For we have seen that 'raw feels' can be dissociated from them. These dissociations become particularly (but not uniquely) obvious when you consider the bodily senses (itches, tingles, feelings of fatigue, drowsiness, and the like), as we did in Chapter 18. These lack intentionality just about as generally as conscious percepts of the external world possess it. Complementing this evidence for conscious experience without intentionality, there is other evidence (for example, Groeger's experiment; see Fig. 4.2) that intentionality can operate unconsciously. This 'double dissociation' of intentionality from qualia has far-reaching consequences.

Note in passing that, in keeping with the line that generally demarcates the Hard Problem from 'easier' aspects of mental and neural science, there is reasonably good understanding in principle of how robotic systems interacting with their environment can develop processes of categorisation with all the hallmarks of meaning and intentionality (Chapter 4). In contrast, there is no understanding at all of how such robotic systems (or our own neural systems) might develop qualia.

Lack of intentionality is not confined to conscious percepts of bodily sensations. It can hold also for conscious percepts of the external world (or 'cognitive consciousness', as I called these in Chapters 1 and 17). However, lack of intentionality in cognitive consciousness seems to be confined to cases of brain damage. The relevant handicaps are known as the agnosias. These can affect any of the sensory systems. They consist, precisely, in the *loss* of the meaning that is normally inherently bound to stimuli in the sensory system concerned. So, depending upon the site of the damage to the brain, one may cease to see a pipe or a face as a coherent object (they become instead meaningless sets of lines) or to understand speech (which becomes a meaningless set of noises). The neurologist Oliver Sacks has movingly described a number of cases of this kind in his book, *The Man Who Mistook his Wife for a Hat*. If we put these pathological cases together with the completely

normal cases of the bodily senses, we can safely conclude that intentionality and
conscious perception are fully dissociable.

Another feature often seen as inherent to conscious perception is their setting
in a spatial frame, either allocentric (world-centred) or egocentric (centred on the
observer) or both. But these too are not essential for the bodily senses. Inner body
space is quite separate from the allocentric and egocentric spaces that apply to
consciousness of the external world. And even this special inner body space
does not seem to figure in the conscious experiences of drowsiness, jitteriness or
depression: can you locate these anywhere?

The bodily senses also limit the role that can plausibly be allotted to feature
binding. As we saw when we considered the psychology and neurology of the
binding of features in the perception of the external world (Chapter 15), this
appears to depend critically upon their co-localisation in an egocentric spatial
frame computed in the inferior parietal lobe. But this frame does not play an essential role for the bodily senses. It is not surprising, therefore, that these are not
generally characterised by feature binding. I do not, for example, blend my feelings
of hunger and thirst into a combined superordinate conscious experience (contrast
the combined auditory and visual experience of someone speaking to you). Indeed,
I have been unable to think of a single good example of feature binding among the
bodily senses.

As in the case of intentionality, what is normal in the bodily senses—the absence
of feature binding—can become apparent also in cognitive consciousness of the
external world, but only after brain damage. Consider the striking symptom known
as 'simultanagnosia', part of Balint's syndrome (consequent upon bilateral damage
to the inferior parietal lobe and the resulting loss of the egocentric spatial frame).
If such a patient is presented simultaneously with two stimuli, each consisting of
two visual features, e.g. a blue cross and a red circle, he frequently *mis*binds them,
perceiving only a red cross or only a blue circle (Section 15.2). Thus, binding of
features, even if they are colocalised in space, is erroneous, yet consciousness of the
misbound features persists.

I conclude, therefore, that 'raw feels' are just that. They can occur without any
high-falutin' trappings of intentionality, spatial framework, feature binding or the
like. They can similarly occur in the absence of any manipulation by so-called
executive processes (attention, working memory, decision making and so on),
which figure so prominently in the concept of the 'global workspace' (Chapter 11).
A toothache will make its presence felt despite your best efforts to prevent it. The
synaesthetes described in Chapter 10 cannot turn off their colour experiences in
response to heard words when these get in the way of other things they are trying
to do; and a non-synaesthete can't turn them on with all the executive processes
in the world.

Once qualia are created, it is clear however that they can be put to the service of
a great diversity of cognitive processes—they can be used to construct intentional

objects, like roses or faces or voices, or multimodal scenes, or maps of space; they can be used to communicate complex propositions to others in speech or to yourself in thought; they can (within limits) be attended to or ignored, remembered or forgotten, (here is where executive processes come into their own). But they do not depend upon any of these for their existence. That is why the Hard Problem of consciousness can be reduced to the straightforward question: how does the brain create qualia?

## 20.2 Reduction

Reduction of the Hard Problem to a single question may, I hope, represent an increment in simplicity. But science looks to 'reduction' for much more than this. The bigger hope is to show that phenomena encountered at one level, or better still the scientific laws used to explain them, can be eliminated ('reduced') in favour of phenomena or laws encountered at a more general level. A successful reduction of this kind would show that conscious experiences can be accounted for entirely in terms of principles that operate at the more general levels of biology or physics.

There are two avenues that such a reduction might in principle take. Recall (Chapter 3) that biology in general works by adding to the laws of physics the engineering principles of cybernetics, especially those of feedback and selection by consequences. Recall also that the principles of cybernetics cannot themselves be reduced to the laws of physics—though they must, of course, respect them. Thus reduction of conscious experience might take the form of showing that this can be explained by the laws of physics, or by the principles of cybernetics. If qualia had remained fully entangled with intentionality, the construction of spatial frameworks and so on, we might also have envisaged a case in which the reduction of conscious experience is jointly to physics and cybernetics. But, if what we have to account for is qualia as such ('raw feels'), it seems unlikely that more than one avenue of reduction will be needed—assuming, that is, that reduction is possible at all.

Reduction by the cybernetic route is the aim of functionalism—that is, the doctrine that qualia are nothing more than their associated functions (where a 'function' consists in corresponding sets of inputs from the environment, outputs back to the environment, and information and neural processing lying in between). This doctrine entails that a quale and its associated function are, when all the details are taken into account, identical. So two different qualia cannot be associated with the same function, nor two different functions with the same quale. But there is a probable exception to this rule in the phenomenon of synaesthesia. 'Coloured-hearing' synaesthetes, for example, experience colour qualia in association with both seeing coloured surfaces and hearing spoken words—two radically different functions. Although our experiments on these phenomena (described in Chapter 10) have yet to be followed up by others, I shall assume that both our findings and the inferences we have drawn from them are correct. Since functionalism purports to provide a perfectly general account of conscious experience, this

mistake is to confuse quale w associated functions
* Mistake is also to lump sensory signals w feelings (indicators of need) used for discernment

one negative instance is strong enough to dislodge it in its entirety. So I conclude that qualia cannot be identified with functions, and that the cybernetic route to reduction is closed.

This conclusion has some interesting consequences, especially if one considers it alongside one reached earlier: that qualia and intentionality are doubly dissociable. For (as Harnad's work on the 'symbol grounding' problem illustrates; Chapter 4), there is every reason to expect that familiar cybernetic principles can fully account for meaning and intentionality. However, if these principles cannot account at the same time for qualia, then one may conjecture that the relationships between meanings and the qualia in which meanings come clothed are more or less arbitrary.

There are two separate realms of intentionality to which this conjecture has potential application. In the first—language—it is almost self-evidently true; in the second—perception—it is, in contrast, strongly counter-intuitive.

Take, first, two languages, English and French for example. Although the meanings of *house* in English and *la maison* in French are not identical, they surely overlap to a very large extent. But the qualia that clothe the meaning (the sounds of *house* and of *la maison*)—are totally different. It follows from this almost trivial example that the relationship between meanings and qualia in natural languages is arbitrary. This same flexible relationship between sounds and meanings can be demonstrated also within a single language. Over a half a century ago experiments demonstrated a simple phenomenon known as 'semantic satiation'. Repeat a word over and over again and it will gradually lose its meaning; but you continue to hear its sound. Change in the one does not force change in the other.

Natural languages have evolved a special arrangement to mediate the relationship between meanings (semantics) and the sounds (phonetics) that clothe them. Between semantics and phonetics the brain interposes a third layer, that of syntax or grammar. There are many experiments in psycholinguistics, not to mention many unfortunate consequences of brain damage, that demonstrate the relative independence with which each of the three layers operates. So, for example, in the production of language, a meaning accessed in the semantic layer can be converted into more than one word or set of words at the phonetic level; and *vice versa* the comprehension of language can interpret a phonetically analysed input into more than one semantic outcome. The polysemous words used by Tony Marcel in his experiments on priming (described in Section 9.3) are a good case in point.

There is a parallel, here, I think, to the circumstances that make possible Darwinian selection—and therefore the whole of the biological world. As we saw in Chapter 3, the laws of physics and chemistry leave open two possibilities of satisfying energy constraints at each point in the formation of a chain of nucleotides making up a stretch of double-stranded DNA. It is upon this range of different possibilities that natural selection is able to act, by selecting those with better survival value. If there were no flexibility in the allocation of nucleotides to positions in the chain, natural selection could not work. In much the same way, natural languages evolve by flexibly allocating meanings to different sounds. If sound and meaning were inflexibly linked, this evolutionary process also could not work. There would be just one rigid language, restricted perhaps to the kind of onomatopoeia that names a dog a 'bow-wow'.

What would it mean if this same flexibility applied in the sphere of perception? Maybe we could then arbitrarily choose to link Pavarotti singing Verdi's *Bella figlia del amore* with the percept of a swirling set of colours (rather like the old Disney film, *Fantasia*). And that (outside the movies) is clearly impossible. Well, yes, it is impossible for any individual human being to choose to do this (despite the fact that this kind of experience is just what happens to 'coloured-music' synaesthetes). Conscious experiences are givens: as often emphasised throughout this book, they come unbidden, automatically and involuntarily (to coloured music synaesthetes, as to everyone else). I cannot choose to have my experiences other than as they are (except by the trivial expedient of shutting my eyes or burying my ears in the pillow). But there is a different level at which the links between meanings and qualia may—just possibly—be as arbitrary in perception as they are in language. That level is the one of biological evolution.

To see that this is so, let us return to synaesthesia. This phenomenon demonstrates that the same conscious sensation can be produced by two quite different functional routes. A particularly common form of synaesthesia, the one we studied in the experiments described in Chapter 10, is coloured hearing: the perception of colours in response to spoken words. But there are also people who experience colours in response to music, or to pain or taste or sexual orgasm, or who experience tastes in response to shapes and so on (there is a great variety of synaesthetic combinations). Relatively rare as such people are, each of them is nonetheless proof that the relationship between qualia, on the one hand, and functions or meanings, on the other, is not immutable. Given this, might not Mother Evolution have allocated qualia to perceptual modalities (or to entities within modalities) differently from the way in fact (for most of us, most of the time) she did? In this context, I am struck by the fact that the sensory modality that figures most frequently in synaesthetic experience—that of trichromatic colour—is the very one that, in humans, has evolved most recently. It is almost as though there happened to be a spare set of qualia lying around and Evolution kept trying them out till she found one set of functions to which they made a particularly good fit: the perception of surfaces that reflect light differently as a function of wavelength[1].

---

[1] This passage elicited from John Mollon the following comment, too late to be properly considered in the book but too interesting to lose. 'The ancestors of the mammals were tetrachromatic, in that they had four cone pigments, as most birds do today. (The proof is the homology between the gene sequences in modern birds and those in modern lampreys.) So—and I adopt your discourse only for this present purpose—the unused qualia might not be ones that had never previously been used, but ones that had been used before but discarded during the long night of the early mammals.'

Thus, at the evolutionary level, the relationship between perceptual qualia and functions may possess at least some of the flexibility that holds in ordinary language between qualia (phonetics) and meanings (semantics). This line of thought casts the Hard Problem in an interesting new light. What appears to be missing in the relationship between percepts and functions is a level corresponding to syntax in language. Might a solution to the Hard Problem consist in the discovery of a kind of syntactical engine to which, on the one side, functions slot in and, on the other, qualia fall out? (This, indeed, is one way of thinking of the bizarre quantum-mechanical theory of consciousness developed by Penrose and Hameroff; see Chapter 16.)

This 'arbitrariness' conjecture—that there is flexibility in the fit between meanings and qualia—also has implications for understanding the arts. These all necessarily involve qualia. At any rate, I cannot imagine an art form that communicates itself entirely unconsciously (which is not to say that the arts do not, like every other human activity, draw heavily also upon unconscious processing). But the degree to which they involve meaning is much more variable. Novels in prose depend strongly on meaning; poetry, song and representational painting are pretty well balanced between meaning and qualia; while abstract art and non-vocal music depend almost exclusively on qualia.

In this last case, I am tempted to delete the 'almost'. I can detect no meaning at all in a Mondrian painting (see Plate 7.2), nor in a Bach fugue or in Lennie Tristano's quartet of 1949 playing *Judy*. If at this point you are desperate to find meaning, you will be inclined to grasp at the sense of religious peace in the Bach or the gentle tranquillity of the Tristano. But there are numberless other pieces of religious or tranquil music. Their differences in style and quality just don't turn on these vague 'meanings'. What they do turn on is a combination of qualia and syntax—melody, harmony, fugal structure, timbre, rhythm and so on. For music has a syntax of its own: the rules that relate one sequence of sounds (whatever sounds they might be) to another so as to make up a fugue or a series of Be-Bop variations on a theme. These rules are not themselves qualia. You can discern them in the written score, as well as in the sounds made by the instruments on which the score is played. Thus, like the syntactical rules of language, the rules of music are independent of any particular instantiation in qualia. But, unlike language, music dispenses with semantics. (That is why it is so difficult to apply to music the notions of either representation or signal, as discussed in Chapter 5.) The sheer existence of music-without-meaning, not to mention its powerful aesthetic effects, is further testimony to the independence of qualia from function.

The flexibility of fit between meanings and qualia is apparent also in art forms like poetry or song which balance meaning and qualia relatively equally. *Fair daffodils, we weep to see you haste away so soon* and *Gather ye rosebuds while ye may, Old Time is still a-flying* (both by Robert Herrick) mean, for all practical purposes, exactly the same thing, as do countless other variations, in many languages, on the old

Latin tag *Tempus fugit*. You can replace them all (if you really want to) by 'human life is short'. It is the qualia (the sounds, the metre, the images of flowers, of movement, and so on) that make each different, and some more treasured than others. The quality of poetry lies in its qualia (pun intended) and, to be sure, in their goodness of fit with the meaning. But if this fit were strongly determined, there would be no room for the poetry.

Such speculations are, I hope, permissible in a final chapter. But it is time to return to the main lines of the argument. By undermining functionalism, we have ruled out cybernetics as a possible route by which to reduce consciousness to the existing corpus of biological principles (a move, you should be warned, that is in flagrant defiance of mainstream contemporary science and philosophy). That leaves the laws of physics as the only alternative. We shall consider this route later.

*(handwritten margin note: missed the turn!)*

## 20.3 The function of conscious experience

The previous section was devoted to undermining the idea that qualia and functions have necessary relationships. Thus the title of this section—'the function of conscious experience'—may come as a surprise. But it addresses a different issue. Conscious experience exists in at least one biological species: our own. The general principles of Darwinian selection, therefore, require conscious experience to have a survival value. That value must (again by general Darwinian argument) lie in a functional contribution to the survival of the individual or to the reproduction of his genes (or both). So, accepting that the particular allocation of qualia to functions is not rigidly determined (as functionalism properly speaking would have it), we nonetheless need to ask the question: in what way does the sheer existence of qualia (however they happen to be allotted to functions) aid survival? This situation is by no means unusual. The properties of a protein need to be explained in terms of its physics and chemistry; but its abundance in a particular species is explained in terms of its contribution to Darwinian fitness. In the same way, we can seek to explain the existence of qualia and their linkage to specific functions in a given species by way of the contribution this arrangement makes to Darwinian fitness, while nonetheless seeking a quite different explanation (as yet unknown) of the properties of qualia as such.

If we are to provide even a half-way satisfactory sketch of the Darwinian side of this story, there are a number of facts we must keep firmly in mind.

First, most of the behaviour which *appears* to be closely associated with conscious experience in fact runs off with no intervention from consciousness at all (see Chapter 2). In some cases, the lack of associated conscious experience is total, to the point that one is not aware even of the fact that the brain is controlling it, or sometimes that it is occurring at all. The control by the brain of body temperature or pupil size, in response to internal metabolic factors or changes in external ambient light, are cases in point. In other cases (e.g. riding a bicycle), you are conscious of doing something, but not remotely of the way in which you do it. In still other cases, you have a pretty good idea of what you are doing and, to some extent, of how you are doing it, but in fact it is all done before your conscious awareness comes into being. Pressing a button the moment you see an *X* in a stream of letters is a familiar laboratory example of this kind. So, whatever function conscious experience discharges, it affects only a portion of our overall abilities to operate in the world.

Second, conscious experience, even when it does accompany function, invariably occurs too late to affect rapid on-line behaviour. I have repeatedly used the example of competition tennis to make this point. Escape from a hungry lion will have often been a similar evolutionary example, and one with dramatic influence upon natural selection. Usually this lateness of conscious experience is by about a tenth to a quarter of a second, but sometimes it is much slower still—pain is an excellent example and emotional turmoil, as in anxiety or depression, another.

Third, there is another way in which conscious experience works on a much slower time base than does unconscious processing. The brain accomplishes a great deal of unconscious processing within a few tens of milliseconds. But conscious processing does not begin to get off the ground until a stimulus has persisted for around 30 milliseconds. So, if a visual stimulus (a word or a face, for example) is presented for 30 milliseconds and then 'backwardly masked'—that is, followed by another, longer-lasting visual stimulus that overlays the first—it is not normally consciously perceived, even though other tests can demonstrate that it was unconsciously analysed (for an example using masked faces, see Section 11.2). Related phenomena have been demonstrated in recordings from single neurons in the monkey brain made by Edmund Rolls and Martin Tovee at Oxford, also using masked and unmasked faces. If a face was presented to the monkey for as little as 20 milliseconds and not followed by a mask, cells (in a region of the temporal lobe corresponding to the human face-selective area) fired continuously for two or three hundred milliseconds. Under these conditions, a human observer would have full conscious perception of the face. However, if the face was presented for 20 milliseconds but now followed immediately afterwards by a mask, the face-selective neurons fired for only 20–30 milliseconds and the rate of firing was much reduced. A human observer would have very little conscious perception of the face under these conditions. We may infer, then, that conscious perception requires a minimum duration of continuous firing in the pool of neurons that generates it. From these experiments it seems that this minimum duration lies somewhere between 30 and 200 milliseconds. In a complementary fashion, once conscious awareness of a stimulus has been achieved, its effects last longer than those exerted by the same stimulus detected unconsciously. So, for example, Greenwald's experiments on semantic priming (Section 9.3) demonstrated that a masked prime exerts its effects for less than 100 milliseconds but the same prime unmasked, for up to 400 milliseconds.

Fourth, most conscious experience is of what we naturally take to be (and philosophers who believe in direct realism—perception of the world just as it is—continue to take to be) a real world external to ourselves. However, a vast array of evidence from psychology and neuroscience compels the conclusion (long ago reached in any case by other philosophers) that the external world as we experience it is entirely constructed by the brain (constrained, to be sure, by information emanating from a real, but unperceived, external world). There is evidently very good agreement between the world constructed by the brain and the real external world, or we would not be as good as we are at using the perceived world as a guide to action. This concordance is the result of natural selection for survival. Similarly, there is very good agreement between the way your brain and mine construct the external world, or we would lack a consensual basis for social inter-action and language; though there are, to be sure, some major discrepancies between the worlds inhabited by different people, as in the familiar example of colour blindness or the less familiar but more striking one of synaesthesia. This general inter-subjective agreement in the construction of our worlds is again guaranteed by natural selection. We are a highly cooperative species. The ability to communicate with each other about action directed towards the common denominator of our several, individually constructed, models of the external world is another essential aid to survival.

The fifth fact we need to bear in mind amalgamates the slow time base of conscious experience with its ability to construct the perceived world. The inter-actions that take place unconsciously between a behaving subject and his environ-ment are fast-moving and fast-changing. Consciousness, in contrast, constructs an external world in which the changes are smoothed out. To take an example, suppose you (or some of your monkey forebears) are moving rapidly between trees in dappled sunlight looking for fruit and berries. Each of your movements changes the scene before you, the angle from which you see it, the wavelengths of light reflected from the surfaces of the leaves and fruit, the amount and location of the shade from the trees, and so on. If you are picking a berry, your brain takes into account, on a time base of a few milliseconds, each such change (and many others too) in guiding and re-guiding your reach and grasp. Your retina is all the while updating its computations of the visual scene, a few photons at a time. Yet your conscious perception is of a stable world populated by trees and fruit, stubbornly retaining their unchanging colours, shapes and locations despite this all-embracing, moment-by-moment confusion. It is by way of these smoothing operations that the constructed perceived world takes on its semi-permanent appearance. Notice that, if there is something foreordained about the occupation by consciousness of this particular time scale, we have no idea what it is. We could conceivably have evolved in such a way that our conscious perceptions took place on the same rapid time scale that guides unconscious action. It is, however, a fact about our consciousness it that it does not work on that time scale. So perhaps there is something about the processes that create consciousness that do in fact require it to operate slowly.

In seeking for a survival value for consciousness we need to take all these facts into account. It is no use, for example, postulating a function for conscious experience in the guidance of rapid action; for such actions are completed before we are aware we are carrying them out. Similarly, it is no use postulating a function for conscious experience that is most manifest in the power to *imagine* a place when we are *not* there; for a much more salient aspect of conscious experience is the power to *construct* the place when we *are* there.

Before going on to seek to satisfy these requirements we need to ask whether it makes sense to seek a survival value for consciousness at all. For there is a well-known and well-defended view that conscious experience may be an epiphenomenon, devoid of causal effects in its own right (as distinct from causal effects exerted by the neural activities that give rise to it).

We have considered this view carefully at several points in the book, concluding that there are good reasons to dismiss it. But these reasons were largely of a general nature. So, for example, I argued that language, science and aesthetic appreciation— an argument strengthened in the previous section—would all be impossible in the absence of the conscious constructs that make up the perceived world (Section 9.2). These, I think, are undeniably major causal consequences of the existence of conscious experiences. But they fall short of demonstrating that conscious experiences play a causal role in the functioning of the brain that produces them, and *as* it produces them—what I called in Section 9.3 'ongoing causal efficacy'. Given the lateness of conscious experience, coupled with the abundant evidence that such experience is always the outcome of a prior chain of unconscious brain processes, the lack of evidence for an ongoing causal efficacy of consciousness in the brain is perhaps not surprising. But it *is* worrying. For it leaves open the possibility that, insofar as the ongoing activities of the brain are concerned, conscious experience is indeed epiphenomenal. Its apparently causal effects may be analogous to those exerted by an external aide mémoire (Section 9.1): the brain can achieve much more with the aide mémoire than without it; but the aide mémoire is itself causally inactive. The case may be the same for conscious experience.

There are, however, a few experimental results which indicate, albeit not unequivocally, that conscious experience may have ongoing causal efficacy. Without being able to resolve the issue, I therefore concluded in Chapter 9 that we should proceed on the assumption that consciousness does indeed play a full causal role in the natural world. That assumption is difficult to fit without conceptual confusion into the closed causality of natural science. However, Searle's conceptual model (Section 4.2) of how the macro-properties of systems can emerge from the micro-properties of their elements offers a way in principle to achieve this fit— with the proviso that no detailed application of his model to consciousness has ever yet been proposed.

So what survival value can be found for consciousness, within the constraints outlined above?

To answer this question I have proposed that consciousness acts as a late detector of error. Chapters 7 and 8 set this proposal out in detail, ground that we shall not cover here again. As summarised in Chapter 8, the proposal includes the following claims. Conscious experience serves three linked functions:

1. It contains a model of the relatively permanent features of the external world; and the model is experienced as though it *is* the external world.
2. Within the framework afforded by this model, features that are particularly relevant to ongoing motor programs or which depart from expectation are monitored and emphasised.
3. Within the framework afforded by the model, the controlled variables and set-points of the brain's unconscious servomechanisms can be juxtaposed, combined and modified; in this way, error can be corrected for future occasions of action.

Points (2) and (3) together constitute the 'late error detection' that gives consciousness its initial (phylogenetically speaking) survival value. The model of the external world (point 1) provides an essential medium in which late error detection can operate.

The lateness of conscious experience—the fact that this follows after its behavioural function has already been accomplished unconsciously—finds a natural account in the functioning of the 'comparator' (see Fig. 7.1) whose operation serves to detect error. The comparator predicts the next likely state of the world, as this will be detected by the brain's sensory systems (located for the most part in the neocortex and thalamus—hence 'thalamocortical' systems); and it compares this prediction to the actual state of the sensory world. All this is done unconsciously. What enters consciousness then consists of the results of the comparison. As already noted, the entry into consciousness picks out for special emphasis departures from prediction (events that have occurred but weren't predicted to occur, or events that were predicted to occur but did not), and those predicted events that are of particular importance for the achievement of current goals. This process of comparison takes time; an estimate based upon the circuitry proposed to underlie it gives a value of the order of 100 milliseconds. This duration is broadly in line with the temporal properties of conscious experience.

As analysed in Chapter 18, the comparator system makes use of two types of error signals: extrinsic and intrinsic.

'Extrinsic error' signals tell you that *something is wrong*, but they provide only very general information as to what that something is. Paradigmatic examples are pain, nausea and dizziness. Extrinsic error signals are communicated by the bodily senses— those that carry information principally about the state of the body as distinct from the state of the external world. As noted above (and in Chapter 18), such signals lack intentionality—a more precise way of saying that the information they convey is very general. The bodily senses are phylogenetically old and depend for their computation, correspondingly, on rather ancient structures in the brain stem. These senses are believed by some scientists (Antonio Damasio and Jaak Panksepp among them) to have constituted the first step in the evolution of conscious perception.

I reject that hypothesis, on two grounds. The first is that error detection would have been of little survival value until it could be juxtaposed with information allowing the error to be corrected. For that to be possible, the construction of a model of the external world is a prerequisite, and this is computed in higher brain regions that evolved later. Second, and consistent with the first reason for rejection of the Damasio–Panksepp hypothesis, human neuroimaging research shows that the conscious experience of pain (a key modality of bodily sensation) is associated with activity, not in the phylogenetically ancient brain stem, but in the more recently evolved neocortex (especially, the anterior cingulate gyrus).

However, my rejection of the Damasio–Panksepp hypothesis is tempered. With respect to the first ground for rejection, conscious perception of inner bodily states might initially have evolved for purposes other than error correction in action programs directed at the external world. It is commonplace for a biological feature to have an initial survival value that differs considerably from the one it attains at a later stage of evolution. With respect to the second ground for rejection, it is commonplace also in the development of the brain for higher and later-evolving structures to inhibit or otherwise control the activities of structures performing related functions at a lower level of the neural hierarchy. So, at an earlier stage in phylogenesis, the brain stem may have initially discharged functions associated with conscious experience only to lose these, or lose their association with conscious experience, at a later stage. However, these possibilities seem less likely than the one accepted in Chapter 18: that the bodily senses did not achieve the ability to enter conscious experience until the distance senses (olfaction, touch, audition and vision) developed the capacity to construct a conscious model of the external world. At that point, the bodily senses were co-opted into the comparator system to serve as extrinsic signals of error.

'Intrinsic error', by contrast, consists in the outputs of the comparator itself: that is, the detection of departure from prediction. This is the heart of my proposal. The major survival value of conscious experience consists in this ability to detect error and to correct it. Intrinsic error signals convey rather precise information as to what has gone wrong. To put essentially the same point differently: the manner in which intrinsic error signals are computed automatically confers intentionality upon them. In addition, their manner of computation necessarily links the conscious experience of the moment to both the past and the future. Error can be detected only in the light of a prediction as to the next likely state of the (constructed) external world; and this prediction can be made only in the light of past experience (stored as memories) of what took place when you were last in circumstances similar to those now in place. Hence the link to the past. Detection of the error occurs after the unconsciously operating motor program has already gone wrong. Its correction, therefore, has to apply to the future running of the motor program. Hence the link to the future.

These aspects of conscious experience are well captured by Gerald Edelman's felicitous term, 'the remembered present'. For the detection of intrinsic error to be possible, there needs to be a model of the external world as it was, as it is, and as it is projected to be. Such a model has to be on a more enduring time base than the fleeting intercourse that is sufficient for the rapid action of a servomechanism. Thus, all the glorious richness and complexity of the perceived world is put together, so to speak, as 'the one discharge from [sin and] error' (T. S. Eliot, *Little Gidding*).

## 20.4 Where does the brain create qualia?

It is one thing to propose a survival value for conscious experience, but quite another to suggest how the brain produces it. Here we reach the hardest part of the Hard Problem. I simplified the situation somewhat by taking it on trust (Chapter 4) that any solution to the problem of how the brain creates qualia would bring along at no extra cost a solution to the problem of how it reads them. It is likely to be a long time before it is known whether this trust is misplaced!

I have rejected the functionalist route (that qualia are identical to the input–output functions with which they are associated), seductive as it nonetheless is. Yet the consequences of that rejection have barely begun to be felt. All existing hypotheses about the empirical basis of consciousness—including my own, as just summarised—are functionalist in spirit, either explicitly or (as in the Penrose–Hameroff quantum-mechanical theory considered in Chapter 16) by way of covert assumption. Thus the demise of functionalism—if demise it be—will necessitate a whole new approach to theory construction.

If we abandon functionalism, the only other place to seek a natural-science account of qualia lies in the non-system properties of the brain. These might be properties of the brain that are specifically neural or biological, or properties that stem from the physics and chemistry that are common to all matter.

Our story is short so far as the first of these is concerned. So far as I know, no-one has yet proposed *any* kind of theory of how the non-system *biological* properties of the constituent cells of the brain—their biophysics or biochemistry—might give rise to qualia. The nearest anyone has come to this is the search by Christof Koch for genes whose expression might characterise only those cells in the brain that participate in what he and Francis Crick call the 'neural correlates of consciousness'. And that of course is not a theory, nor in any case has the search for such genes yet discovered any. For the most part, neuroscientists have been content to join the functionalist camp and to suppose that qualia are the inevitable result of certain types of behavioural or cognitive function. Thus all they do is add to the functionalist bestiary descriptions of the brain systems that mediate these functions.

The essential functionalist correlational game can then be played out at two parallel levels: correlations between qualia and behavioural or cognitive functions, as studied in the psychological laboratory; and correlations between qualia and neural systems studied by neurophysiology or neuroimaging. But, no matter how detailed these three-way correlations become, it is unlikely that they will by themselves lead to an understanding of how the brain creates qualia. Nor can they by themselves address the question whether the same functions, discharged by systems other than brains (a digital computer, say, or a computer-controlled robot), would remain correlated with the same—or any—qualia. The major (though not, so far as I know, stated) difference between cognitive scientists and neuroscientists who both pursue the functionalist agenda is that the former by and large say 'yes' in answer to this question and the latter, 'no'. Neither answer has any substantive empirical or theoretical foundation.

This is not to say that the search for the neural correlates of consciousness is a waste of time. On the contrary, it is likely to prove the most fruitful activity in the contemporary empirical science of consciousness. For a successful delineation of the necessary and sufficient neural events underpinning the entry into consciousness of specific contents (as in the search for the correlates of visual consciousness, reviewed in detail in Chapter 13) will build the data base that will in turn nourish the imagination of some future theoretician. Indeed, this is already happening, with the consequence that some of the debates that have hitherto been fought only on philosophical ground are rapidly entering the scientific laboratory.

As we saw in Chapters 11–15, the starting intuitions of those who seek the neural correlates of consciousness differ to a striking degree. At one extreme Dan Dennett and Marcel Kinsbourne scorn the notion that there could be any unit short of the entire brain that could be the site of conscious experience; at the other lies Semir Zeki's hypothesis that (sufficient) activity in, say, the colour-selective region of the visual system, V4, is necessary and sufficient for the experience of colour. In between, hypotheses like those proposed by Changeux and Dehaene and by Edelman and Tononi call upon networks that are very widely distributed but nonetheless clearly delimited from the brain as a whole. It is undoubtedly premature to bring closure to this debate; however, certain conclusions can already be reached.

The whole brain can certainly be excluded as the neural correlate of conscious experience. There are two reasons for this. First, there are classes of behaviour which require a very considerable degree of neural processing but which remain unconscious. These include, for example, the visual action systems described in Chapter 2 and the procedural learning discussed in Chapter 14. We may reasonably infer, therefore, that the neural activity that underpins these classes of behaviour does not participate in the neural correlate of consciousness. Second, the brain may suffer a variety of often quite extensive forms of damage without compromise of conscious experience.

The various proposals for a 'global neuronal workspace' seek the neural basis of conscious experience in complex networks that communicate between different regions by way of long-axoned tangential projections spanning much of the neocortex (see Chapter 12). They all have in common a strong focus upon the prefrontal cortex. Vital as is this region (which has grown particularly large in the human species) for the control of complex behaviour (by way of so-called 'executive functions'), there are strong reasons to doubt that it plays a critical role in the neural correlate of conscious experience.

To begin with, this is one of the parts of the brain that can sustain massive damage without apparent change in conscious experience as such. Second, those aspects of conscious experience for which there is evidence of strong prefrontal involvement are, by and large, to do with the 'private' space of consciousness (Chapter 1)—functions like imagining, directing covert attention, subvocal rehearsal, mental problem-solving, and the like. These are important features of conscious life. However, they pale into insignificance against the vast arena of the 'public' conscious experience of the external world. I suspect that, if we can once understand how the brain creates public experience, explanation of the private space of consciousness will fall out as a simple derivative. Third, there have been a number of reports of neuroimaging experiments in which conscious experience has *not* been accompanied by activity in the prefrontal cortex. When it has been so accompanied, the specific prefrontal regions activated have been very diverse. This diversity is comprehensible in light of the diversity of the executive functions that the prefrontal cortex discharges, especially in relation to the private space of conscious experience. Thus the neuroimaging results, whether negative or positive, fail to indicate a special role for the prefrontal cortex in conscious experience as such.

One way of understanding conscious experience is as an amalgam between 'top-down' and 'bottom-up' processing. This point of view has been strongly and cogently urged by Ray Jackendoff, who proposes an 'intermediate-level' theory of consciousness (Chapter 14). This holds that one is not normally aware of sensation unaffected by conceptual interpretation, nor of pure conceptual structure, but only of an admixture of the two that optimises their mutual fit. The conceptual structure results from top-down processing, sensation from bottom-up processing, and conscious experience results at the point where these two forms of processing meet. This analysis seems generally to be true of cognitive consciousness of the external world, but not of many (perhaps any) of the bodily sensations. This is another way of saying that the latter more often than not lack intentionality. Still, it is worth pursuing Jackendoff's hypothesis as it applies to cognitive consciousness.

There are two regions of the forebrain which can plausibly be seen to supply the necessary top-down processing for cognitive consciousness: the prefrontal cortex, as in the global workspace models considered above, and the hippocampal system. I have proposed that the latter is the neural substrate of the comparator system that underlies the late detection of error and so provides conscious experience with its evolutionary survival value (see above). Note, however, that the suggestion that the hippocampus is a neural substrate of conscious experience is conceptually distinct from the comparator function that it is proposed to serve. It could be correct that the selection of the contents of consciousness is achieved by a comparator system, but that this function is not discharged by the hippocampus; or that the hippocampus plays an important role in conscious experience, but this has nothing to do with a comparator system (and of course both parts of the hypothesis could be wrong). I am now, in fact, inclined to the view (in retreat from the position I held when I first proposed this hypothesis in 1995) that the hippocampal system does not discharge the comparator function on its own.

My reasons for this retreat include the fact that, like the prefrontal cortex, extensive damage to the hippocampal system is compatible with the maintenance of apparently normal conscious experience (but see the description of the patient, Clive Wearing in Chapter 14). Also like the prefrontal cortex, the hippocampus has not been shown in neuroimaging studies to display activity consistently in association with conscious experience. One might discount this negative evidence on methodological grounds. Specifically, neuroimaging experiments depend upon a subtraction of the activity observed during a control condition from that observed during an experimental condition. The subject of the experiment is necessarily consciously aware of *something* or other during both these phases of the experiment. Thus, if the hippocampus (or indeed the prefrontal cortex) is responsible for the selection of the contents of consciousness, it will be active in both phases, and this activity will be subtracted out of the results. This would be a reasonable defence, were it not for the fact that there is now good neuroimaging evidence for involvement of the hippocampus in a more restricted aspect of conscious experience, namely, the recollective experience of episodic memory (Chapter 14).

But other neuroimaging results suggest that a more substantial retreat is required, not only from my hypothesis but from all those that give too great a role in conscious experience to top-down processing. For these results (reviewed in Chapter 13) offer good support for Zeki's hypothesis that visual conscious experience can result from activity in just one module of the visual perception system, with little if any additional activity in either higher cortical regions responsible for executive functions or lower parts of the visual system. So, under at least some circumstances, activity in V4 is sufficient to produce an experience of colour, activity in V5, an experience of motion, and so on. A particularly dramatic example of this kind is Dominic ffytche's study of the neuroimaging correlates of hallucinations occurring in patients with the Charles Bonnet syndrome. Complex hallucinations, e.g. of faces or objects, were accompanied by activity in just the region of the fusiform gyrus (part of the ventral stream of the visual perception system) specialised for that type of visual percept, with no additional activity in the prefrontal cortex (the hippocampal system was not included in the description of the results).

It is always dangerous in science to rely upon negative results, and never more so than in the case of neuroimaging experiments. Nonetheless, results of this kind require us to take seriously the possibility that qualia are far more independent of cognitive influences from top-down processing than has hitherto seemed likely. This conclusion, drawn from neuroimaging experiments, is pleasingly congruent with the one drawn in the first section of this chapter on quite different grounds. I concluded there that 'raw feels' are just that. They can occur without any of the trappings of intentionality, spatial framework, feature binding or the like. They can similarly occur in the absence of any manipulation by executive processes (attention, working memory, decision making etc). I did not hold this view when I started writing this book. But the cumulative effects of a variety of different kinds of observation now appear to require its adoption. An important task for future experimentation will be to see whether the same pattern emerges from neuro-imaging experiments investigating senses other than vision, from which the exist-ing data are almost entirely drawn. Subject to the judgement to be passed by such future experiments, it seems reasonable for now to conclude that separate types of qualia (such as colours, visual motion, scents, pain, and so on) each result from activity in a circumscribed neocortical region that is specialised in the analysis of the corresponding type of information.

This conclusion, of course, does not mean that qualia are not then subject to manipulation by executive processes. Thus, there is no reason not to accept a role for the prefrontal cortex or hippocampal system in, as it were, putting conscious experiences constructed in sensory neocortex through the hoops of selective atten-tion or working memory, or to the service of problem solving or conflict resolution. Among such top-down processes, I continue to see the comparator as holding pride of place, since so many features of conscious experience seem to make better sense in the light of this hypothesis (see Chapters 7 and 8). The most likely brain region to discharge this function remains the hippocampal system in its wider sense (Chapter 14). As we have seen, the evidence is that the hippocampus itself plays a more circumscribed role: underpinning the recollective experience of episodic memory. In this sense, the hippocampus may resemble, in its relation to conscious experience, one of the specialised modules of the visual perception system. That is, just as activity in V4 may be sufficient for the experience of colour, so activity in the hippocampus may be sufficient for the experience of an autobiographically authenticated episodic memory. Note, however, that even this circumscribed role is, in at least three respects, of special significance.

First, episodic memory is multimodal. So the hippocampus is one region where all the senses can apparently come together into a single, unified conscious experience. Indeed, the hippocampus is so far the only region known to play such a multimodal role in conscious experience. It outdoes even the thalamus (where virtually all sensory inputs converge on their way to the neocortex) in the range of the modalities it represents, since it (but not the thalamus) receives direct olfactory input.

Second, in an important recent study, Kreiman, Koch and Fried recorded the activity of single neurons in the human brain (the recordings were made in epileptic patients prior to surgery so as to map the functional state of the brain). An important commonality emerged in the way that hippocampal neurons respond to recalled and perceived stimuli, respectively. The patients were shown pictures and then asked to imagine what they had just seen. Some hippocampal neurons (and also some in adjacent regions of the wider hippocampal system) responded to both the seen and the imagined stimuli, and with the same specificity for the type of material depicted or imagined (faces, objects, spatial lay-outs, etc.). In a single modality, then, the hippocampus is active in much the same way when a stimulus is recalled or when it is perceived. It is an important task for future research to determine what happens in the brain when the conscious experiences of perceived or recalled colour, shape, sound, scent etc all come together in a unified scene. Is this binding problem solved simply by the juxtaposition of neural activity in each of the specialised regions, or does some additional region take on the responsibility of binding them all together? If there is indeed such an additional region, the hippocampal system remains, in my view, a strong candidate.

Third, if the survival value of conscious experience lies, as I have suggested, in the late detection of error and its correction for future action, then (as set out in Chapter 14), this is just the type of function in which context-specific memories of the kind mediated by the hippocampus play a crucial role.

## 20.5   Enter quantum mechanics

Slowly but surely we are being led to some surprising conclusions, including quite a few that I did not anticipate when I started writing this book. To be sure, each has been cushioned, quite properly, with *caveats*. Still, let us now accept them and try to plot a way forward.

Crucially, we have ditched functionalism. Our search now, therefore, is for a physical basis of qualia irrespective of the functions to which they are attached. Work on the neural correlates of consciousness, especially the visual kind, suggests that this search is best conducted in relation to each elemental feature of which, at any one time, the total multimodal conscious scene is made up—features such as colour, motion, faces, tones, scents and so on. Correspondingly, and in agreement with a hypothesis first enunciated by Zeki and ffytche, it seems that the physical basis for each of these elements may lie within a relatively circumscribed region of the neocortex—V4 for colours, V5 for motion, and so on. Presumably, once qualia were first made available for natural selection in this limited manner, the brain was then able to use them to construct the model of the external world, along with the mechanisms for late error detection and correction which, if my comparator hypothesis is right, provided the survival value for further evolution.

A key reason for ditching functionalism is the demonstration, discussed in detail in Chapter 10, that colour experience can be induced synaesthetically by auditory stimuli, and that this experience depends upon activity in V4 just as does the more common non-synaesthetic experience of colour resulting from visual stimulation. If we can trust these arguments, it follows that there must be something about V4 which gives rise, *under appropriate conditions*, to the experience of colour; and that this something does not necessarily lie in those connections which embed V4 in the wider functional systems of the brain.

These inferences raise the question: what are these 'appropriate conditions'? Might they pertain, for example, to V4 isolated in a Petri dish? There is, of course, no way as yet of giving a rational answer to this question, since we lack either a theory of how brain tissue generates conscious experience or any means of detecting conscious experience in an isolated piece of tissue, supposing it to exist there. But it should not be taken for granted that the answer is 'no'. The notion that an isolated piece of brain tissue might sustain conscious experience is no more fantastical *per se* than the notion that a system, like a computer, made of quite different materials might do so. Yet the latter is taken for granted by probably the majority of functionalists; and these are the dominant force in today's science and philosophy of consciousness.

One might have hoped that there would by now be at least some kind of a theoretical model of how the specifically neural or biological properties of neural tissue could create qualia. But none has yet been put forward. Unless and until such a model is proposed, the only remaining avenue lies in the laws of physics and chemistry.

A model starting from these laws can in principle take two forms.

The simpler one would leave unchanged the laws of physics and chemistry as we at present know them. Such a model would then need to show how, at a particular level of complexity of organisation (organisation, that is, of brain cells as such, not of the cybernetic systems in which these participate), physical laws lead inevitably to the occurrence of qualia. An analogy would be the way in which the laws of physics, present in the universe before there were any molecules, give rise later in cosmic evolution to the huge variety of chemical forms and interactions. If Lehar's model (Chapter 16) were to succeed in explaining the properties of conscious perception by invoking the principle of harmonic resonance, this would be such a case. However, neither that model nor others which share with it a broad family resemblance, such as Köhler's model based upon electrical fields

(Chapter 16), have made any headway either in passing the test of experiment or in showing how the postulated physical substrates of perception (harmonic resonance, electrical fields, etc.) could generate qualia.

Alternatively, no such new arrangement of the existing laws of physics and chemistry will turn out to be possible. The fundamental laws of physics themselves will need supplementation. It is difficult to see how new fundamental laws could come into play only during biological evolution, or they would not be fundamental. So it is probably inevitable that any theory which seeks to account for consciousness in terms of fundamental physical processes will involve 'panpsychism'. That is to say, it will be a theory in which the elements of conscious experience are to be found pretty well in everything, animate or inanimate, large or small. To most people this prospect will seem even less palatable than that of consciousness in computers or brain slices. But the state of our ignorance in this daunting field is so profound that we should rule out nothing *a priori* on the grounds of absurdity alone. Bear in mind the absurdity of quantum mechanics!

The best worked out theory of this more complex kind is the quantum mechanical model proposed by Roger Penrose and Stuart Hameroff. This model was presented in considerable detail in Chapter 16. Here, therefore, I shall be brief, asking only whether it brings us any closer to a meaningful solution to the Hard Problem than do the other approaches considered in this book.

There are, I think, two ways in which 'Penroff' theory (as Max Velmans and I took to calling it at the end of a gruelling three-day conference) does perhaps represent at least a small advance over the other contenders.

The first arises from its very panpsychism. By postulating that the processes that go to create qualia were there all along, one finesses the problem of the evolution of consciousness as such. One now has to consider only the evolution of complex organisms and the uses to which qualia can then be put—a much more tractable problem. Furthermore, Penroff theory does this while deftly avoiding paying the expected price of panpsychism—having every atom, stick and stone share in conscious experience. The theory achieves this seductive outcome (as explained in detail in Section 16.7) by arranging that the conditions which create qualia are found in nature *only* in highly developed cells of just the kind found in brains—and this despite the fact that the processes responsible for the creation of qualia have been biding their time since the universe began.

The second way in which Penroff theory may represent a conceptual advance is that it sketches a way in which qualia might actually be produced by, as distinct from merely correlated with, processes in the physical universe. Qualia, according to the theory, exist potentially (as '*proto*conscious' entities) from all time as possible particular constellations of variables (edge length, spin, etc.) embedded in space-time at the Planck scale. They are then selected as fully conscious qualia by quantum-mechanical processes, operating within specific structures inside nerve cells, that cause the collapse of superpositions of sets of protoconscious qualia onto the finally chosen conscious set (see Chapter 16 for details). This is not yet a full account of how physical processes might create qualia. For that, we would need in addition a proposal specifying the rules and mechanisms by which any particular constellation of Planck-scale variables gives rise to (or is identical with) any particular quale. Penroff theory does not yet offer such a proposal.

The chances that Penroff theory represents a correct description of real processes in the brain are remote in the extreme. Like the Giants attacking the Gods on Mount Olympus, it piles Pelion upon Ossa in an accumulation of separate hypotheses, all equally unlikely and each occupying a different conceptual level in a dizzying progression from the fundamental physics of quantum gravity and quantum mechanics to the specifics of neuroanatomy and neurophysiology. But at least some of these hypotheses are experimentally testable. And the theory has the supreme merit that it genuinely takes the Hard Problem seriously. It is an attempt to account for qualia, not just to dismiss them, nor to explain something else only tangentially related to them. Nonetheless, there will be few yet ready to buy into its panpsychic—indeed, Platonic—founding assumptions, in which qualia permeate the universe waiting for our brains to access them.

## Last words

We started this book lacking a viable theory of consciousness. We lack it still. But the first and often most important step in any form of construction is to clear the ground. In that respect, I believe, real progress is being made. We have two thousand years of testimony that the problem of consciousness will not yield to the purely verbal tools of philosophy. It is time to try instead the approach of natural science. But the edge of this approach has so far been blunted by a series of unexamined and untested assumptions. These have prevented the most important experimental questions from ever being asked, let alone finding answers.

Some of these assumptions are held most strongly by the folk psychologist to be found in each and every one of us. These include the assumptions that make up the *conscious narrative* (Chapter 2)—the illusion that much, much more of behaviour is controlled by conscious experience than is in fact the case; and the assumption of *direct realism*—that the world we consciously perceive is out there, just as we perceive it. Other assumptions are much more likely to be found in the thinking of professional scientists and philosophers. These include *epiphenomenalism*—that conscious experience can have no causal effects in its own right; and *functionalism*—that a thorough-going analysis of behavioural and neural functions is all that is needed to account *ipso facto* for conscious experience. These assumptions do not come as a package—those of the conscious narrative and epiphenomenalism, for example, directly contradict one another. However, if you shared any of them when you started this book, I hope to have shaken your faith. For it is only when they are abandoned that the true lines of the scientific Hard Problem of consciousness begin to become clear.

No theory yet proposed is up to the mark as a solution to the Hard Problem. But some of the right questions are now being asked, and relevant data are beginning to come in. And, not for the first time, it already seems likely that the eventual scientific solution to the problem will be far more surprising than any of the philosophical speculations that have gone before.

# References

Aleksander, I. (2000). *How to build a mind.* Weidenfeld and Nicolson, London.

Baars, B. J. (1988). *A cognitive theory of consciousness.* Cambridge University Press, Cambridge.

Baddeley, A. D. (1976). *The psychology of memory.* Basic Books, New York.

Baddeley, A. (2002). The concept of episodic memory. In *Episodic memory: new directions in research* (ed. A. Baddeley, M. Conway and J. Aggleton), pp. 1–10. Oxford University Press, Oxford.

Balleine, B. and Dickinson, A. (1998). Consciousness—the interface between affect and cognition. In *Consciousness and human identity* (ed. J. Cornwell), pp. 57–85. Oxford University Press, Oxford.

Banks, G., Short, P., Martinez, J., Latchaw, R., Ratliff, G. and Boller, F. (1989). The alien hand syndrome: clinical and post-mortem findings. *Archives of Neurology*, **46**, 456–9.

Baron-Cohen, S., Harrison, J., Goldstein, L. H. and Wyke, M. (1993). Coloured speech perception: is synaesthesia what happens when modularity breaks down? *Perception*, **22**, 419–26.

Berthier, M., Starkstein, S. and Leiguarda, R. (1988). Asymbolia for pain: a sensory-limbic disconnection syndrome. *Annals of Neurology*, **24**, 41–9.

Bisiach, E and Luzzatti, C. (1978). Unilateral neglect of representational space. *Cortex*, **14**, 129–33.

Blackmore, S., Brelstaff, G, Nelson, K. and Trościanko, T. (1995). Is the richness of our visual world an illusion? Transsaccadic memory for complex scenes. *Perception*, **24**, 1075–81.

Blakemore, C. and Greenfield S. (ed.) (1987). *Mindwaves.* Basil Blackwell, Oxford.

Blood, A. J. and Zatorre, R. J. (2001). Intensely pleasurable responses to music correlate with activity in brain regions implicated in reward and emotion. *Proceedings of the National Academy of Science USA*, **98**, 11818–23.

Bolton, D. and Hill, J. (1996). Mind, meaning, and mental disorder: the nature of causal explanation in psychology and psychiatry. Oxford University Press, Oxford.

Broadbent, D. E. (1958). *Perception and communication.* Pergamon Press, London.

Burgess, N., Jeffery, K. J. and O'Keefe, J. (ed.) (1999). *The hippocampal and parietal foundations of spatial cognition.* Oxford University Press, Oxford.

Castelo-Branco, M., Goebel, R., Neuenschwander, S. and Singer, W. (2000). Neural synchrony correlates with surface segregation rules. *Nature*, **405**, 685–9.

Chalmers, D. (1996). *The conscious mind: in search of a fundamental theory.* Oxford University Press, New York.

Changeux, J.-P. and Dehaene, S. (1989). Neuronal models of cognitive function. *Cognition*, **33**, 63–109.

Chen, W., Kato, T., Zhu, X. H., Ogawa, S., Tank, D. W. and Ugurbil, K. (1998). Human primary visual cortex and lateral geniculate nucleus activation during visual imagery. *NeuroReport*, **9**, 3669–74.

Clark, A. (1997). *Being there: putting brain, body, and world together again*. MIT Press, Cambridge, Mass.

Cohen, M. S., Kosslyn, S. M., Breiter, H. C., DiGirolamo, G. J., Thompson, W. L., Anderson, A. K., Bookheimer, S. Y., Rosen B. R. and Belliveau, J. W. (1996). Changes in cortical activity during mental rotation: a mapping study using functional MRI. *Brain*, **119**, 89–100.

Cowey, A. and Stoerig, P. (1999). Spectral sensitivity in hemianopic macaque monkeys. *European Journal of Neuroscience*, **11**, 2114–20.

Craig, A. D. and Bushnell, M. C. (1994). The thermal grill illusion: unmasking the burn of cold pain. *Science*, **265**, 258–60.

Craig, A. D., Reiman, E. M., Evans, A. and Bushnell, M. C. (1996). Functional imaging of an illusion of pain. *Science*, **384**, 252–5.

Crick, F. H. C. (1994). The astonishing hypothesis: the scientific search for the soul. Scribner, New York.

Cumming, B. G. and Parker, A. J. (1997). Responses of primary visual neurons to binocular disparity without depth perception. *Nature*, **389**, 280–3.

Damasio, A. (1999). *The feeling of what happens*. Harcourt, San Diego.

Dawkins, R. (1997). *Climbing mount improbable*. Penguin Science, London.

Dehaene, S. and Naccache, L. (2001). Towards a cognitive neuroscience of consciousness: basic evidence and a workspace framework. *Cognition*, **79**, 1–37.

Dennett, D. C. (1991). *Consciousness explained*. Little, Brown, Boston.

Dennett, D. C. and Kinsbourne, M. (1992). Time and the observer: the where and when of consciousness. *Behavioral and Brain Sciences*, **15**, 183–247.

Dimberg, U., Thunberg, M. and Elmehed., K. (2000). Face to face: unconscious emotional communication. *Psychological Science*, **11**, 86–9.

Donald, M. (2002). *A mind so rare*. Norton, New York.

Driver, J. and Vuilleumier, P. (2001). Perceptual awareness and its loss in unilateral neglect and extinction. *Cognition*, **79**, 39–88.

Edelman, G. M. and Tononi, G. (2000). *A universe of consciousness: how matter becomes imagination*. Allen Lane, London.

Ekman, P. and Friesen, W. (1976). *Pictures of facial affect*. Consulting Psychologists Press, Palo Alto, CA.

Eldridge, L. L., Knowlton, B. J., Furmanski, C. S., Bookheimer, S. Y. and Engel, S. A. (2000). Remembering episodes: a selective role for the hippocampus during retrieval. *Nature Neuroscience*, **3**, 1149–52.

ffytche, D. H. and Zeki, S. (1996). Brain activity related to the perception of illusory contours. *NeuroImage*, **3**, 104–8.

ffytche, D. H., Howard, R. J., Brammer, M. J., David, A., Woodruff, P. and Williams, S. (1998). The anatomy of conscious vision: an fMRI study of visual hallucinations, *Nature Neuroscience*, **11**, 738–42.

Fodor, J. (1979). *The language of thought.* Harvard University Press, Cambridge, Mass.

Friedman-Hill, S. R., Robertson, L. C. and Treisman, A. (1995). Parietal contributions to visual feature binding: evidence from a patient with bilateral lesions. *Science*, **269**, 853–5.

Frith, C. (1995). Consciousness is for other people. *Behavioral and Brain Sciences*, **18**, 682–3

Gaffan, D. (1994). Scene-specific memory for objects: a model of episodic memory impairment in monkeys with fornix section. *Cognitive Neuroscience*, **6**, 305–20.

Gallagher, S. and Shear, J. (ed.) (1999). *Models of the self.* Imprint Academic, Thorverton UK.

Geldard, F. A. and Sherrick, C. E. (1972). The cutaneous 'rabbit': a perceptual illusion. *Science*, **178**, 178–9.

Ghirardi, G.C., Rimini, A. and Weber, T. (1986). Unified dynamics for microscopic and macroscopic systems. *Physical Reviews D*, **34**, 470–91.

Goebel, R., Khorram-Sefat, D., Muckli, L., Hacker, H. and Singer, W. (1998). The constructive nature of vision: direct evidence from functional magnetic resonance imaging studies of apparent motion and motion imagery. *European Journal of Neuroscience*, **10**, 1563–73.

Goebel, R., Muckli, L., Zanella, F. E., Singer, W. and Stoerig, P. (2001). Sustained extra-striate cortical activation without visual awareness revealed by fMRI studies of hemianopic patients. *Vision Research*, **41**, 1459–74.

Gray, J. A. (1987). *The psychology of fear and stress*, 2nd edn. Cambridge University Press, Cambridge.

Gray, J. A. (1995). The contents of consciousness: a neuropsychological conjecture. *Behavioral and Brain Sciences*, **18**, 659–722 (including commentary and reply).

Gray, J. A. and McNaughton, M. (2000). *The neuropsychology of anxiety* (2nd ed.). Oxford University Press, Oxford.

Gray, J. A, Chopping, S, Nunn, J., Parslow, D., Gregory, L., Williams, S., Brammer, M. J. and Baron-Cohen, S. (2002). Implications of synaesthesia for functionalism: theory and experiments. *Journal of Consciousness Studies*, **9** (12), 5–31.

Greenfield, S. (2000). *The private life of the brain.* Allen Lane, London.

Greenwald, A. G., Draine, S. C. and Abrams, R. L. (1996). Three cognitive markers of unconscious semantic activation. *Science*, **273**, 1699–702.

Gregory, R. L. (1997). *Eye and brain: the psychology of seeing.* Princeton University Press, Princeton.

Groeger, J. A. (1988). Qualitatively different effects of undetected and unidentified auditory primes. *Quarterly Journal of Experimental Psychology*, **40A**, 323–39.

Grush, R. (2001). Self, world and space: on the meaning and mechanisms of egocentric and allocentric spatial representation. *Brain and Mind*, **1**, 59–92.

Gur, M. and Snodderly, D. M. (1997). A dissociation between brain activity and perception: chromatically opponent cortical neurons signal chromatic flicker that is not perceived. *Vision Research*, **37**, 377–82.

Hadjikhani, N., Liu, A. K., Dale, A. M., Cavanagh, P. and Tootell, R. B. (1998). Retinotopy and color sensitivity in human visual cortical area V8. *Nature Neuroscience*, **1**, 235–41.

Haggard, P. and Eimer, M. (1999). On the relation between brain potentials and the awareness of voluntary movements. *Experimental Brain Research*, **126**, 128–33.

Hameroff, S. (2001). Consciousness, the brain, and spacetime geometry. In *Cajal and consciousness: scientific approaches to consciousness on the centennial of Ramon y Cajal's Textura* (ed. P. C. Marijuan), Annals of the New York Academy of Science, **929**, 74–104.

Harnad, S. (1990). The symbol grounding problem. *Physica*, **D42**, 335–46.

Harnad, S. (2002). Turing indistinguishability and the blind watchmaker. In *Evolving consciousness* (ed. J. Fetzer), pp. 3–18. John Benjamins, Amsterdam.

He, S., Cavanagh, P. and Intriligator, J. (1996). Attentional resolution and the locus of visual awareness. *Nature*, **383**, 334–7.

Hobson, P. (2002). *The cradle of thought*. Macmillan, London.

Howard, R. J., ffytche, D. H., Barnes, J., McKeefry, D., Ha, Y., Woodruff, P. W., Bullmore, E. T., Simmons, A., Williams, S. C., David A. S. and Brammer, M. (1998). The functional anatomy of imagining and perceiving colour. *NeuroReport*, **9**, 1019–1023.

Hsieh, J.-C., Ståhle-Bäckdahl, M., Hägermark, Ö, Stone-Elander, S., Rosenquist, G. and Ingvar, M. (1995). Traumatic nociceptive pain activates the hypothalamus and the periaqueductal gray: a positron emission tomography study. *Pain*, **64**, 303–14.

Huk, A. C. and Heeger, D. J. (2002). Pattern-motion responses in human visual cortex. *Nature Neuroscience*, **5**, 72–5.

Humphrey, N. K. (1974). Vision in a monkey without striate cortex: a case study. *Perception*, **3**, 241–55.

Humphrey, N. (1983). *Consciousness regained*. Oxford University Press, Oxford.

Hurley, S. (1998). *Consciousness in action*. Harvard University Press, Cambridge, Mass.

Hurley, S. (2004). The shared circuits hypothesis: a unified functional architecture for control, imitation, and simulation. In *Perspectives on imitation: from neuroscience to social science*, vol. 1 (ed. S. Hurley and N. Chater). MIT Press, Cambridge, Mass.

Hurley, S. and Noë, A. (2003). Neural plasticity and consciousness. *Biology and Philosophy*, **18**, 131–168.

Jackendoff, R. (1987). *Consciousness and the computational mind*. MIT Press, Cambridge, Mass.

Jeannerod, M. (1999). The 25th Bartlett Lecture. To act or not to act: perspectives on the representation of action. *Quarterly Journal of Experimental Psychology*, **52A**, 1–29.

Kandel, E. R., Schwartz, J. H. and Jessell, T. M. (2000). *Principles of neural science* (4th ed.). McGraw-Hill, New York.

Kinsbourne, M. (1987). Mechanisms of unilateral neglect. In *Neurophysiological and neuropsychological aspects of spatial neglect* (ed. M. Jeannerod), pp. 235–58. North-Holland, Amsterdam.

Klein, I., Paradis, A. L., Poline, J. B., Kosslyn, S. M. and Le Bihan, D. (2000). Transient activity in the human calcarine cortex during visual-mental imagery: an event-related fMRI study. *Journal of Cognitive Neuroscience*, **12**, Suppl. 2, 15–23.

Kleiser, R., Wittsack, J., Niedeggen, M., Goebel, R. and Stoerig, P. (2001). Is V1 necessary for conscious vision in areas of relative cortical blindness? *NeuroImage*, **13**, 654–61.

Koch, C. and Crick, F. C. R. (2000). Thoughts on consciousness and neuroscience. In *The cognitive neurosciences*, 2nd edn. (ed. M. S. Gazzaniga), pp. 1285–94. MIT Press, Cambridge, Mass.

Koch, C. and Crick, F. C. R. (2001). The zombie within. *Nature*, **411**, 893.

Köhler, W. (1969). *The task of Gestalt psychology.* Princeton University Press, Princeton NJ.

Kolers, P. A. and von Grünau, M. (1976). Shape and color in apparent motion. *Vision Research*, **16**, 329–35.

Kosslyn, S. M., Thompson, W. I., Kim, I. J. and Alpert, N. M. (1995). Topographical representations of mental imagery in primary visual cortex. *Nature*, **378**, 496–8.

Kreiman, G., Koch, C. and Fried, I. (2000). Imagery neurons in the human brain. *Nature*, **408**, 357–61.

Kumari, V., Gray, J. A., Honey, G. D., Soni, W., Bullmore, E. T., Williams, S. C., Ng, V. W., Vythelingum, G. N., Simmons, A., Suckling, J., Corr, P. J. and Sharma, T. (2002). Procedural learning in schizophrenia: a functional magnetic resonance imaging investigation. *Schizophrenia Research*, **57**, 97–107.

Lamme, V. A. F., Zipser, K. and Spekreijse, H. (1998). Figure-ground activity in primary visual cortex is suppressed by anaesthesia. *Proceedings of the National Academy of Science USA*, **95**, 3263–8.

Lehar, S. (2003). The world in your head: a Gestalt view of the mechanism of conscious experience. Lawrence Erlbaum, Mahwah NJ.

Lehar, S. (2003). Gestalt isomorphism and the primacy of subjective conscious experience: a Gestalt Bubble model. *Behavioral and Brain Sciences*, **26**, 375–444.

Libet, B. (1985). Unconscious cerebral initiative and the role of conscious will in voluntary action. *Behavioral and Brain Sciences*, **6**, 529–66.

Logothetis, N. (1998). Single units and conscious vision. *Philosophical Transactions of the Royal Society B*, **353**, 1801–18.

Mack, A. and Rock, I. (1998). *Inattentional blindness*. MIT Press, Cambridge, Mass.

Macphail, E. (1998). *The evolution of consciousness*. Oxford University Press, Oxford.

Maguire, E. A. (2002). Neuroimaging studies of autobiographical event memory. In *Episodic memory: new directions in research* (ed. A. Baddeley, M. Conway and J. Aggleton), pp. 164–80. Oxford University Press, Oxford.

Maguire, E. A., Gadian, D. G., Johnsrude, I. S., Good, C. D., Ashburner, J., Frackowiak, R. S. and Frith, C. D. (2000). Navigation-related structural change in the hippocampi of taxi drivers. *Proceedings of the National Academy of Science USA*, **97**, 4398–403.

Marcel, A. J. (1980). Conscious and preconscious recognition of polysemous words: locating the effect of prior verbal context. In *Attention and performance VIII* (ed. R. S. Nickerson), pp. 435–57. Lawrence Erlbaum, London.

Mattingley, J. B., Rich, A. N., Yelland, G. and Bradshaw, J. L. (2001). Unconscious priming eliminates automatic binding of colour and alphanumeric form in synaesthesia. *Nature*, **410**, 580–2.

Mayes, A., Isaac, C. L., Holdstock, J. S., Hunkin, N. M., Montaldi, D., Downes, J. J., MacDonald, C., Cezayirli, C. and Roberts, J. N. (2001). Memory for single items, word pairs, and temporal order of different kinds in a patient with selective hippocampal lesions. *Cognitive Neuropsychology*, **18**, 97–123.

McCrone, J. (1999). *Going inside: a tour round a single moment of consciousness*. Faber and Faber, London.

Mechsner, F., Kerzel, D., Knoblich, G. and Prinz, W. (2001). Perceptual basis of bimanual coordination. *Nature*, **414**, 69–73.

Mellet, E., Petit, L, Mazoyer, B., Denis, M. and Tzourio, N. (1998). Reopening the mental imagery debate: lessons from functional anatomy. *NeuroImage*, **8**, 129–39.

Merikle, P. M. and Joordens, S. (1997). Parallels between perception without attention and perception without awareness. *Consciousness and Cognition*, **6**, 219–36.

Merikle, P. M., Joordens, S. and Stolz, J. A. (1995). Measuring the relative magnitude of unconscious influences. *Consciousness and Cognition*, **4**, 422–39.

Merikle, P. M., Smilek, D. and Eastwood, J. D. (2001). Perception without awareness: perspectives from cognitive psychology. *Cognition*, **79**, 115–34.

Michaels, C. F and Carello, C. (1981). *Direct perception*. Prentice-Hall, Englewood Cliffs NJ.

Milner, A. D and Goodale, M. A. (1995). *The visual brain in action*. Oxford University Press, Oxford.

Mishkin, M., Suzuki, W., Gadian, D. G. and Vargha-Khadem, F. (1999). Hierarchical organisation of cognitive memory: interactions between parietal and hippocampal systems in space and memory. In *The hippocampal and parietal foundations of spatial cognition* (ed. N. Burgess, K. J. Jeffery and J. O'Keefe), pp. 290–302. Oxford University Press, Oxford.

Mollon, J. D. (1999). Color vision: opsins and options. *Proceedings of the National Academy of Science USA*, **96**, 4743–5.

Moutoussis, K. and Zeki, S. (2002). The relationship between cortical activation and perception investigated with invisible stimuli. *Proceedings of the National Academy of Sciences, USA*, **99**, 9527–32.

Nagel, T. (1974). What is it like to be a bat? *Philosophical Review*, **4**, 435–50.

Nagel, T. (1986). *The view from nowhere*. Oxford University Press, Oxford.

Neisser, U. (1976). *Cognition and reality*. Freeman, New York.

Nunn, J. A., Gregory, L. J., Brammer, M., Williams, S. C. R., Parslow, D. M., Morgan, M. J., Morris, R. G., Bullmore, E. T., Baron-Cohen, S. and Gray, J. A. (2002). Functional magnetic resonance imaging of synesthesia: activation of V4/V8 by spoken words. *Nature Neuroscience*, **5**, 371–5.

O'Craven, K. M. and Kanwisher, N. (2000). Mental imagery of faces and places activates corresponding stimulus-specific brain regions. *Journal of Cognitive Neuroscience*, **12**, 1013–23.

O'Keefe, J. and Nadel, L. (1978). *The hippocampus as a cognitive map*. Clarendon Press, Oxford.

Panksepp, J. (1999). *Affective neuroscience*. Oxford University Press, Oxford.

Penrose, R. (1989). *The emperor's new mind*. Oxford University Press, Oxford.

Penrose, R. (1994). *Shadows of the mind*. Oxford University Press, Oxford.

Phillips, M. L., Young, A.W., Senior, C., Brammer, M., Andrew, C., Calder, A. J., Bullmore, E. T., Perrett, D. I., Rowland, O., Williams, S. C. R., Gray, J. A. and David, A. S. (1997). A specific neural substrate for perceiving facial expressions of disgust. *Nature*, **389**, 495–8.

Phillips, M. L., Williams, L. M., Young, A. W., Russell, T., Herba, C. M., Heining, M., Andrew, C., Bullmore, E. T., Brammer, M. J., Williams, S. C. R., Morgan, M. and Gray, J. A. (2004). Differential neural responses to overt and covert presentations of facial expressions of fear and disgust. *NeuroImage*, **21**, 1486–98.

Polanyi, M. and Prosch, H. (1975). *Meaning*. University of Chicago Press, Chicago.

Pribram, K.H. (1971). Languages of the brain: experimental paradoxes and principles in neuropychology. Prentice-Hall, Englewood Cliffs, NJ.

Ramachandran, V. S. and Blakeslee, S. (1998). *Phantoms in the brain*. Morrow, New York.

Ramachandran, V. S. and Hubbard, E. M. (2001). Psychophysical investigations into the neural basis of synaesthesia. *Proceedings of the Royal Society of London B*, **268**, 979–83.

Rees, G., Kreiman, G. and Koch, C. (2002). Neural correlates of consciousness in humans. *Nature Reviews in Neuroscience*, **3**, 261–70.

Rees, G., Wojciulik, E., Clarke, K., Husain, M., Frith, C. and Driver, J. (2000). Unconscious activation of visual cortex in the damaged right hemisphere of a parietal patient with extinction. *Brain*, **123**, 1624–33.

Regan, B. C., Julliot, C., Simmen, B., Viénot, C., Charles-Dominique, P. and Mollon, J. D. (2001). Fruits, foliage and the evolution of primate colour vision. *Philosophical Transactions of the Royal Society B*, **356**, 229–83.

Rizzolatti, G., Fadiga, L., Fogassi, L. and Gallese, V. (1999). Resonance behaviors and mirror neurons. *Archives Italiennes de Biologie*, **137**, 85–100.

Robertson, L. C. (2003). Binding, spatial attention and perceptual awareness. *Nature Reviews in Neuroscience*, **4**, 93–102.

Rolls, E. T. and Tovee, M. J. (1994). Processing speed in the cerebral cortex and the neurophysiology of visual masking. *Proceedings of the Royal Society of London B*, **257**, 9–15.

Sacks, O. (1986). *The man who mistook his wife for a hat*. Picador, London.

Searle, J. R. (1980). Minds, brains, and programs. *Behavioral and Brain Sciences*, **3**, 417–24.

Searle, J. R. (1983). *Intentionality: an essay in the philosophy of mind*. Cambridge University Press, Cambridge.

Searle, J. R. (1987). Minds and brains without programs. In *Mindwaves* (ed. C. Blakemore and S. Greenfield), pp. 209–33. Basil Blackwell, Oxford.

Shallice, T. (1988). *From neuropsychology to mental structure*. Cambridge University Press, Cambridge.

Simons, D. J. and Levin, D. T. (1998). Failure to detect changes to people during real-world interaction. *Psychonomic Bulletin and Review*, **5**, 644–9.

Stickgold, R., Malia, A., Maguire, D., Roddenberry, D. and O'Connor, M. (2000). Replaying the game: hypnagogic images in normals and amnesics. *Nature*, **290**, 350–3.

Stoerig, P. and Cowey, A. (1992). Wavelength discrimination in blindsight. *Brain*, **115**, 425–44.

Tootell, R. B. H., Reppas, J. B., Dale, A. M., Look, R. B., Sereno, M. I., Malach, R., Brady, T. J. and Rosen, B. R. (1995). Visual motion aftereffect in human cortical area MT revealed by functional magnetic resonance imaging. *Nature*, **375**, 139–41.

Treisman, A. (1998). Feature binding, attention and object perception. *Philosophical Transactions of the Royal Society B*, **353**, 1295–306.

Tulving, E. (2002). Episodic memory and common sense: how far apart? In *Episodic memory: new directions in research* (ed. A. Baddeley, M. Conway and J. Aggleton), pp. 269–87. Oxford University Press, Oxford.

Van Essen, D. C., Anderson, C. H. and Felleman, D. J. (1992). Information processing in the primate visual system: an integrated systems perspective. *Science*, **255**, 419–23.

Vargha-Khadem, F., Gadian, D. G. and Mishkin, M. (2002). Dissociations in cognitive memory: the syndrome of developmental amnesia. In *Episodic memory: new directions in research* (ed. A. Baddeley, M. Conway and J. Aggleton), pp. 153–63. Oxford University Press, Oxford.

Velmans, M. (1991). Is human information processing conscious? *Behavioral and Brain Sciences*, **14**, 651–69.

Velmans, M. (2000). *Understanding consciousness*. Routledge, London.

Velmans, M. (2003). Preconscious free will. *Journal of Consciousness Studies*, **10**(12), 42–61.

Virley, D., Ridley, R. M., Sinden, J. D., Kershaw, T. R., Harland, S., Rashid, T., French, S., Sowinski, P., Gray, J. A., Lantos, P. L. and Hodges, H. (1999). Primary CA1 and conditionally immortal MHP36 cell grafts restore conditional discrimination learning and recall in marmosets after excitotoxic lesions of the hippocampal CA1 field. *Brain*, **122**, 2321–35.

von der Heydt, R., Peterhans, E. and Baumgartner, G. (1984). Illusory contours and cortical neuron responses. *Science*, **224**, 1260–2.

Vuilleumier, P., Sagiv, N., Hazeltine, E., Poldrack, R. A., Swick, D., Rafal, R. D. and Gabrieli, J. D. (2001). Neural fate of seen and unseen faces in visuospatial neglect: a combined event-related functional MRI and event-related potential study. *Proceedings of the National Academy of Science USA*, **98**, 3495–500.

Wegner, D. M. and Wheatley, T. (1999). Apparent mental causation: sources of the experience of will. *American Psychologist*, **54**, 480–92.

Weiskrantz, L. (1997). *Consciousness lost and found*. Oxford University Press, Oxford.

Weiskrantz, L., Cowey, A. and Hodinott-Hill, I. (2002). Prime-sight in a blindsight subject. *Nature Neuroscience*, **5**, 101–2.

Williams, T. H., Gluhbegovic, N. and Jew, J.Y. *The human brain*, Chapter 5. *http://www.vh.org/adult/provider/anatomy/BrainAnatomy/TOC.html*

Wilson, B. A. (1999). *Case studies in neuropsychological rehabilitation* (Chapter 6, pp. 72–87). Oxford University Press, New York.

Woolf, N. J. and Hameroff, S. (2001). A quantum approach to consciousness. *Trends in Cognitive Sciences*, **5**, 472–8.

Zeki, S. (2003). The disunity of consciousness. *Trends in Cognitive Sciences*, **7**, 214–8.

Zeki, S. (1993). *A Vision of the brain*. Blackwell Scientific Publications, Oxford.

Zeki, S. (1999). *Inner vision*. Oxford University Press, Oxford.

Zeki, S. and ffytche, D. H. (1998). The Riddoch syndrome: insights into the neurobiology of conscious vision. *Brain*, **121**, 25–45.

Zeki, S., Watson, J. D. G. and Frackowiak, R. S. J. (1993). Going beyond the information given: the relation of illusory visual motion to brain activity. *Proceedings of the Royal Society of London B*, **252**, 215–22.

Zohar, D. and Marshall, I (1993). *The quantum society*. Bloomsbury, London.

# Index